Collections and Recollections

A Search for World Legacies of Ethnic Dress

Dorothy Owen Knop

Jane Benson, Illustrator

Welred Books, Inc.
P. O. Box 401
Youngtown, Arizona 85363

Library of Congress Cataloging-in-Publication Data

Knop, Dorothy Owen, 1911-
        Collections and Recollections: A Search for World Legacies of Ethnic Dress.
        ISBN 0-9646786-0-8 (P)
        1.Costume. 2.Travel.

Acknowledgements

It all began with a desire to see the world and an interest in all of the people in it. Then came a wish to share both the experiences and the acquisitions of ethnic dress.

My late husband, Herman Knop, known as Ham to his friends, insisted that he had lots to keep him busy and that he liked TV dinners, and he didn't like to shop. So, in spite of my own twinge of a guilty conscience at leaving him alone, off I would go on another glamorous shopping trip with Jo. Ham was a good and helpful reader, and I greatly appreciate his interest and encouragement.

Josephine Pionkowski is my patient, agreeable, go-anywhere friend of many years. Jo and I are kindred spirits; we both love to travel and to shop. Between us we have raised five children and have 14 grandchildren. We were ready to follow our dreams.

Jane Benson, illustrator extraordinaire, added graphic beauty to my words, making them come alive. My gratitude to her is unbounded for allowing me to tap her rare and wonderful illustrative talent for this book.

Carol Secord, ASU teacher, writer and editor, gave extensive editorial assistance and encouragement. She and her husband, Ronald Secord, also formatted the book. Without her there would have been no book.

Veronika Barnes, whose sharp eye made for a sharper product, was invaluable as a very capable proofreader.

My family, Owen, Dave, Sally, and grandchildren, Rick, Jim, Alan, Christy, Dina, Molly, Andy and Kara have been supportive and patient listeners.

Elizabeth Marsh, Collection Manager at the Sun Cities Museum of Art, has organizational ability that made it possible to find anything anytime.

Merilyn E. Ulrich, who has been a freelance editor of screenplays, television scripts and books for more than 20 years, read the manuscript and wrote such encouraging words that she lifted my lagging spirits with her enthusiasm.

FOREWORD

I visited the Sun Cities Museum of Art during a showing of authentic costumes from around the world. Dorothy Knop, who had collected and donated to the museum much of what was displayed, took me on a tour of the room that actually seemed more like a tour of the world.

Dorothy's travels have included more than 100 countries and have filled six passports. She has journeyed with the focus and purpose of acquiring authentic ethnic costumes from around the world. Her extensive travels began 30 years ago and have taken her to some countries repeatedly. For instance, she has returned to Guatemala 13 times.

"The story of mankind is written in the clothing that has developed because of the climate of an area and the education and lifestyle of the people," Dorothy explains. She loves to travel and to search in out-of-the-way places for authentic, ethnic dress, not that which is manufactured for the tourist trade. She senses that many cultures throughout the world are turning their backs on traditional ways. Her own passion for preserving cultural awareness has been a major motivator as she has traveled, studied and collected these prize examples.

Even in that one afternoon at the museum, I was exposed to more history, geography and cultural awareness than I could have absorbed from several books. We traveled the world, seeming to meet a Sumatran bride, a Tibetan monk, a Berber dancer, a nomadic Bedouin woman, as well as viewing elaborate authentic examples from India, Korea, Thailand, China, Lapland and on and on. It was fascinating to hear Dorothy's stories of acquisition, each one an adventure tale.

With the encouragement of those who enjoyed the exhibit so much, she embarked on the project of writing this book. It is an excellent 'armchair travel book' for people like me who are just conventional tourists, as the paths that Dorothy has trod are not the usual ones. This book guides the reader through the recollections of her many interesting experiences. It has contributed to my own geographical, cultural and costume awareness in a way no textbook could approach.

by Carol Secord, Editor, Publisher
New Mature Woman Newsletter, Glendale, Arizona

For the past 20 years I have read and edited many scripts and manuscripts, ranging from fantasy to true crime. Many are time consuming and often not very interesting. All have had numerous errors which kept my pencil flying over the pages. Not until I read Dorothy's delightful and well written book did I find a manuscript that was all pleasure and no work!

Not only are the costumes depicted authentic and intricate, but the adventures of Dorothy and company are heartwarming and humorous. What an accomplishment!

It is a once-in-a-lifetime journey that can be shared by everyone. You too can travel the world and experience through Dorothy's eyes the rare beauty of each country's native costumes and the unique way in which she acquired them.

by Merilyn E. Ulrich, Freelance Editor
Assistant Manager, Waldenbooks, Sun City, Arizona

CONTENTS

In this book, in order to encircle the world in as orderly and reasonable a fashion as possible, we begin at the San Blas Islands in the Caribbean Sea, off the coast of Panama in Central America, and end in Mexico, also bordered by the Caribbean.

Since there are dozens of fine American Indian museums, we have made no attempt to compete with them in this collection. The concentration, instead, has been on the ethnic dress of much of the rest of the world.

180° 160°W 140°W 120°W 100°W 80°W 60°W 40°W 20°W
80°N
ARCTIC CIRCLE
ALASKA (U.S.)
60°N
CANADA
40°N
NORTH PACIFIC OCEAN
UNITED STATES
MIDWAY IS. (U.S.)
NORTH ATLANTIC OCEAN
ST. PIERRE & MIQUELON (FRANCE)
BERMUDA (U.K.)
TROPIC OF CANCER
HAWAII (U.S.)
20°N
MEXICO
BAHAMAS
CUBA
DOMINICAN REPUBLIC
PUERTO RICO (U.S.)
JAMAICA HAITI
BELIZE
ST. KITTS & NEVIS
ANTIGUA & BARBUDA
ST. LUCIA
GUATEMALA HONDURAS DOMINICA
BARBADOS
EL SALVADOR NICARAGUA GRENADA
ST. VINCENT & THE GRENADINES
COSTA RICA
TRINIDAD & TOBAGO
PANAMA
VENEZUELA
SURINAME
COLOMBIA
FRENCH GUIANA (FRANCE)
EQUATOR
GALAPAGOS IS. (ECUADOR)
ECUADOR
GUYANA
0°
KIRIBATI
BRAZIL
TOKELAU IS. (N.Z.)
PERU
WESTERN SAMOA AMERICAN SAMOA (U.S.)
FRENCH POLYNESIA (FRANCE)
COOK IS. (N.Z.)
BOLIVIA
FIJI NIUE (N.Z.)
20°S
TONGA
TROPIC OF CAPRICORN
PARAGUAY
SOUTH ATLANTIC OCEAN
PITCAIRN I. (U.K.)
EASTER ISLAND (CHILE)
CHILE
ARGENTINA
URUGUAY
40°S
CHATHAM IS. (N.Z.)
SOUTH PACIFIC OCEAN
FALKLAND IS. (U.K.)
SOUTH GEORGIA (U.K.)
SOUTH SANDWICH ISLANDS (U.K.)
60°S
ANTARCTIC CIRCLE
80°S
180° 160°W 140°W 120°W 100°W 80°W 60°W 40°W 20°W
ARCTIC
GREENLAND (KALAALLIT NUNAAT) (DENMARK)
ICELAND
FAROE IS. (DENMARK)
IRELAND
PORTUGAL
AZORES IS. (PORTUGAL)
MADEIRA IS. (PORTUGAL)
MOROCCO
CANARY IS. (SPAIN)
WESTERN SAHARA (MOROCCO)
MAURITANIA
CAPE VERDE
SENEGAL
GAMBIA
GUINEA-BISSAU GUINEA
SIERRA LEONE
LIBERIA
EQUATOR
SAO TOME
ASCENSION (U.K.)
TRISTAN GROUP

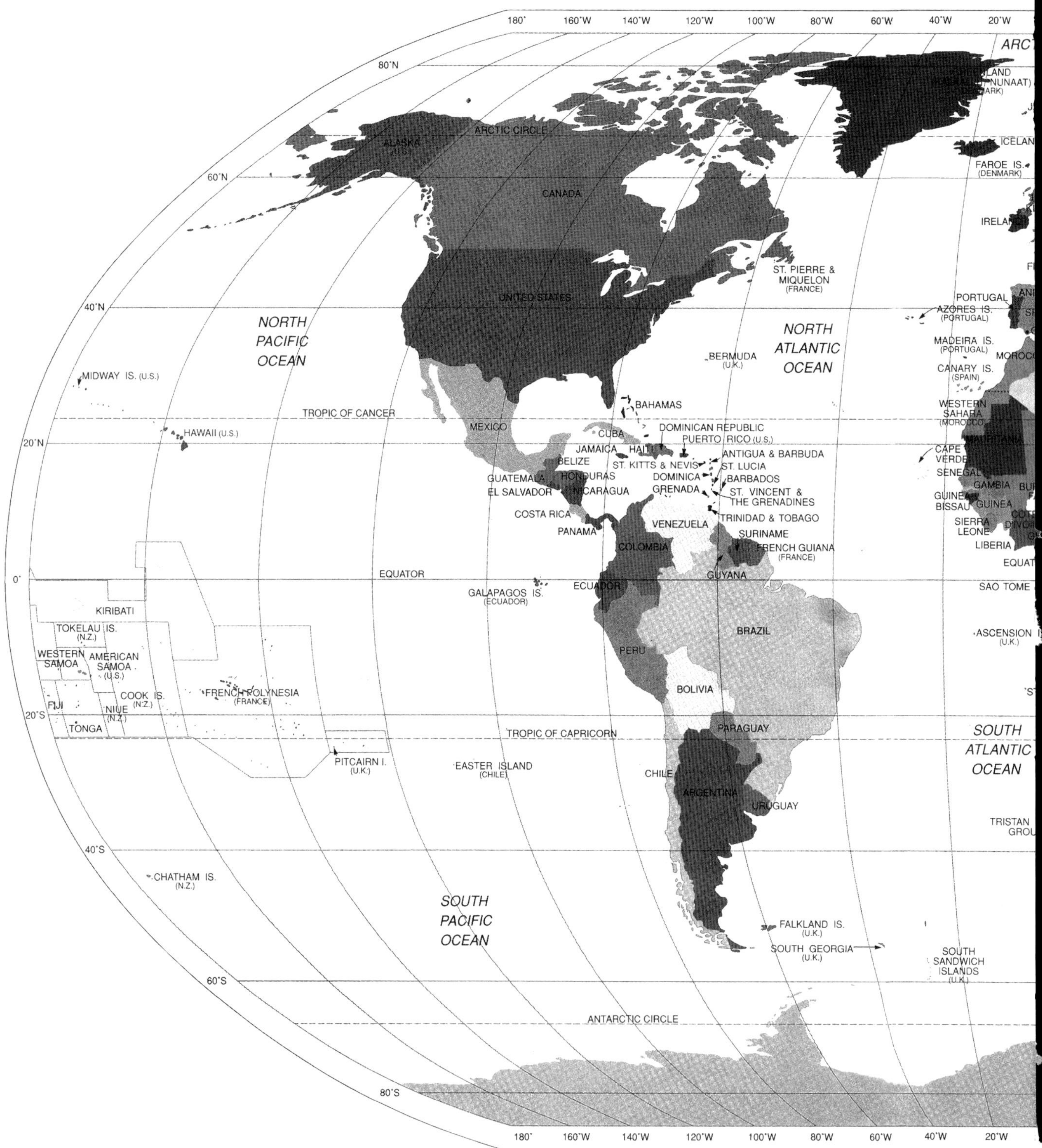

vi

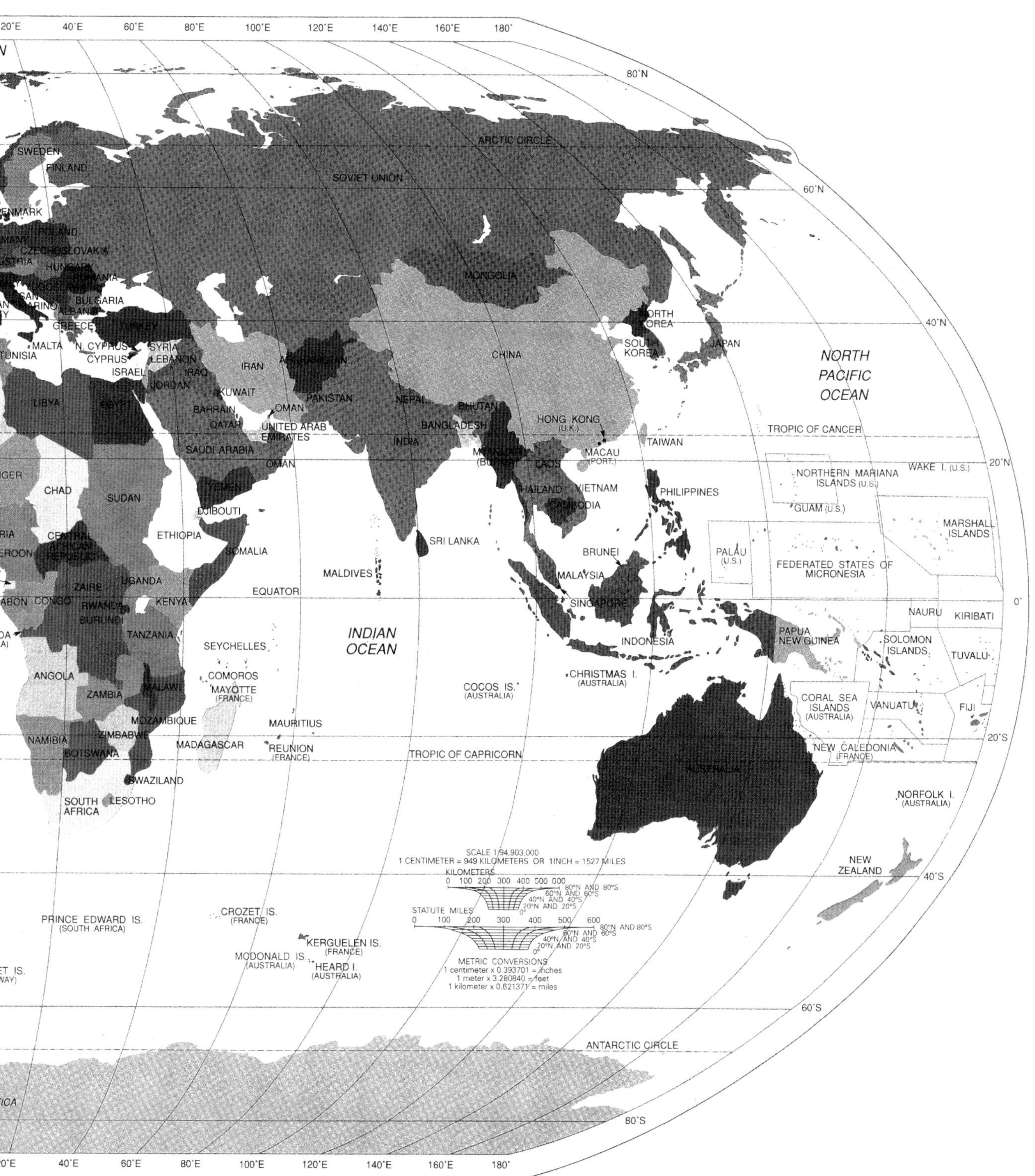

20°E
40°E
60°E
80°E
100°E
120°E
140°E
160°E
180°
80°N
ARCTIC CIRCLE
60°N
SWEDEN
FINLAND
SOVIET UNION
DENMARK
POLAND
GERMANY
CZECHOSLOVAKIA
AUSTRIA
HUNGARY
ROMANIA
MONGOLIA
YUGOSLAVIA
BULGARIA
SAN MARINO
ALBANIA
GREECE
TURKEY
NORTH KOREA
40°N
ITALY
MALTA
N. CYPRUS
SYRIA
SOUTH KOREA
JAPAN
TUNISIA
CYPRUS
LEBANON
IRAN
AFGHANISTAN
CHINA
NORTH
ISRAEL
IRAQ
JORDAN
PACIFIC
LIBYA
EGYPT
KUWAIT
OMAN
PAKISTAN
NEPAL
BHUTAN
OCEAN
BAHRAIN
UNITED ARAB
BANGLADESH
HONG KONG
QATAR
EMIRATES
INDIA
(U.K.)
TROPIC OF CANCER
SAUDI ARABIA
MYANMAR
MACAU
TAIWAN
20°N
NIGER
OMAN
(BURMA)
LAOS
(PORT.)
CHAD
SUDAN
YEMEN
THAILAND
VIETNAM
WAKE I. (U.S.)
NORTHERN MARIANA
DJIBOUTI
CAMBODIA
PHILIPPINES
ISLANDS (U.S.)
GUAM (U.S.)
NIGERIA
CENTRAL
ETHIOPIA
SOMALIA
MARSHALL
CAMEROON
AFRICAN
SRI LANKA
ISLANDS
REPUBLIC
BRUNEI
PALAU
FEDERATED STATES OF
ZAIRE
UGANDA
MALDIVES
(U.S.)
MICRONESIA
GABON
CONGO
RWANDA
KENYA
MALAYSIA
EQUATOR
0°
BURUNDI
SINGAPORE
NAURU
KIRIBATI
TANZANIA
INDIAN
PAPUA
SEYCHELLES
INDONESIA
SOLOMON
OCEAN
NEW GUINEA
ISLANDS
TUVALU
ANGOLA
COMOROS
CHRISTMAS I.
ZAMBIA
MALAWI
MAYOTTE
COCOS IS.
(AUSTRALIA)
CORAL SEA
(FRANCE)
(AUSTRALIA)
ISLANDS
VANUATU
MOZAMBIQUE
MAURITIUS
(AUSTRALIA)
FIJI
NAMIBIA
ZIMBABWE
20°S
BOTSWANA
MADAGASCAR
REUNION
TROPIC OF CAPRICORN
NEW CALEDONIA
SWAZILAND
(FRANCE)
AUSTRALIA
(FRANCE)
SOUTH
LESOTHO
NORFOLK I.
AFRICA
(AUSTRALIA)
NEW
ZEALAND
40°S
PRINCE EDWARD IS.
CROZET IS.
(SOUTH AFRICA)
(FRANCE)
KERGUELEN IS.
(FRANCE)
BOUVET IS.
MCDONALD IS.
(NORWAY)
(AUSTRALIA)
HEARD I.
(AUSTRALIA)
60°S
ANTARCTICA
ANTARCTIC CIRCLE
80°S
20°E
40°E
60°E
80°E
100°E
120°E
140°E
160°E
180°
SCALE 1/94,903,000
1 CENTIMETER = 949 KILOMETERS OR 1INCH = 1527 MILES
KILOMETERS
0 100 200 300 400 500 600
80°N AND 80°S
60°N AND 60°S
40°N AND 40°S
20°N AND 20°S
0°
STATUTE MILES
0 100 200 300 400 500 600
80°N AND 80°S
60°N AND 60°S
40°N AND 40°S
20°N AND 20°S
0°
METRIC CONVERSIONS
1 centimeter x 0.393701 = inches
1 meter x 3.280840 = feet
1 kilometer x 0.621371 = miles

Seeds of an Obsession are Planted

How did it all begin . . . my flights into fancy, which led to an obsession to see the whole world and to get to know its people? It began during the early years of my marriage, which coincided with the depths of the Great Depression, in the early 1930's. Everyone knew then that two could live as cheaply as one. At least all of the popular magazines tried to prove it.

But three posed some problems. When a baby came along in those days, women were supposed to stay home and be mothers. We were lucky that my husband had a job. It didn't pay much, but he was able to work overtime, and some months we were almost able to come out even. Overtime meant 12 hours a day, seven days a week. But we did not feel sorry for ourselves. We were healthy, and all our friends were in a similar situation.

We were more fortunate than some. We owned a Victrola. So while I hand-laundered baby clothes, boiled diapers to hang out to dry in Chicago's unpredictable weather, or ironed my husband's shirts by the hour, I wasn't really there at all. I had flown away on the strains of "The Hawaiian Wedding Song" to magic isles of sunlit beaches, rolling surf and gently rustling palm trees.

Our Chicago was not a clean place in which to live, because our apartment was on a busy street. That faded kitchen linoleum looked clean only when hand-scrubbed with a brush and soapy water, but I wasn't on my knees performing an unpleasant task. The strains of that beautiful Kashmiri song, "Pale Hands I Loved," had wafted me to a gaily decorated houseboat floating in a sea of waterlilies on Lake Dal in the Vale of Kashmir, surrounded by a misty ring of snow-covered mountains.

My imagination was as unhampered by distance as it was by reality. I sat on the stone steps of a mighty river and watched barges deliver bodies to be cremated before sending their ashes to be sanctified by burial in the Holy Ganges. And there, gleaming in all of its magnificence, was the Taj Mahal, a monument to the love for a woman who died giving birth to her 13th child. Oh, the romance of it all in that land of enchantment, India!

Scraping carrots and peeling potatoes for our often-nightly meal of stew wasn't a chore, because I was sailing into Shanghai Harbor on a "Slow Boat to China." Our gangplank was surrounded by rickshaws, pulled by human bearers wearing large pointed straw hats. Walking on the Great Wall of China, I could distinguish smoke signals from fires in the watchtowers, the kind of communication used around 200 B.C.

Many years have now passed, but unlike some dreams, mine turned into reality. There was no 'empty-nest syndrome' to overcome when my youngest child flew the coop - literally, as a Pan American Airlines stewardess. I was ready to fly, too.

Did reality live up to my imagination? Indeed, yes! Now, whenever I hear "The Hawaiian Wedding Song" or "Slow Boat to China," I am once again transported, not to the countries I longed to see, but to that apartment on Chicago's northwest side, where I was young and the world was mine. "Slow Boat to China" is still my favorite tune.

A Collection Begins

During my travels I fell in love with the ethnic dress of the natives. I became aware that in some lands, especially Asia, Southeast Asia, the Middle East and parts of Central and South America and Africa, clothing worn was very much like that worn centuries ago.

Folk customs resist change, but costumes do not last for years undamaged as clay pots and iron tools can. While in many countries traditional treasures are handed down from parents to children, their life is finite. Although costumes are still worn for festivals and important events, the influence of Western fashion through television and tourism is strong, and a great deal of ethnic beauty is disappearing from the world.

It was not possible for me to search individual attics and storerooms, but I soon learned that museums are very proud of their country's culture. Curators were more than willing to advise me when asked, and tour guides are usually well-educated and knowledgeable about the dress and customs of their people.

When it became known that the final result of our efforts would be on display in a museum in the United States, the eagerness of everyone involved to put together a masterpiece of ethnic authenticity was exciting and heart-warming.

The examples of timeless fashions still available for purchase today created so much attention when I brought them home, that invitations to display them came often. At first regular models were used, but it soon became evident that the dress of a particular country was enhanced by the grace and beauty of the natives of that country.

Coeds from the International Club of the University of Colorado volunteered to model at a show given for the benefit of the university library. The program was well received and great fun for everyone. I knew I was on the right track when an Afghan girl said to me, "We were all surprised and thrilled when we saw that everything you have is well chosen and properly put together. We love wearing our country's clothing, but it makes us a little homesick."

My obsession for traveling and collecting was heightened by this remark, and increased interest from local museums was also encouraging. There are not many decades left to obtain materials from ways of life that may soon cease to exist.

This study is incomplete at best, but I hope you will enjoy my contribution to the fascinating world of ethnic dress.

It All Began With a Needle

Man began wearing clothes over 100,000 years ago. Like food, shelter and his family, it has always been one of his basic needs. Costume, or to use the correct term, ethnic dress, is not just body covering. The history of a civilization and its people can be found in the study of clothing, which is worn for protection, status, adornment and ritual ceremonies.

The Bible tells us that the first body covering was worn by Adam and Eve. Aprons of leaves were followed by animal skins. This analysis agrees with that of anthropologists who tell us that early dress consisted of leaves, woven reed and a type of fabric called tapa, which is made from the bark of the mulberry tree. The bark is softened with water and then beaten with a mallet into cloth. It is still worn today on some of the islands of the Pacific Ocean.

A bone needle was found in a burial site that has been estimated to be 25,000 years old. This date corresponds with the fourth and last glacial period. Within that same time frame controlled fire was discovered in China. With the needle to sew skins together and the knowledge of the safe use of fire, man was ready to handle climate changes. From the Magdalenian period, 17,000 B.C., to 11,000 B.C., bone needles with eyes have been found in large quantities in graves.

Anthropologists can determine many things about man from his clothing . . . his sex, his occupation, his wealth, influence and power, his religious beliefs, his language, his place within his culture and his identity in general.

Magdalenians were among the first known nomadic people. They followed reindeer, wild horse and bison herds. Life became easier with abundant food, allowing more leisure for aesthetics and the arts. The famous cave paintings in the Grotte de Lascaux in France and the Altamira Caves in northern Spain are products of this period. They show figures in stitched fur garments which are not unlike those worn by modern Eskimos.

The expression "Clothes make the man" has been true since the dawn of history. The first adornment was probably painted on man's body in colors that represented the earth, with red for air, blue for sky, yellow for fire and white for water. The designs had tribal meanings. Patterns were carved on stone, metal, wood and pottery. Next came necklaces of lions' claws, horn, ivory or bone amulets, and capes of animal skins. All of this undoubtedly contributed to man's feeling of strength and virility, showing that he was a mighty hunter.

When textiles replaced animal skins, an important industry developed. Weaving may be the oldest of the arts. Learning to make yarn from flax, cotton and animal wool and weaving it into cloth took thousands of years. Flax has been under cultivation for at least 10,000 years, and there is evidence that woolen textiles were known in southern Turkey since 6000 B.C. By 3000 B.C., cotton was grown in the Indus River Valley, and by 2600 B.C., the Chinese Empress Hsi-ling Shih had learned the art of raising silkworms by unraveling and joining the strands, or filaments, of their cocoons and twisting them into silk thread.

With the development of textiles, designs were transferred to them in the form of embroidery. Metals were used like embroidery, and in some cultures stones are believed to have magic powers. Symbols that could be easily understood were invented. While each cultural group had its own folklore, legends and myths, there were often patterns between these groups that have universal themes. The circle is one of the oldest of all symbols. It and the interlocking spiral represented the rebirth of man; later these became serpents and dragons. The circle, the disk or the rosette may also symbolize the sun or the universe. Triangles became stars, and the "Tree of Life" meant the center of the world or the binding together of heaven and earth.

Early Greece, Rome, Egypt and Persia greatly influenced the development of clothing, as did wars and conquests, weather, materials and methods of their creation and customs.

In the beginning fabric was draped or wrapped around the body. A simple sleeveless tunic followed. The man's garment came just to or above the knee, and the woman's tunic was long, and later worn bloused. Slaves wore breechcloths. As civilization advanced class differences increased, and upper classes dressed to show their social status and rank. Peasant style remained remarkably unchanged until the 15th century, when the bodice, apron and trousers became popular.

Linen could be worn only by priests and used as burial wrappings for the Pharaohs in ancient Egypt. Egyptians and Chinese considered anyone who wore wool a barbarian, and Turks, Central Asians and some Europeans considered any man who wore silk to be weak and effeminate. However, this attitude changed when silk began arriving in Rome from China by way of the 4,000 mile "Old Silk Road." By 47 B.C., crowds witnessing Julius Caesar's triumphant entry into Rome were astonished to see canopies of silk stretched overhead. By 14 A.D., there was such a clamor for this beautiful fabric that it sold for its weight in gold.

Many changes in the way of making clothing and the materials used have come during the last 200 years. One of the catalysts of the Industrial Revolution was the need to produce textiles cheaply, quickly and in large quantities.

The significance of color cannot be overlooked. It has played an important part in clothing and embroidery. In Europe and the United States black is the color of mourning. In China and India, white is the color of grief. In many areas of the Far East yellow is used for death, but in early Chinese dynasties it was the color of royalty, and blue was for commoners. A hapless peasant could lose his head for wearing yellow. Syrians and Armenians wore light blue for mourning, and in Iran the color of withered leaves was used for that purpose. Everywhere in Asia, red is the color of happiness, life and love, and is used for wedding attire in many countries.

Fine examples of traditional dress are still worn for festivals and religious celebrations and important social events. Masks and formal dress for holy days were often thought to become possessed with the spirits of the gods or of animals. Animal skins are worn in cold countries, reindeer skins in Lapland, yak wool and leather in Mongolia, Tibet and Siberia. Alpaca and llama wools are woven into clothing in the altiplano of Bolivia and Peru.

Not very long ago in Guatemala, Central America, there were 200 different Mayan Indian tribes, each wearing, with pride, the costumes of their ancestors. Men, women and children could be seen trotting barefoot along the road, each family wearing its own hand-loomed textile in the color favored by the tribe.

No, costume is not just body covering. Its study makes an important contribution to the history of man.

Sea-Fever

I must go down to the seas again, to the lonely sea and the sky,
And all I ask is a tall ship and a star to steer her by;
And the wheel's kick and the wind's song and the white sail's shaking,
And a gray mist on the sea's face, and a gray dawn breaking.

I must go down to the seas again, for the call of the running tide
Is a wild call and a clear call that may not be denied;
And all I ask is a windy day with the white clouds flying,
And the flung spray and the blown spume, and the sea-gulls crying.

I must go down to the seas again, to the vagrant gypsy life,
To the gull's way and the whale's way, where the wind's like a whetted knife.
And all I ask is a merry yarn from a laughing fellow-rover,
And quiet sleep and a sweet dream when the long trick's over.

John Masefield

Chapter One

Isles of Enchantment

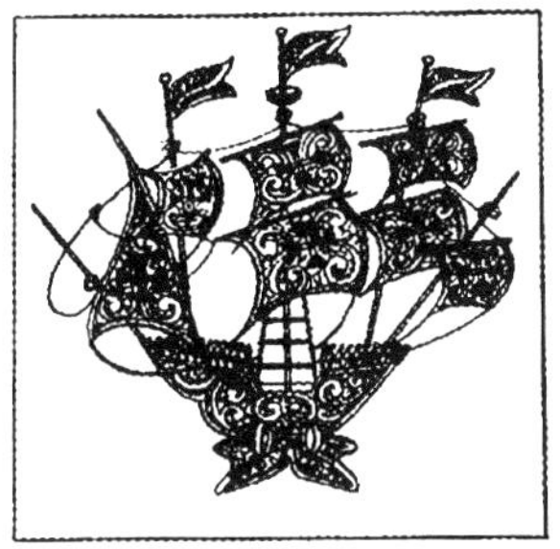

San Blas
Hawaii
New Zealand
Lamu
East and South Africa

The San Blas Islands

The territory of San Blas is administratively part of the province of Colón of the Republic of Panama. It is 360 islands near the Archipelago de las Mulatas, off the northeast coast of Panama, in the Caribbean Sea. The natives of the islands are the Cuna Indians. They speak Chibchan, an unwritten language. Once, they occupied the central region of what is now Panama and the neighboring San Blas Islands. Now, 25,000 Cunas live on the islands, while 1,200 live on the mainland.

In the 16th century the Cunas were an important group, living in villages under chiefs who had considerable power. Agriculture was slash and burn, and trade was carried on by canoe along the coast. European contact destroyed this political superstructure, and in modern times they live in small villages and are dependent upon fishing and hunting for subsistence. The society is matriarchal, with the line of inheritance passing through the women.

Mola Blouses of the Cuna Indians

Mola blouses evolved during the Victorian period. Older molas, or `grandmother molas,' are scarce, due to deterioration in tropical weather conditions. Few exist dating back to before the 1920's. Girls start working on molas at the age of seven or eight, and there is intense rivalry to see who can be the most imaginative. A mola is a rectangular, many-colored, hand-stitched panel worn by all Cuna women and girls on the front and back of their blouses. They are approximately 14 by 16 inches in size, and the embroidery is a type of reverse appliqué. Every mola is a personal statement, but quality molas have particular characteristics. There is continuity of thought, with an identifiable theme in the design and impressive detail, such as whiskers or eyelashes. Thread and cloth must match in color, and rick-rack should be made by hand. Fine stitches are neatly placed. Poplin is the background cloth, and should not be pieced. Cigar-shaped slots should be no more than 3/32 of an inch wide.

The Smithsonian Institute declared molas to be pre-Columbian art, and their importance is increasing in the art world. Good molas are becoming difficult to find because of the many ships now making the islands a port of call. Not all the molas tourists find are of top quality. The molas in the collection were purchased from the Cuna Indians in the San Blas Islands. From Panama City we took a small plane to the largest island and then traveled by boat.

This cow mola is one of the finest the collector has ever seen. The head of the cow is well executed, with a flower dangling from its mouth. It is probably the older of the two molas because of its more subdued coloring, although both have a background color of red with blues, greens and yellows. The square designs on the collar and the bits of embroidery and hand-made rick-rack are exquisitely stitched. The top of the blouse is a bright yellow synthetic fabric.

An excellent donkey mola has cigar slots which are not as narrow as those on the cow mola, and the colors are a bit bright for some tastes, but the design is wonderful. Looked at one way it is that of two donkeys, and from a different perspective it is a very large head of a fanciful figure. The beautiful workmanship and the symmetry of the design make this mola noteworthy. The blouse itself is made of a blue material with a leaf design.

The blue and gold calico skirts are sarongs, with differing designs. The scarves, worn as headshawls, are red and yellow, with a fish design in the center of each square. Many yards of shell, shark's teeth and colored bead necklaces are wound around the wrists and ankles, and Costa Rican coins are strung into pieces of jewelry. The nose ring was a real find.

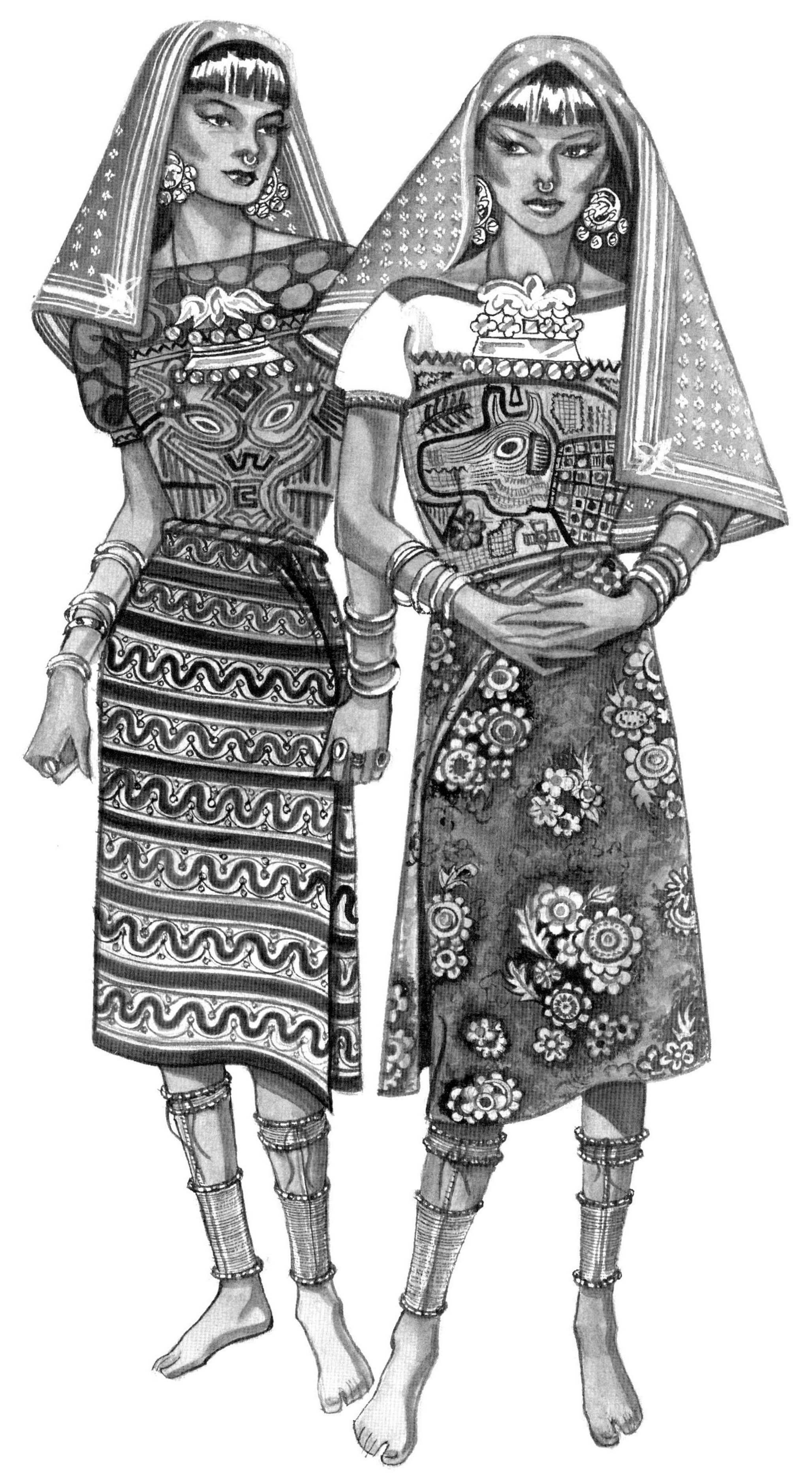

A life on the ocean wave,

A home on the rolling deep,

Where the scattered waters rave,

And the winds their revels keep!

Like an eagle caged I pine

On this dull, unchanging shore:

Oh! give me the flashing brine,

The spray and the tempests' roar.

Epes Sargent

Hawaii

The United States acquired the Hawaiian Islands in 1898 by annexation, and they entered the Union as the 50th state in 1959. These islands lie in the North Pacific Ocean, 2,400 miles from San Francisco. They are over 6,400 square miles in land area, smaller than the state of New Jersey, with a population a little more than the state of New Hampshire. The state consists of the tops of a chain of submerged volcanic mountains, which form eight major islands and 124 small islets, stretching in a 1,500-mile crescent. Although these islands lie in the tropical zone, the average temperature in Honolulu is 71.9 F in the coolest month and 78.4 F in the warmest. Famous for their climate, their luxuriant tropical foliage, superb beaches and some of the world's most glamorous hotels, the islands are a tourist's paradise. If visitors arrive at the Big Island of Hawaii at the right time they can even see spectacular volcanic eruptions. Early Hawaiians believed that the active volcano Kilauea, on this island, was the home of a family of fire deities headed by the goddess Pele. Whenever Pele stomped her feet in anger, the earth quaked.

Around 400 A.D., the first Hawaiians were thought to have migrated from the Marquesas Islands. For nine centuries they continued their contacts with other Polynesian islands, particularly Tahiti. They developed an elaborate calendar and navigational methods, and their huge outrigger canoes are considered technical wonders today. From the arrival of the canoes to the visit of Captain Cook there are fascinating stories to be told. Powerful chiefs and priests emerged and conflicts not unlike the feudal struggles in Europe took place. In 1778 Captain James Cook, in his search for a passage between the Atlantic and Pacific Oceans, landed on Kauai Island, naming it part of the Sandwich Islands. He returned the following year and was killed by local inhabitants. In the early 19th century whaling fleets began wintering in Hawaii, and by 1820 the first of 15 companies of missionaries arrived, bringing their families with them. By mid-century the Hawaiians had a written language, frame homes, horse-drawn vehicles, schools and churches. American civilization and religious beliefs irrevocably changed Hawaiian culture.

After the death of King Kamehameha I, his favorite wife, Queen Kaahumanu, became premier to his successor. She instigated many reforms and urged the new king to abolish traditional taboos and to welcome the Christian missionaries from New England. She worked closely with the first group of women who arrived and was even baptized. An island king and his queen visited London and died there from measles. The pineapple business developed on a huge scale, as did that of macadamia nuts. The sadness of Pearl Harbor came, and finally, the happy assumption of statehood. Hawaii has a fascinating history and an extraordinary collection of races and peoples, Polynesian, Asian, European and American.

One of our most delightful recollections is a barefoot stroll on the beach at dusk in Waikiki with members of our family, who were living in Hawaii. We stepped over a low stone fence, helped ourselves to a seat on the sand and watched the after-dinner entertainment that was in progress on the patio of a nearby hotel. Hula dances were performed to the accompaniment of Hawaiian ukeleles, playing songs of the islands. Pele's Fire Dance ended the program. No one worried about our cost-free enjoyment. Everyone goes to Hawaii to relax, and does so!

Hawaiian Princess Kaiulani Tutu

James Jarvis, a journalist from Boston, wrote in 1837:

"A few white women had followed their adventurous missionary husbands hither, and with their Parisian hats and boots, despite much domestic discomfort, made quite a social oasis amid the general dirt and barbarism. . . A white woman in full toilet was still a sufficient curiosity to attract a crowd. Consequently, if one went out, she was soon surrounded by a cortege of men and maidens, more or less in a state of nudity, all bent upon studying the fashions with an eagerness proportionate to their own want of clothing."

The gowns of these missionary wives were admired and copied by the islanders, particularly since their Queen Kaahumanu was one of the first to acquire one. Because some of the Hawaiian ladies were of generous proportions, the dresses were often shorter in front, resulting in a train, or 'holoku,' in the back. Trains were all the rage in the mid 1800's.

The 'Grandma MuuMuu' or 'Tutu' is of red cotton with a narrow stripe of tiny white dots. It is a long tunic with a wide flounce around the bottom. There is a high neck with a white cotton yoke at the front and back, which comes to a point. Narrow, white eyelet ruffling trims the neck and outlines the yoke. The cuffs of the long, tight sleeves and the top of the flounce at the bottom of the skirt have the same ruffled trim. These dresses, just like the tutus of 1820, were very popular at the time we visited Hawaii. They are perfect for teas and lawn parties.

Flower crowns worn around the head are called a 'wili wili,' pronounced, 'veely-veely.' They are usually made with hedge flowers and woven onto 'ti' leaves. The earrings are 'kukui,' or candle nuts, hand sanded and polished in the islands. They are from the state tree and were regarded by the early Hawaiians as a symbol of royalty.

This charming tutu was found in a shop called The Princess Kaiulani. Princess Kaiulani was the daughter of A.S. Cleghorn, a successful Honolulu merchant who married the sister of King Kalakaua in 1898. The princess later became heir-apparent. Robert Louis Stevenson tried to persuade her to visit Scotland, but found her loath to leave her islands. He wrote:

Forth from her land to mine she goes,
The island maid, the island rose,
Light of heart and bright of face:
The daughter of a double race.
Her islands here, in southern sun,
Shall mourn their Kaiulani gone,
And I, in her dear banyan shade,
Look vainly for my little maid.
But our Scots Islands far away
Shall glitter with unwonted day,
And cast for once their tempest by
To smile in Kaiulani's eye.

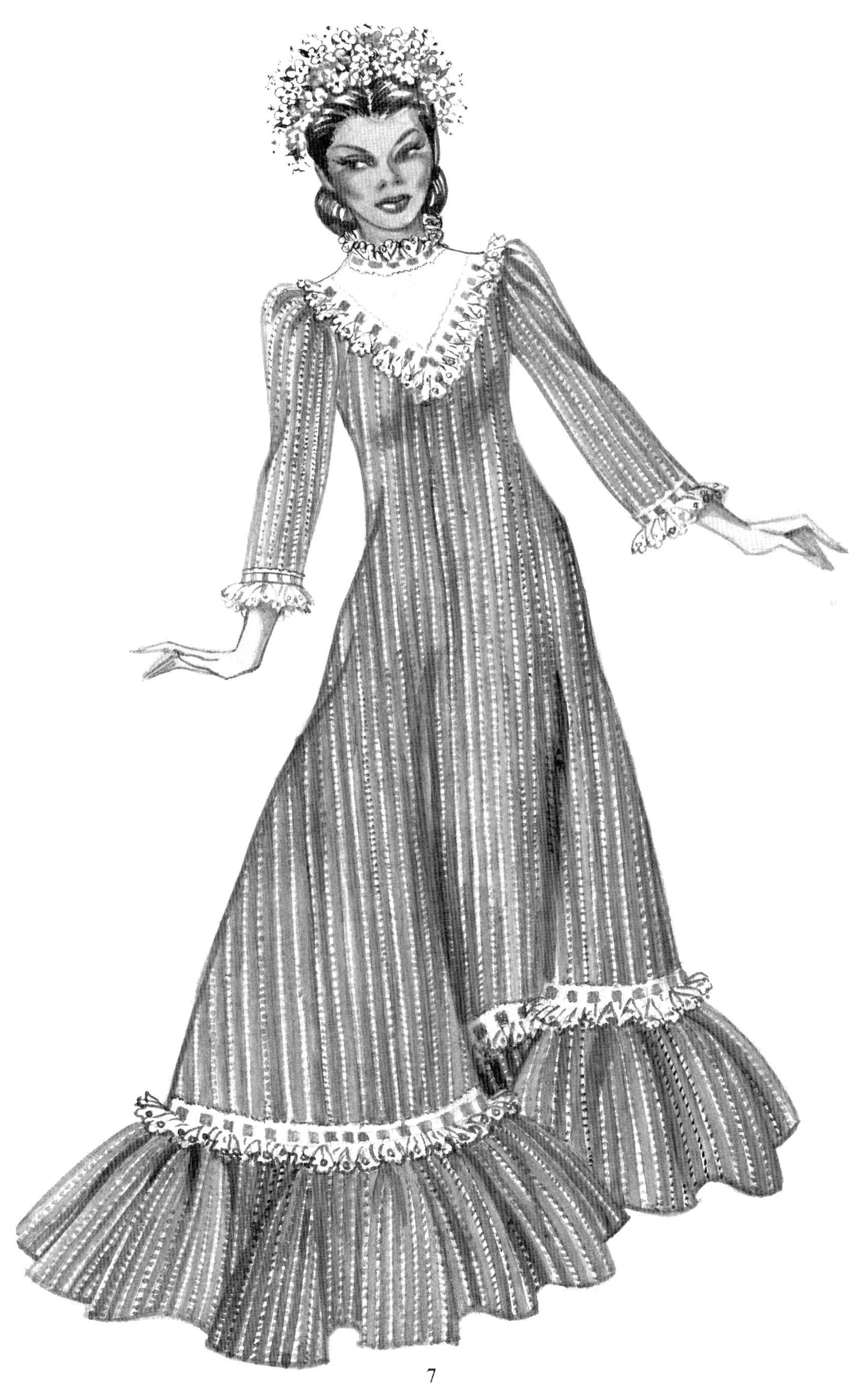

New Zealand

New Zealand is an island nation in the southwestern Pacific with two main islands, North Island and South Island, plus Stewart Island, the Chatham Islands and the Ross Dependency, which is in the Antarctic. The total land area is about the size of Colorado, with the same population. There are more sheep than people in New Zealand. Each of the main islands is hilly and mountainous. South Island has glaciers and 15 peaks over 10,000 feet in altitude. The fjords here compare in beauty with those of Norway. The North Island mountains are volcanic in origin, with active volcanoes in a wide belt of thermal activity.

It is an independent member of the British Commonwealth, with a parliamentary democracy whose head of state at the present time is Queen Elizabeth II, represented by a governor general. The capital is Wellington, on North Island. The ethnic groups are British and Maori, and the religions are Anglican, Presbyterian and Roman Catholic. The Maoris are mostly Mormon. The currency is the dollar, and literacy is 99 percent.

The Maori people reached New Zealand from the eastern Pacific before and during the 14th century. Although they resisted early foreign settlement, Captain James Cook explored the coasts in the late 1760's, and European colonies flourished. British sovereignty was proclaimed in 1840. The Maori Wars ended in 1870 with a British victory, and in 1907 the colony became a dominion. The native Maoris now number about nine percent of the total population.

Maori Woman's Ceremonial Dress

Rotorua, a city on North Island where this dress was found, is in the heart of the thermal belt, and its homes are heated with natural steam. There are hot springs, boiling pools of mud and spouting geysers. Amazing firefly caves are entered by boat. When lights are turned off thousands of tiny, flickering, pinpoints of light can be seen.

A large proportion of Rotorua's population is Maori. A school has been set up here to teach the young people to scrape the reeds which are used to make the skirt of this costume. Weavers show them how to fashion the blouse and the headband, using traditional designs, which are always geometrical and have names and meanings. For example, a downward zig-zag pattern denotes the sea.

There are 116 reed lengths to this skirt. It is a yard wide, 21 inches long, and is banded at the top by a woven length of grasses. It is worn knee length, by either men or women. The bodice and matching headband are woven from hand-loomed wool in red, black, yellow and white. A piece of cotton weaving is sewn into a short, red, sleeveless shift that is held up by black woolen braided shoulder straps. The 'tiki,' or locket, a greenstone fetish design, was originally a fertility symbol but has become New Zealand's good luck charm.

Maori dancing and music are Polynesian in style. The dancers are barefoot and swing the poi balls with skill and gusto. These balls are made of cellophane, with hand-braided silk yarn ropes and yellow-fringe handles. It takes a lot of practice to swing them properly, without getting them wound around the other or oneself.

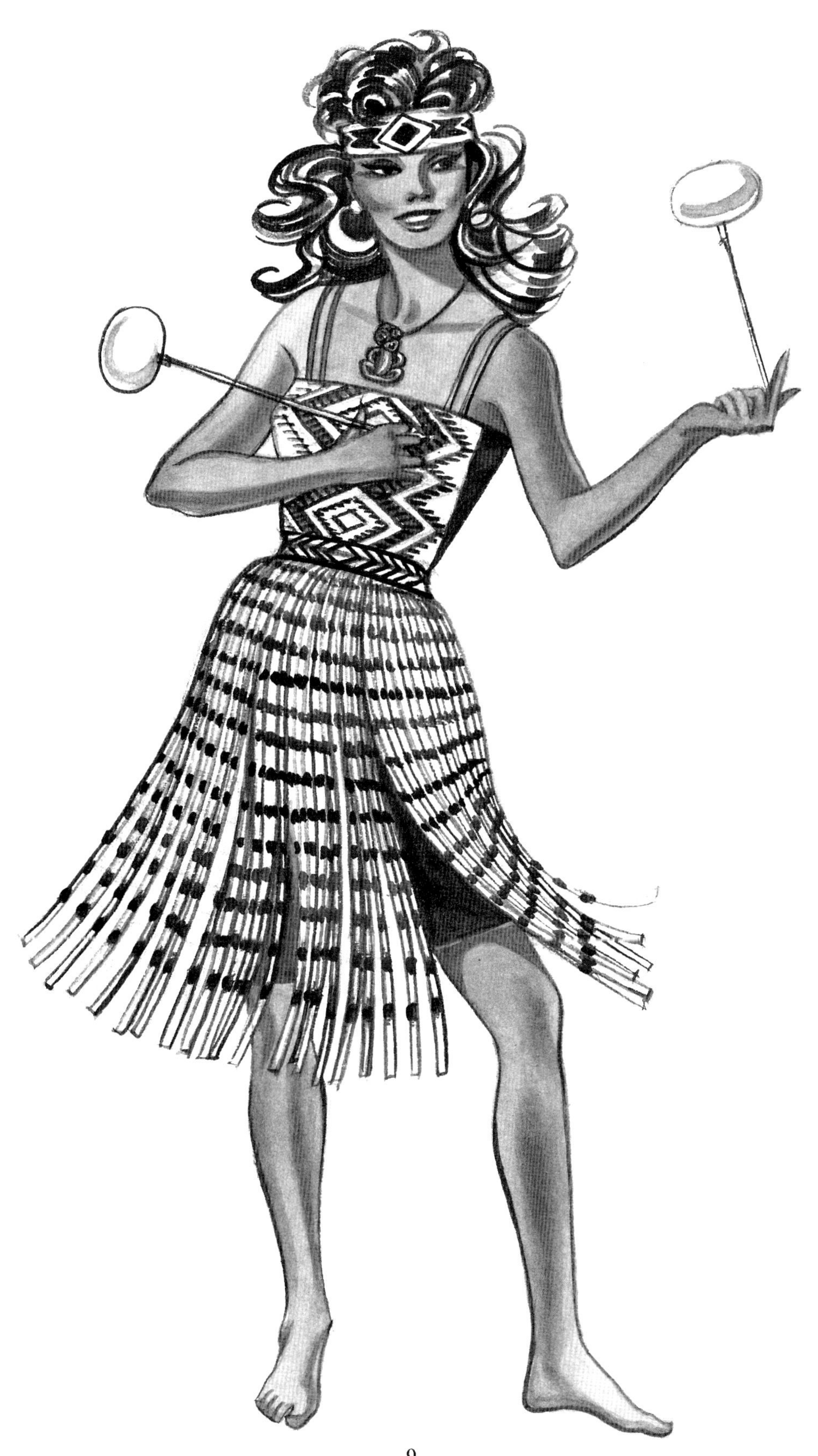

Lamu Island

Lamu is an island in the Indian Ocean off the coast of East Africa, about 150 miles northeast of Mombasa, Kenya. Administered now as part of the Coast Province of Kenya, it was a former Persian colony and later belonged to Zanzibar. Until the 19th century it rivaled Mombasa as a market for gold, spices and slaves. This island is of great value to historians because its customs have been frozen for centuries. It is often called 'The land where time has stood still.' It was an age-old trade route for India, the Malays and Arabia, and the Arab influence is still strong. Most of the people are Muslim, and the official language is Swahili, which is more than a language; it is also a society. Lamu is showing signs of coming into the modern age. It now has electricity, unless an elephant on the mainland knocks down a critical pole. The practice of covering the women's faces while in public is still observed and modern girls, like all well-bred women on Lamu, must wear their bui-buis while out-of-doors. These garments, with their long, black folds, cover their faces and bodies. They are worn until the girls cross on the ferry to Kenya, to go to school in Nairobi. In Kenya women do not veil their faces, so the bui-buis are rolled into balls and put away until they return to Lamu at holiday time.

Woman's Bui-bui and Khanga

A bui-bui is a floor-length, black coat-like garment made of a synthetic fabric, sewn on both sides, but open halfway down the front. Attached to the garment is a large piece of the same material to be wrapped skillfully around the woman's head and face. The 60-inch by 43-inch sarong worn under the bui-bui is called a 'khanga.' Its background is bright red, with eight large circles printed in navy, white and red and a six-inch border surrounding the entire sarong. It is worn tightly wrapped into a sleeveless tunic with a pleat on the left side. The top ends are tied into a knot and tucked into the garment so that it fits properly, falling to the floor in a straight line. At the back, above the bottom border, printed on a white strip is the Swahili motto "Ukweli ni dawa ya urongo," which means "Truth is the medicine of lies." Khangas are not only worn as dresses inside the home, they also serve as nightdresses for both men and women.

The valuable silver jewelry was collected with great diligence by Linda Donley. There are four rings worn on the left hand. The square earrings are made from melted-down coins. The silver tube-like talisman case carries, rolled up inside, an inscription from the Koran. It is tied on the wrist with a silk cord. There are 10 thin, handmade silver bracelets. A woman of Lamu carries her wealth in silver on her body and may wear as many as 200 of these bracelets at one time. The finest piece is the stunning, handcrafted silver necklace called a 'mkufu,' from Yemen.

How did we get this wonderful costume? We became acquainted with Linda Donley while on safari in Kenya, Tanzania and Uganda. She had been sent by the Smithsonian Institute to help in the organization of the Lamu Museum. She agreed to assemble and mail this costume to me. In a letter which accompanied the costume, Linda wrote that her success in finding the precisely appropriate parts of this ethnic dress made it very difficult to part with, rather than keeping it for the new museum. But she had promised!

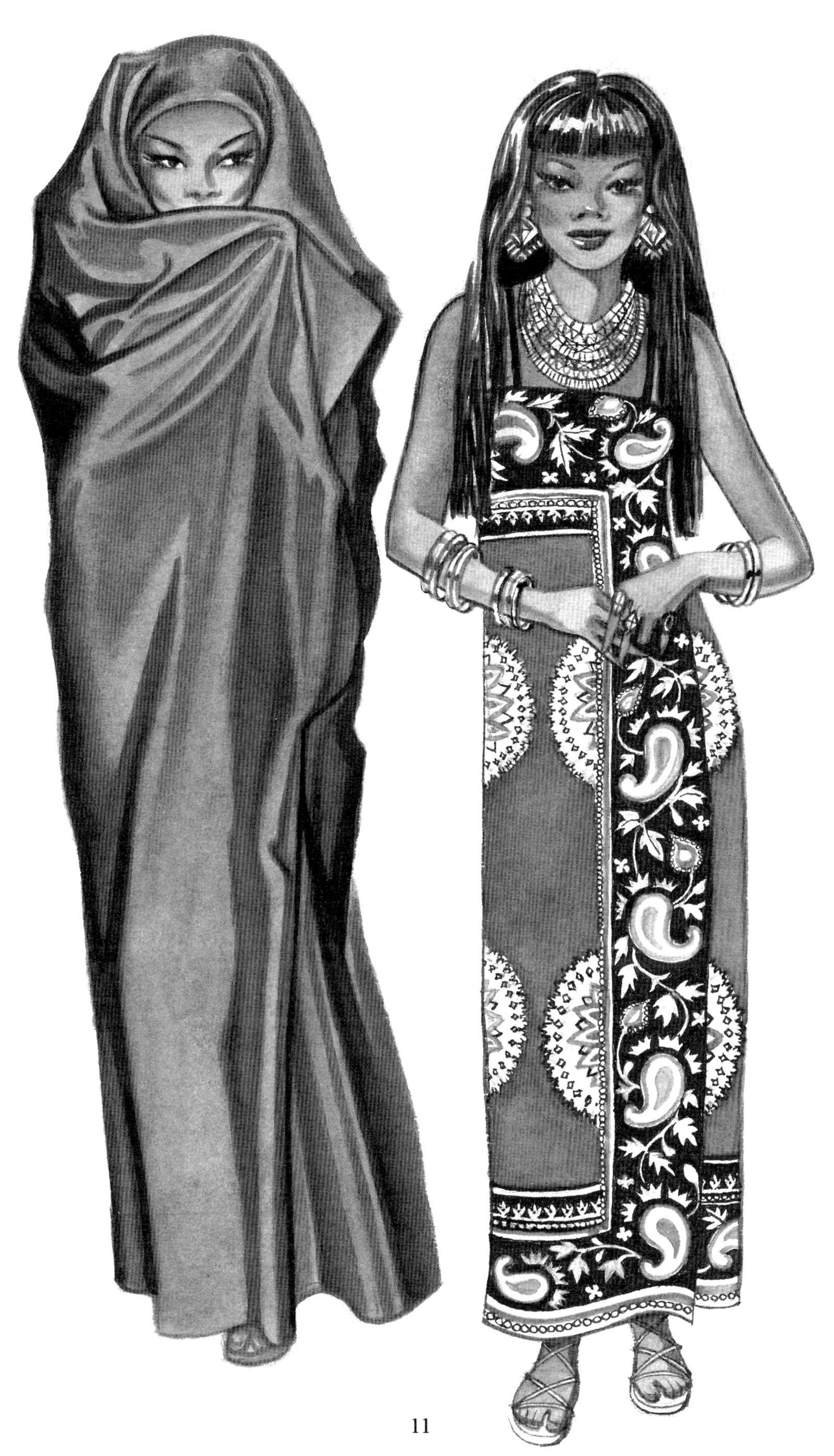

East and South African Panorama

Kenya, which borders on the Indian Ocean, is slightly smaller than Texas, with a population of 28 million. The capital is Nairobi and official languages are Swahili and English. Its currency is the shilling, and literacy is 50 percent. The dominant religions are Christian and Muslim. We drove through Nairobi's 45-square-mile game park, and observed a sky full of flamingos at the Nakuru Bird Sanctuary. We experienced elephant-viewing at dinner on an open terrace about 100 yards from a waterhole. Over fresh linen tablecloths, set with fine British china and silver, we ate our grilled steaks and hot rolls while watching a baby and two adult elephants squirting water at each other. This was game watching 'in the wild'. . . British style.

On the Masai-Mara Game Reserve, noted for its black-maned lions, we were chased by Masai men, dressed only in long, orange-red cloaks. Their bodies were dyed with ocher clay and decorated with colored beads and disks. They ran after our bus, cloaks flying, brandishing long spears, shouting what must have been threats in Swahili. Our guide seemed unperturbed. He hadn't given them enough of a tip for our picture-taking, and they were letting us know. Other highlights included Mt. Kilimanjaro, as beautiful as we'd imagined, The Ark, a comfortable lounge with its worm's-eye view of animals and two nights at the Mt. Kenya Safari Club, with its stately peacocks, decorating the spacious lawns. At Mt. Kenya Game Farm wild animal orphans are raised with loving care.

Tanzania, on the coast of East Africa, south of Kenya and Uganda, is twice the size of California. It was a slave trading center for many years. Its currency is the shilling, and literacy is 85 percent. The capital is Dar-es-Salaam. The religions are Christian and Muslim. A thrilling sight was watching the migration of thousands of wildebeests, zebras and giraffes in Serengeti National Park, which has the world's largest concentration of game. At Lake Manyara National Park lazy tree-climbing lions were stretched out on high limbs, safe from predators. Olduvai Gorge is a 30-mile-long ravine, the home of prehistoric man and animals, covering a time span from two million to 15 thousand years ago.

Uganda, in east central Africa, is slightly smaller than Oregon. The capital is Kampala, the currency the shilling, and literacy is 52 percent. The religions are Christian and Muslim. We stayed in a rustic hotel in Entebbe on the shores of Lake Victoria. We heard shrieking sounds in the night, and were told by waiters at breakfast that Sabena (Belgium) Airline pilots were chasing the hotel's maids around. On a trip in small boats up the White Nile to Murchison Falls, we were eyed by hippos and crocodiles.

Zimbabwe, formerly Rhodesia, in southern Africa, is slightly larger than Montana. The capital is Harare, the monetary unit the dollar, and literacy is 67 percent. The religions are tribal belief, with a Christian minority. We saw the perpetual rainbow through the mist that veils Victoria Falls, which the natives call "Smoke Does Sound."

South Africa is about twice the size of Texas. Its capital is Capetown, currency the rand, literacy 99 percent, and the religion Christian. Modern, sophisticated Capetown, on the shores of the Cape of Good Hope, is overlooked by Table Mountain. The Blue Train from Capetown to Johannesburg is one of the most luxurious of all railways. We counted 16 pieces of silver at each dinner table setting. As we approached Pretoria, the administrative capital of South Africa, we saw a lavender haze around the city. It came from thousands of jacaranda trees in full bloom.

Chapter Two

Island Hopping in Southeast Asia

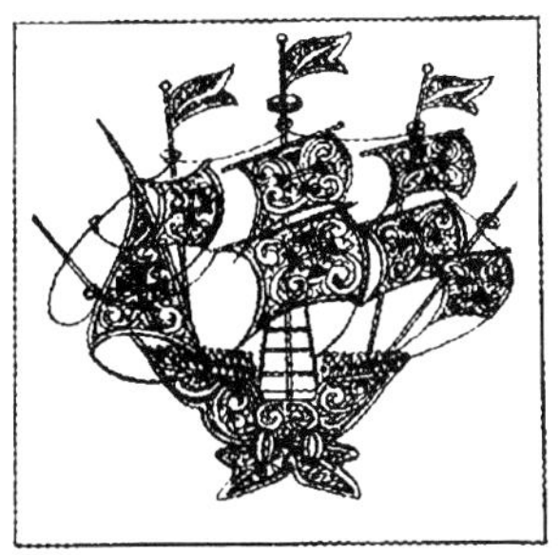

Indonesia
Singapore
Malaysia
Philippines

Republic of Indonesia

Indonesia forms an archipelago of 17,000 islands, southeast of Asia, along the equator, covering an area of 741,052 square miles. The population is more than three-quarters the population of the United States. The capital is Djakarta, on the island of Java. Currency is the rupiah, and literacy is 85 percent. Malay is the official language, and the religion is 87 percent Muslim. President Suharto has been head of state since 1968, and in 1993 was re-elected to a sixth term of five more years.

Hindu and Buddhist civilizations reached Indonesia from India 2,000 years ago. By the 16th century Islam had become prominent. In the 17th century the Dutch became the most important European trading power, and by the early 20th century all of the country was united under one rule, that of the Dutch. After the Japanese occupation from 1942-45, Indonesia became a republic. The Netherlands gave up sovereignty in 1949, and in 1963 a vote by the whole area was promised. In 1969 voting by tribal chiefs favored staying with Indonesia.

Java is the fourth largest island in Indonesia, but it is the most important both politically and economically. Its population density of 1,500 people per square mile is a world record. Jogjakarta, Java's capital, produces many batiks. It is a cottage industry, and the finest of all batiks often originate in this area. Both the tjanting and the tjap types of batik were developed here.

In 800 A.D., one of the greatest Buddhist monuments of all time, Borobudur, was built in central Java. The monument is an enormous pyramid, built around a natural hillock. It is not really a temple, as there is no interior area that can be entered. Eight terraces are crowned by a main stupa (a free-standing monument), and 72 stupas contain statues of Buddha, fenced with perforated stonework. Dutch archeologists restored this magnificent work in the early 1900's.

Kebayas and Kains of Java and Bali

This Javanese 'kebaya,' or blouse, is of machine-made green lace. It has a rolled collar and an insert of the same material at the neck. There are long, tight sleeves. The 'kain,' or sarong, is worn long and is six yards in length. It has a brown background with small black squares with a white dot in one corner of each square. Large 'garudas,' or wings, form a pattern. This is a 'tjap' batik, which looks much like the 'tjanting' batik of the costume from Bali. An expert can tell the difference by two clues, the textile used and the skill of the handwork . . . tjap batiks are more precise. Tjanting batiks are considered worthy of only the finest fabrics. Kains are folded at the top left side of the waist before wrapping so that the length is more manageable and a smoother appearance is achieved. The other end is pleated with odd numbers (5, 7 or 11) of inside pleats which are held in place with paper clips until worn. Wrapping this batik tightly into a smooth-fitting kain with the pleats at exactly the right place is no easy feat for a novice. A long strip of matching material is often wound around the waist so there is is no noticeable gap between the kebaya and kain. Women of these islands are modest. A 'sabai,' a long chiffon scarf, is worn with the long end draped over the inside of the left arm, an important detail in Indonesian dress. This outfit, found in Jogjakarta, is still worn by Javanese women.

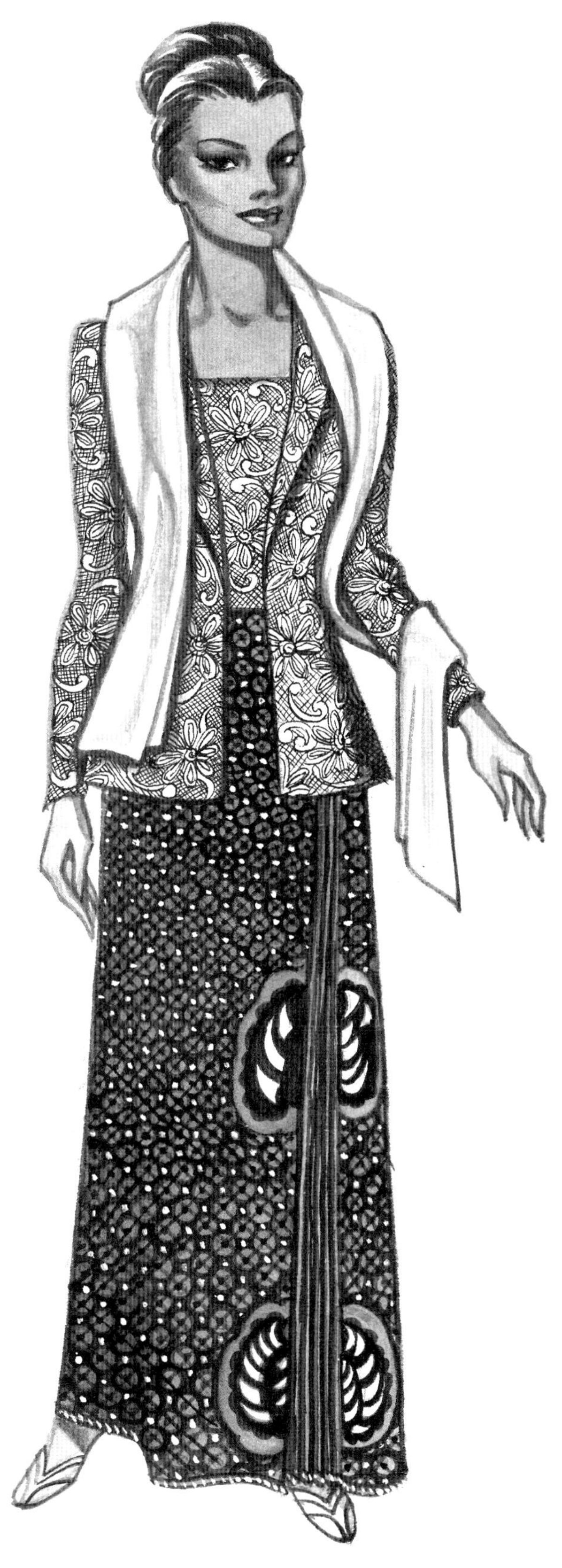

Bali

To many travelers, the best loved of the Indonesian islands is Bali, which is truly a paradise. In the 16th century Islam triumphed over Hinduism in Java. Bali, just a mile from Java by water, became a refuge for Hindu nobles, priests and intellectuals. Beautiful Hindu temples dot the countryside, and there is a profusion of flowers everywhere. The terraced rice fields are backed by mountains. Most of Bali's area of over 2,000 square miles is mountainous. The natives call Bali Peak, which is 10,000 feet in altitude, "The Navel of the World." In the foothills of the mountains, in Ubud, there is a center for European and American artists with a fine museum.

Bali is a country of villages. Each family in a village lives in its own compound, surrounded by earthen or stone walls. The shaded courtyard is divided into three sections, containing a rice granary, cattle shed, sleeping quarters, kitchen and the house temple. The roofs are thatched or made of palm leaves. Balinese life is centered around religion, which is a blend of Hinduism, Buddhism, Malay ancestor worship and beliefs in animism, reincarnation and magic. There is a caste system, but it is not strictly observed, as nine-tenths of the people belong to the lowest caste.

Everyone loves music, poetry, festivals, gambling and dancing. Two of the country's dances are famous - the 'Ketjak,' or Monkey Dance, and the 'Barong Dance.' The Monkey Dance is performed by 100 men and a girl, and it is very amusing, since the men take the part of the monkeys. The Barong Dance represents the eternal struggle between good and evil. Barong is the good spirit and Rangda, the evil one. The good spirit banishes the evil one at the end of the dance.

My husband took a moving picture of this dance, or so I thought. When developed, it turned out to be an entire reel of a little Balinese girl in the audience. She was possibly four years old and imitated every move of the star dancer. The photographer had fallen in love with the child and forgotten all about the performance.

A treasured memory of Bali is the wonderful chorus of frogs that live in the ponds among huge waterlilies. Every evening as the sun goes down the frogs talk to each other, or sing, or whatever frogs do to communicate. It certainly cannot be called 'croaking,' as it is so melodic.

Balinese Costume

The kebaya of this costume was found at the Bali Beach Hotel in Denpasar, the capital of Bali. It is white and dainty, with delicate, white embroidery around the neck and down the front, coming to points below the waist. A silver pin fastens the garment at the neck. Silver is more prized than gold on this island. The sarong, or kain, was found in a museum in Singapore. It is a tjanting batik, which is numbered and has a name, "Taman Sari of the Sultan's Castle." The textile base is a fine poplin imported from Holland. The design, wings in shades of cream and brown, has a background of brown with touches of black. The belt is six yards long, and is orange and silver, firmly woven so that it has a very stiff texture and can be wrapped tightly to hold the kain in place. Over the blouse, sarong and belt a long, soft-textured 'sabai,' or shawl, is doubled lengthwise and worn in the proper fashion.

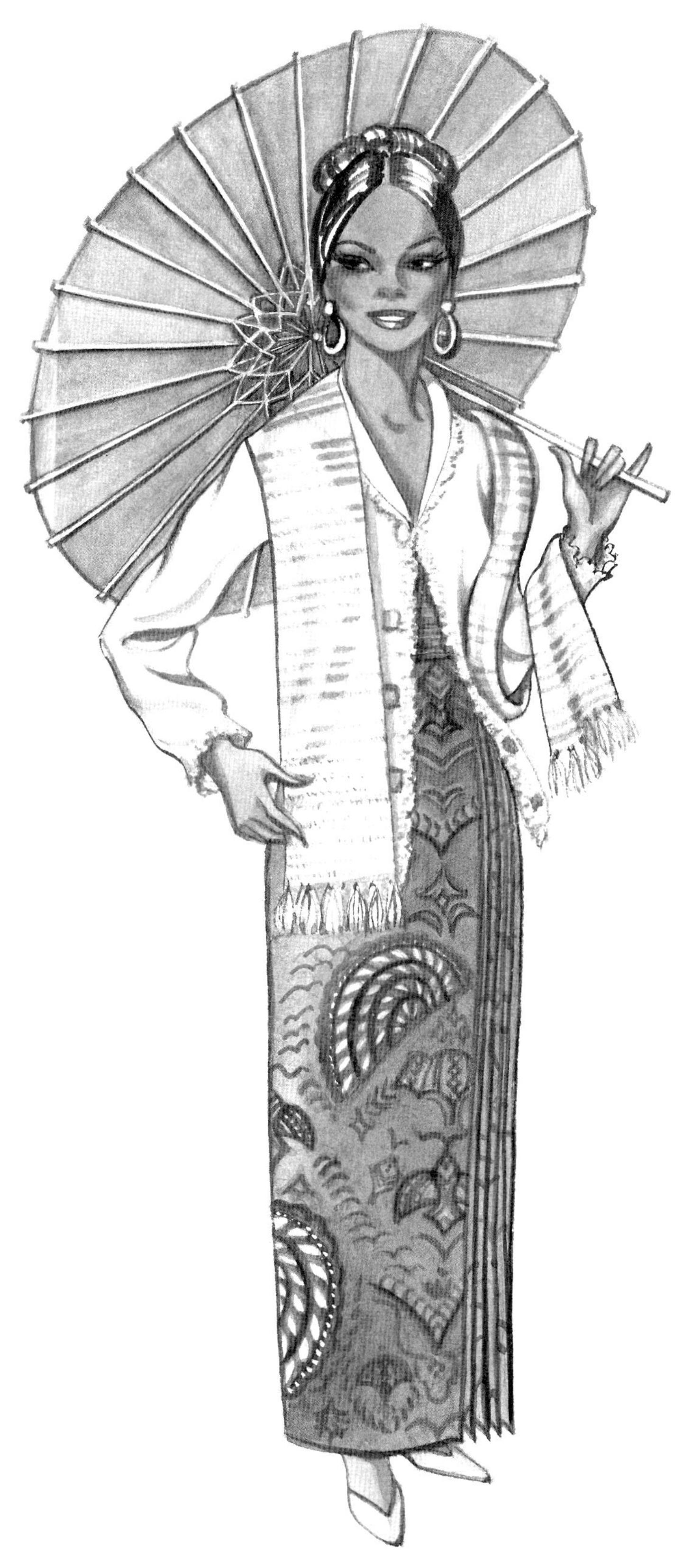

A Bit about Batiks

The art of making batiks is truly one of the world's great crafts, and worthy of understanding and appreciation. This art has flourished in Indonesia for centuries, except for a short period before 1817, at which time Sir Stamford Raffles' efforts caused a revival of interest in this craft.

In Indonesia batiks are usually made of poplin, imported from Holland or England, although some are on silk or voile, and very old ones were made on homespun. The most valuable pieces are waxed by hand with a 'tjanting,' which resembles a small, wooden pipe. It sometimes takes several months to produce one sarong-length batik in this way. The tjanting is giving way to the `tjap,' which is a metal block with a ribbon design on the underside. The block is dipped into hot wax and stamped onto the fabric. This is heavy work, done by men. Both sides of the cloth have to match exactly, so this is a painstaking process, but a skilled tjap printer can create about 20 sarong-lengths in a day.

After the wax is put on the cloth, it is allowed to harden, and the fabric is dipped into the dye. The wax is then removed, with that part of the cloth which had been covered with wax still uncolored. It is possible for the layman to tell the difference between a hand and tjap print by the perfection of the latter design, as hand printing is less exact. Many fine pieces are a combination of both methods. It took a year to complete the tjanting batik given by President Suharto as a gift to President Reagan.

Some designs have been used for generations, and many have names. They are interwoven with the history and culture, and the nobility developed their own motifs, much as did the English their crests and the Scottish clans their tartans.

Sumatra

Jo and I took a special side trip to Sumatra, the second largest island in Indonesia. Except in the highlands, the climate is hot and moist. It is the people and customs that make this island so interesting. Sumatra and Borneo are both less modern and sophisticated than most of the large islands of Indonesia. Animal life on Sumatra includes orangutan, elephant, rhinoceros, wild boar, tiger, tapir and civet cat. In Bukittinggi there is a city park where monkeys live freely, swinging through the trees.

The Minangkabaus are the largest ethnic group on the island. They are the world's largest matrilineal society, passing property through female lines. The eldest daughter inherits, but must share with her sisters. Each Minangkabau man and woman maintains permanent membership in the longhouse of his or her mother, even after marriage. Most Sumatrans are Muslim, and this matrilineal society is rare in the Muslim world of male dominance. The Muslim women of Indonesia do not, however, cover their faces.

More than one-third of the Bataks, an ethnic group in central Sumatra, are Lutheran Christians. The Lutheran Church there is the largest in Asia. A lasting memory from this trip was the harmonizing of Jo and our Batak guide. They were both Lutheran, both had excellent voices, and as we drove around Sumatra they sang the miles away with beautiful songs they both knew. Music provided a delightful cultural bridge.

October 1 was Liberation Day, celebrating freedom from the communists. We were near Lake Toba, in Batak country, and caught in groups of hundreds of parading children. They appeared to be about the age of our high school students, dressed from head to toe in snowy white, the boys in shorts, the girls in pleated skirts. We had seen them emerging from the most primitive of huts along the way, wearing these dazzling white clothes that must have been beaten clean on the rocks of Lake Toba. It was natural to compare their appearance with that of U.S. high school students.

In another area we saw a small girl, perhaps eight or nine years of age, carrying a baby about half her size on her back and leading another small child by the hand. The baby started to slip off her back, and we watched with horror, caught in traffic and unable to help. The little girl skillfully adjusted her burden and continued on her way. We all agreed that those babies must receive lots of bumps.

Many of the people we met were Dutch, returning on a holiday to the land where their parents had lived when Indonesia was under Dutch control. Evenings at the Lake Toba Hotel were filled with music and dancing. All Sumatran men seem to have beautiful voices. We heard two superb concerts at Lake Toba, as fine as we have heard anywhere in the world. And later there was Dutch dancing, which is very lively. Everyone joined in.

The only first-class Sumatran hotel we stayed in was in Padang. The Mariani Internationale is very small, but expertly run and full of Javanese treasures. Mariana, the owner, had a collection of 200 kebayas and kains in silks, velvets and gold and silver woven textiles. She modeled them for us, but would not part with even one. However, she did help us find our baju panjang and jewelry. It has been a constant source of wonder that when finding a good example of ethnic dress with proper accessories seemed beyond hope, something usually happened that helped accomplish the impossible.

Sumatran Baju Panjang

This costume is from West Sumatra, near Padang. The knee-length tunic and the shawl are made of a synthetic, silky, peach-colored fabric with hand-embroidered flowers in colors of a deeper peach, yellow, light and dark red and gold. The large shawl, with hand-tied silk fringe, is worn over the left shoulder and fastened at the right side of the waist. The sarong is a deep orange hand-loomed textile, interwoven with silver. A wide silver panel is folded, forming the front of the sarong. This textile was woven on a footloom, much like those found in Guatemala.

Crowns, wedding chains and necklaces are very difficult to find unless one is prepared to order them in solid gold from a jeweler in the area where the ethnic dress originates. We were very grateful to the owner of the Mariani Internationale Hotel for putting us in touch with a family who was willing to part with such important and memorable articles as those worn in the wedding of their daughter. This jewelry was gold-dipped, but nonetheless very special.

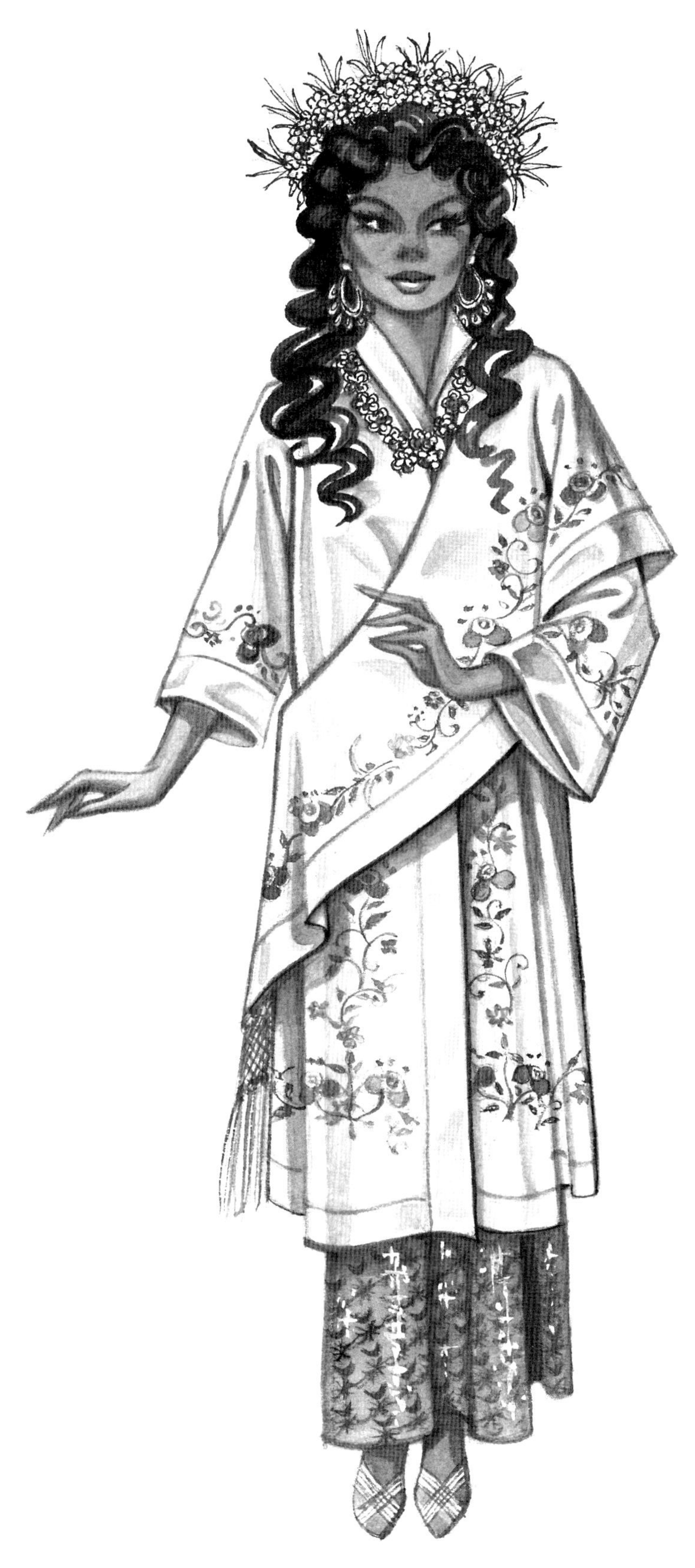

Republic of Singapore

Singapore is the capital of the island state of Singapore, which includes 40 nearby islets, covering an area of 247 square miles. The population estimate in 1992 was 2,859,000. It is located off the tip of the Malay Peninsula in Southwest Asia. This is a strategic position between the Indian Ocean and the South China Sea, and this city is one of the world's great commercial centers.

Singapore is called 'Instant Asia' because of the cultures brought to it by immigrants from all parts of Asia. It is a free port. The currency is the Singapore dollar, there is 87 percent literacy, and the main religions are Buddhism, Taoism, Muslim, Hinduism and Christianity.

Sir Thomas Stamford Raffles founded Singapore in 1819. It was a British colony until 1959, when it became autonomous within the British Commonwealth. In 1963 it joined with the Federation of Malaysia, until two years later when Singapore became a separate nation.

This modern city is very beautiful, with parks and flower-lined highways. There are many modern hotels, and 40-story buildings are being built on the ocean floor, for lack of space. It is very clean, and is kept so by stringent rules. Just throwing a cigarette out of a car window or discarding chewing gum on the sidewalk subjects one to a very heavy fine. It is wise to obey all laws in Singapore.

Uniform of Flight Attendant of Singapore Airlines (SIA)

Balmain, a Parisian designer of note, was chosen to adapt the Indonesian kebaya and kain to the world of modern flight. The Indonesian design is on cotton and is a roller print. The background color is a medium dark blue with an all-over design of red, blue and green flowers and brown leaves. Each flower and leaf is outlined by a narrow brown band with white dots. There is a narrow border in a geometric design around the neck, front closing and hipline hem of the kebaya and around the bottom of the kain.

The dainty kebaya, or blouse, has been made into a fitted jacket with a round neck and three-quarter-length sleeves. The sarong, or ankle-length skirt, has the accordion pleated closing found all over Indonesia, although the pleating in the uniform skirt is worn at the front of the garment, instead of at the left side.

This uniform was found in a shop in Singapore. It was one of the easiest of the costume searches. The people of the Island State are proud of their airline and its excellent reputation. It is considered by many to be the world's finest.

Since our daughter was a stewardess, the artist decided to put her in the SIA dress.

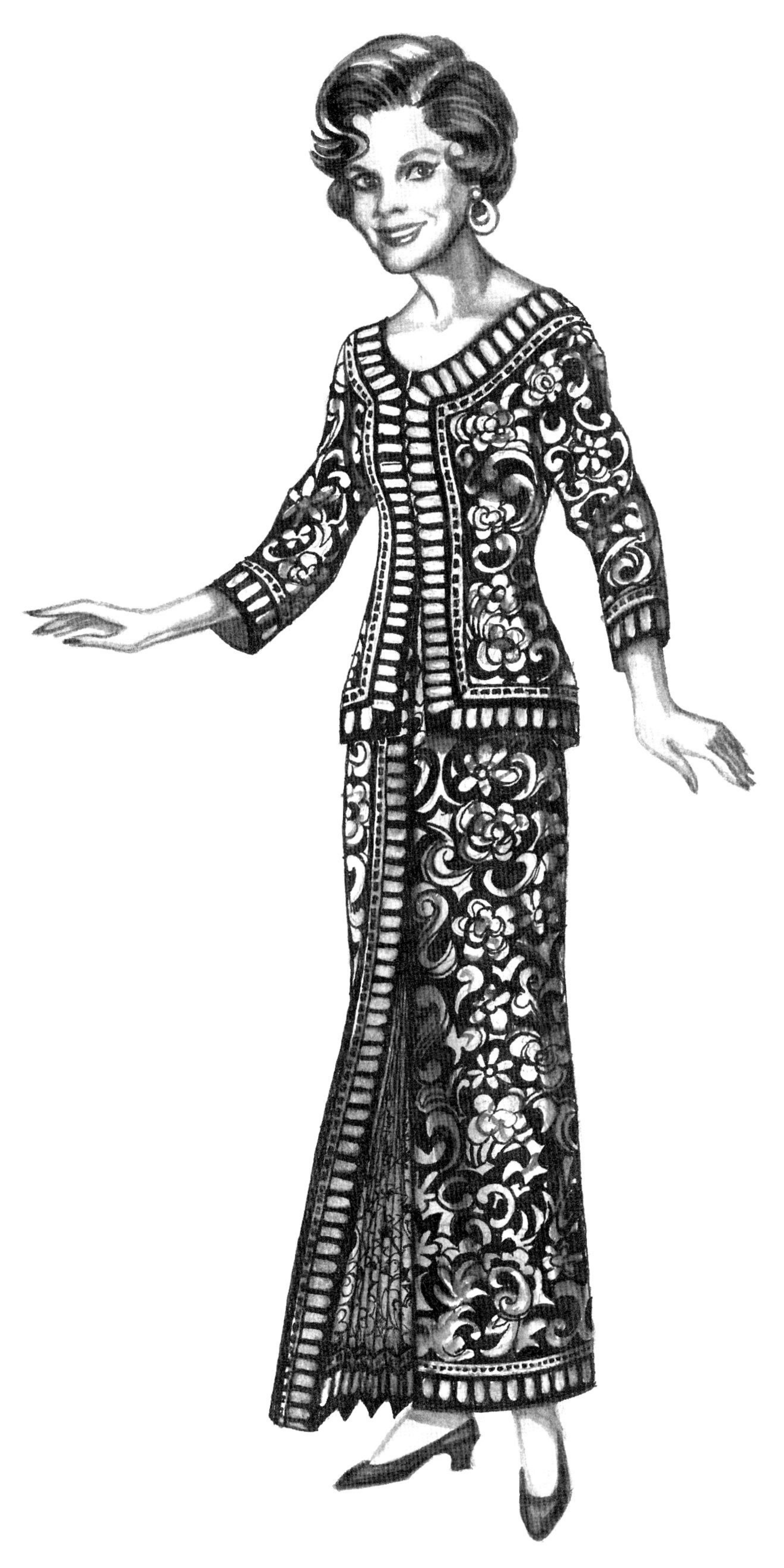

One can pay back the loan of gold,

but one dies forever in the debt

of those who are kind.

Malayan Proverb

Malaysia

Malaysia is a country on the north coast of the island of Borneo, on the southeast tip of Asia. Its total area is about the size of New Mexico, with over 12 times the population of that state. Its capital is Kuala Lumpur (popularly called K.L.), the currency is the dollar and the main religions are Muslim, Hindu, Buddhist, Confucian, Taoist and local. Literacy is 80 percent.

The type of government is a federal parliamentary democracy with a constitutional monarchy. There is a head of state, a head of government and a monarch elected every five years by the Council of Hereditary Rulers of the Malayan states.

European traders appeared in the 16th century, and from then on Malaya was under the Portuguese, the Dutch, and in 1867, the British. Malaya secured its independence in 1957. Six years later Singapore, Malaya, Sarawak (northwest Borneo) and Sabah (north Borneo) established the independent nation of Malaysia, with Singapore preferring autonomy in 1965.

Kuala Lumpur is built where two rivers join, and its name means "Mouth of Two Muddy Rivers." There is so much rubber in Malaysia that it is used in surfacing the streets, making driving very pleasant. The most beautiful of the world's Hilton hotels is said to be in K.L., and we would not dispute this description. It is magnificent!

Kuching, which means 'cat,' is the gateway to a country of rain forests and unexplored ravines. It is the capital and chief port of Sarawak State in East Malaysia, on North Borneo, which is the third largest island in the world. Sir James Brooke, an English explorer, founded Kuching in 1839. He became the ruler of Sarawak, with the title of Raja. He built the town's first European-style house on a jungle bank of the muddy, crocodile-infested Sarawak River. Although the city is mostly Chinese now, the Land Dyaks and Ibans live on the outskirts. There is a Land Dyak longhouse near Kuching, where each family has a separate room in which to eat and sleep. We were told that the Malays in Borneo are all Muslim and still practice purdah, but we saw no veiled women at all. Our guide was Chinese and wore modern clothing.

The Sarawak Museum was a fascinating place, with interesting displays. This was a land of headhunters, with the last head being taken during World War II. Although the Japanese had firearms and the natives only blowguns, it wasn't long before the invaders learned to stay out of the forests and away from the Dyaks. Today, the only headhunters tourists can find are in the Headhunter Bar in the Holiday Inn. The nearest thing to jungle music we heard was "Love Me Tender" and "Danny Boy."

Pinang, formerly Penang, is a beautiful city on the Strait of Malacca. It was founded in 1786 by the British East India Company. Downtown Pinang resembles a British town. Our guide, Selvaraj, said that tourists must not miss the Snake Temple, with hundreds of snakes of all kinds, secreted among altars and rafters. We finally convinced him that finding a Malaysian Airline 'stew's' uniform was more important than dodging snakes. This was the last stop in Malaysia and the prospects of finding that costume were not good. Selvaraj was Indian and his wife Malayan. He said that children of this mixture are remarkably intelligent and that his daughter Sumitra spoke at the age of 72 days, saying "Mama." Of course, we marveled, adding that the father of such a genius would know where to find this costume. It took the whole of an afternoon, but we achieved our goal. Sumitra will go far if she takes after her father.

Uniform of Malaysian Airline (MAS) Flight Attendant

This dress is very similar to that of the Singapore (SIA) flight attendant. The fabric, a cotton roller print, resembles a batik. The background is bright blue with orange, aqua and gold-colored flowers with brown leaves. Each figure in the print is outlined by a narrow brown border with white dots.

The sleeves of the 'kebaya,' or blouse, are wrist length, and there is no border at the bottom of the kebaya, as there is on the SIA uniform. There are pleats in the front of the sarong skirt. The most striking difference between these two uniforms is the neckline. The Malaysian kebaya has a narrow collar which comes nearly to its hem. Inserted into the neckline of this collar is a dickey, which is folded into diamond-shaped designs. Another difference is the narrower decorative band around the bottom of this sarong.

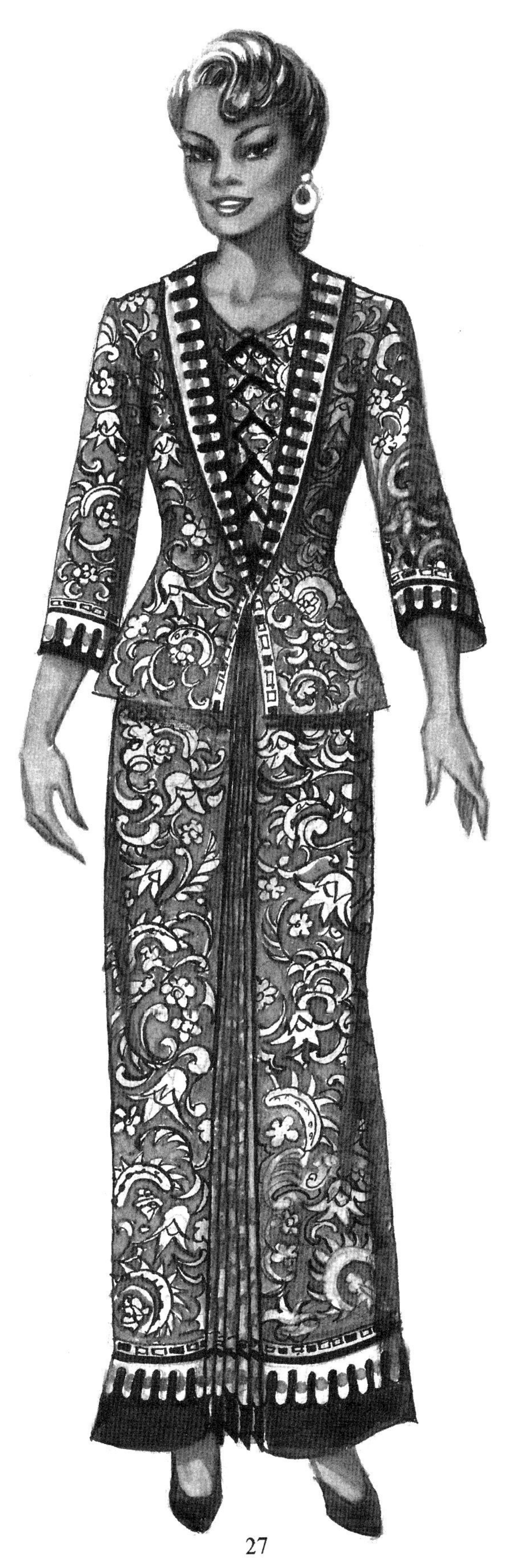

The Republic of the Philippines

The Philippines is an archipelago consisting of some 7,100 islands, stretching 1,100 miles from north to south. The area is slightly larger than that of Arizona, with a population of more than 17 times that state. About 95 percent of the population reside on the largest 11 islands.

Manila, the capital, is on the island of Luzon, the largest and most important of all of the Philippine islands. Manila Bay is known to be the finest harbor in the Far East. The currency is the peso, literacy is 88 percent, and the religions are 83 percent Roman Catholic, nine percent Protestant and five percent Muslim.

The Malay people of the Philippines, whose ancestors probably migrated from Southwest Asia, were mostly fishers, hunters and unsettled cultivators when the islands were first visited by Magellan in 1521. The Spanish founded Manila in 1571, and the islands were named for King Philip II of Spain. They were ceded to the United States in 1898 following the Spanish-American War.

Japan occupied the islands during World War II. When independence was declared in 1946 a republic was established. In 1972 Ferdinand Marcos declared martial law and later proclaimed himself president. In 1983 opposition candidate Benigno Aquino was assassinated, which incited wide-spread demonstrations. Although Marcos was declared the victor in an election in 1986, the widow of the slain Aquino declared herself president. When Marcos fled the country, the U.S. and other nations recognized Córazon Aquino as president.

The Terno

Our guide in Manila was a retired college professor. She spoke perfect English, and she was fascinated by our costume search. She knew how to go about getting exactly the right Philippine terno for the collection. We saw a picture of the dress she had worn when she married a number of years ago. It was like the terno, but had an apron. She explained that this costume used to be worn with an apron, sometimes a shawl and often a train. Today, however, the dress itself, with its exquisite embroidery, is usually worn without other embellishment.

This terno is made of off-white silky pineapple cloth. The colors of the embroidery are peach, pink, blue, yellow and green, in a design of flowers and leaves. It has a bateau neckline and elbow-length sleeves. These sleeves are distinctive in that they form almost a circle, with the embroidery at the outside of the elbow. They are pleated so that they are very stiff and stand up several inches above the shoulder of the dress. Hooks are used to fasten them into the armhole so that they can lie flat when not being worn. There is a narrow belt with a bow at the waistline, and the long skirt has a front and back panel of solid embroidery that measures 30 inches at the hem and narrows to a point a few inches below the waistline.

Women in elite social circles often wear this type dress. Imelda Marcos, widow of the exiled president, wore them constantly. Her ternos were beautiful, but not more so than the one in this collection. (Only slight prejudice admitted.)

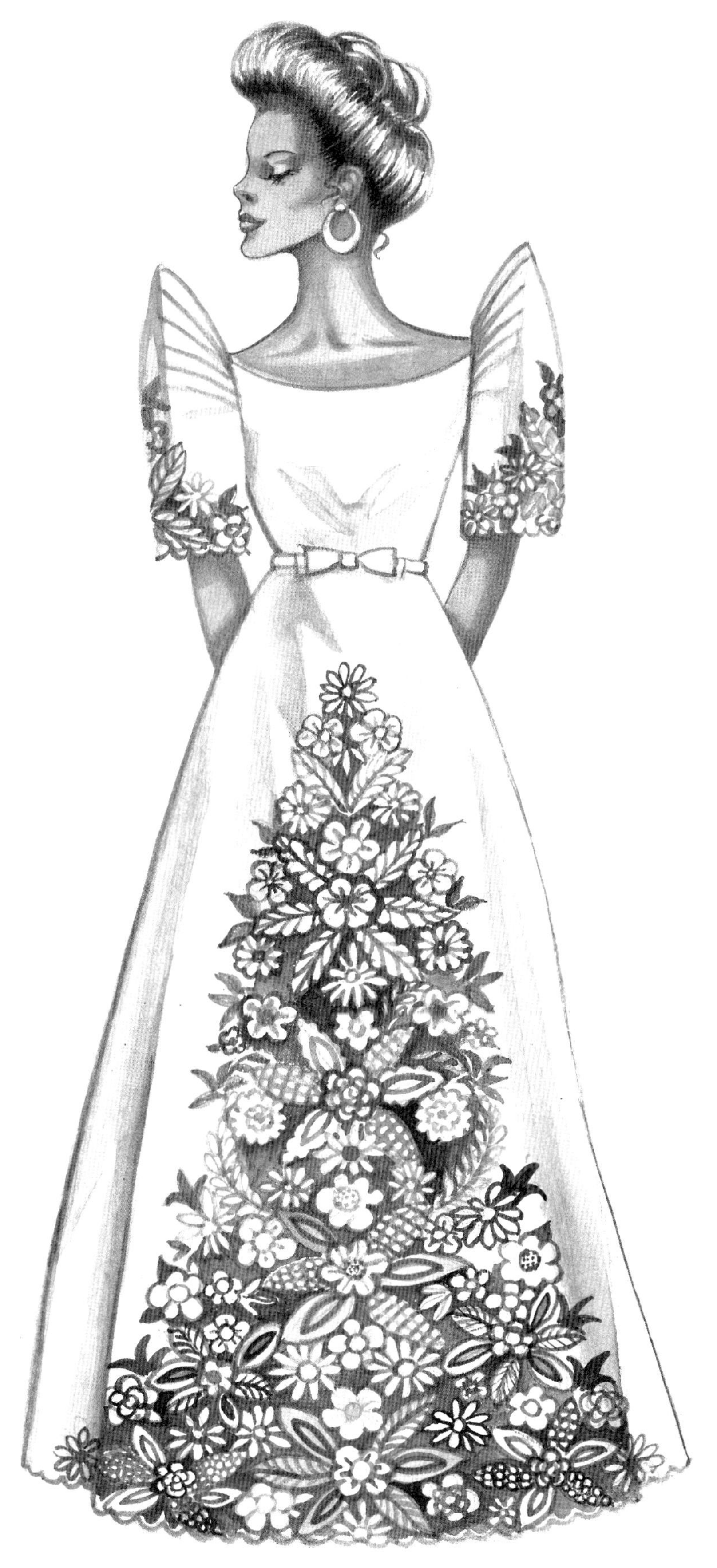

Bontoc, 1981

We landed in Baguio with our hearts in our mouths and our knuckles white. Later we were told that this airport, in a resort area of northwest Luzon, is considered one of the most dangerous in the world because of its short runway.

We had arranged to have a car, driver and guide take us to Bontoc. They were waiting at the airport in their 'jeepney' which had a banner across the back window that we saw on many other cars: General MacArthur's words, "I shall return," in colorful embroidery. We didn't feel unwelcome.

For eight hours we went as far up and down as we did forward. There was ample time to get acquainted with our guide, who spoke English, and our driver, who did not. They were both Igorots, and both spoke Spanish and Tagalog. The Igorot people are found in a mountain province of northern Luzon. They number about 250,000, and two broad distinctions can be made: those who grow wet rice in the high country and those who grow rice in the rain forests of the low country. Both branches were head-hunting warriors until quite recently.

We learned that our guide was Catholic, our driver 'almost' Catholic, which meant he sacrificed a duck on important occasions just to be on the safe side. The guide, the better educated of the two, assured us that he was 'all' Catholic, but when our driver invited us to his home in order to sacrifice a duck to insure our safe return to America, the guide seconded the motion that one could never be too careful. We decided to take our chances and forgo this security. We loved adventure, but were selective. The afternoon was well advanced when we arrived in Bontoc. We got the only room in town with a private bath, running water and electricity. Both of the latter were turned on from 6 to 8 in the evening. The rest of the time 'running water' was a barrel with a large wooden dipper. The only tourists we saw were some hikers with their backpacks.

After an excellent dinner we were taken to an ATO, a meeting place for old men and young boys. Men counsel the boys, who live for several of their teen years in this ATO, just as the girls live in a dormitory. Jo and I have 14 grandchildren between us, and this sounded like an excellent idea. We were anxious to see an ATO.

The guide and driver were waiting for us on the front porch of the hotel, enjoying local brandy. It had been a long wait, so they were a bit unsteady. We were glad to learn that we would walk to the ATO. We followed narrow paths over underground pigpens, where a missed step in the blackness of the tropical night would have sent us plunging six feet to a rock floor, joining the enormous pigs. The guides had flashlights, but the light was not steady. We later agreed that the precarious footing amidst the snuffling and oinking pigs was a bit more adventure than we really wanted.

The ATO was a circular area where two elderly men in breechcloths were surrounded by about a dozen young boys dressed in jeans and T-shirts. All seemed to be awaiting our arrival. We were the only guests. The old men were totally absorbed with our presence, interested in finding out why two elderly ladies would be traveling alone to such a distant land. Jo was a widow, and that they could handle. But when they learned that I had a husband at home, it almost broke up the meeting. My age is always asked in Asian countries. This is considered good manners, evidently, and Jo is always willing to tell anyone who asks. She is only seven years younger than I, but her hair is dark. Written notes were sent from the ATO to our guide who answered them in the same way. The questions about our homeland, our travels and opinions of their country went on for over an hour, while the boys watched in wide-eyed fascination. Each answer elicited much hilarity and loud comments in Tagalog. Of course, there was no way we could know what the guide was telling them. Finally, it was time to leave. A note came asking for $10 apiece. We paid, but felt that it was we who should have have been paid, since we had provided the entertainment.

On our drive back to Baguio and the airport we took a road that was much shorter and comfortably smooth. Why we had to suffer that rocky horror to get to Bontoc is still a mystery. We drove through a tiny town where the driver lived and he repeated his offer to sacrifice a duck to insure our safe journey home. Again we declined, although we were told that we would never forget such an interesting ceremony. That's exactly what we were afraid of.

The final hours of our trip took on a dream-like quality. The rice terraces of Banaue are beyond a doubt one of the most wonderful and breathtaking sights in the world. They are irrigated, steeply contoured, mountain-terraced walls of stone with inward-leaning tops that had been carved out of the sides of the mountains without the aid of metal tools, hundreds of years ago. They are still under cultivation. It has been estimated that, if put end to end, those terraces would stretch halfway around the world. The rice terraces of Banaue well deserve the opinion of many authorities that they are one of the wonders of the present-day world.

Going Home

Occasionally, even carefully laid plans will go astray. My bag, filled with treasures from Indonesia and the Philippines, was the only one to not arrive in Hawaii, where we went through customs. Seeing my distress, a member of the crew said that she had seen a red bag fall from one of the baggage carriers during the loading of the plane in Manila. It was raining hard and visibility was not good, but she knew it was red. My bag was red. The ticket agent at the desk at Philippine Airlines was most considerate and said he would cable Manila immediately. The plane for San Francisco left, but I didn't get on it. We had been flying all night, so a little more time wouldn't hurt. Jo left, as she was going home on a different plane. The airport quieted down. There were only workers cleaning up and a few agents answering phones. One of the remaining was the agent at the Philippine Airlines desk. So I curled up on a few seats and waited for news from Manila. This meant returning often to the long-suffering agent who had sent the cable.

It's easy to lose one's perspective with no sleep for so many hours and a disappointment, so I did the only thing left to do when he hadn't heard. . . I cried, much to the embarrassment of that poor fellow. Tears every half hour for several hours must have been unnerving. I had a feeling that the agent would have gladly sent me anywhere I chose to go, somehow...just so I went!

Ten days later a call came to my home from Philippine Airlines in Honolulu. A red bag fitting the description I gave was there, with no identification. A man's voice said, "It was headed for Timbuktu or somewhere, but I knew it was yours." He even knew my voice!

I said, "How could you possibly know?"

He replied, "Lady, how could I possibly forget?"

What a night, for both of us. The airline was so solicitous; perhaps they thought I had something like my husband's ashes in that bag. They never asked.

The Igorot Woman's Costume

This ethnic dress was obtained with the help of the owner of Bontoc's small hotel and Sister Basil of the Convent of St. Vincent. We were assured that the sarong and belt are of the highest weaving quality.

Sister Basil explained that originally the sarong and belt were all the clothing that was worn, but that Sears Roebuck blouses now complete this outfit. That change began, of course, when the Belgian sisters established a dormitory for the young girls of the area.

The sarong is several yards long and a yard wide and is wrapped tightly into a short skirt. The wide, heavily woven belt with its long, white fringe is also tightly wrapped, holding the sarong in place. Colors in the weaving are red, white and black, with some green. The blouse really is from Sears Roebuck, and the genuine rattlesnake skeleton is worn either as a necklace or a headdress.

The owner and operator of the Bontoc Museum was Sister Basil, who took us on an escorted tour. The history of the Igorot people is eerie and fascinating. Not long before our visit a head had been removed from a member of an unfriendly tribe about forty miles from Bontoc. Head-hunting had been banned by the Americans, but during World War II, the Japanese enemy of the Igorots nonetheless lost some heads. Animal sacrifice, though, is still an important ritual in tribal ancestor worship.

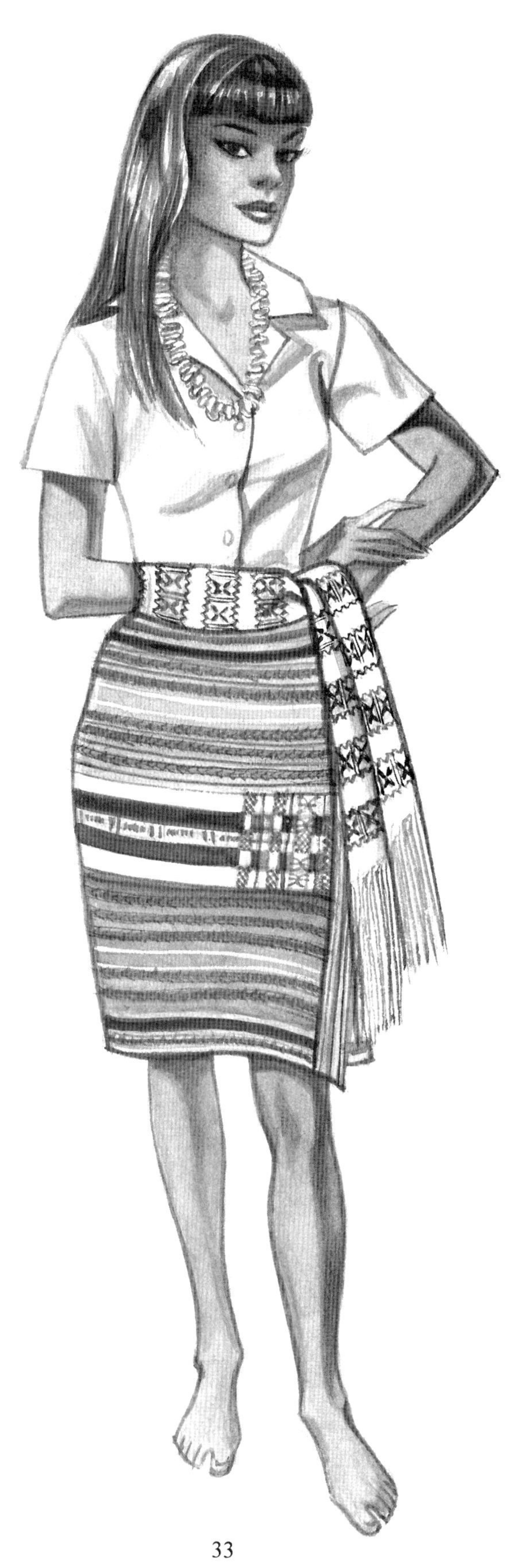

The months and days are the travelers of eternity.

The years that come and go are also voyagers . . .

I, too, for years past have been stirred by the sight of a solitary cloud,

drifting with the wind to ceaseless thoughts of roaming.

Matsuo Basho, 1644-1694

Chapter Three

Oriental Elegance

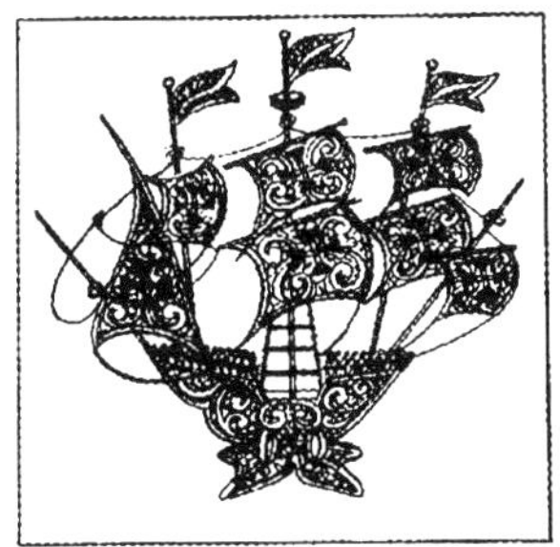

Japan
South Korea
Hong Kong

Japan . . . Nippon

Japan is a crescent-shaped archipelago off the east coast of Asia, separated from Asia by the Sea of Japan. The four main islands are Kyushu, Honshu, Shikoku and Hokkaido. The capital city is Tokyo, located on the island of Honshu. Japan is smaller than California, with a population one-half that of the entire United States. The amazing fact is that the Japanese people are crowded onto only one-fifth the land area of the islands, because the other four-fifths is too mountainous for habitation. The currency is the yen, and the literacy rate is 99 percent. Religions are Buddhism and Shintoism. Most funerals are Buddhist, and most weddings are Shinto. The government is a parliamentary democracy, with the emperor being head of state and the prime minister, head of government.

Earliest records of a unified Japan date from 340 A.D. From the end of the 12th century a feudal system existed for 700 years, dominated by powerful noble families of shoguns, who were military dictators. In 1854 Commodore Perry opened Japan to U.S. trade. After World War II, the United States, with 48 other non-communist nations, signed a bilateral defense agreement restoring Japan's sovereignty, and allowing the U.S. to have military bases on Okinawa. Industrialization began, and Japan emerged as one of the world's most economically powerful countries and a leader in technology.

The educational system of Japan is worthy of mention, because it is so successful. Wherever it is possible to measure educational achievement, the Japanese usually rank first in the world. American universities are considered superior to those of the Japanese, but this is not so at the lower levels. Preschool and kindergarten training are of utmost importance. The entire family centers around helping prepare students for entry into the desired university, as it is seen as determining the success of the rest of the child's life. It is considered a mother's prime job to keep her children at their studies. This puts the student under great pressure to succeed, but study habits become so well established that success is virtually guaranteed.

On one trip from Los Angeles to Tokyo a kindergarten-aged group of about 30 children was on our plane and we did not even realize they were there until we disembarked. They had been to Disneyland. We saw hundreds of very well-behaved groups of children while on a three-day cruise of the Inland Sea during cherry blossom season, which coincides with spring vacation in Japanese schools. The children wore their school uniforms, the small ones wearing little pink caps and following the yellow flags of their teachers or guides. The teenagers also wore their school uniforms, setting these young people apart from the teenagers in many countries.

The Japanese are great world travelers, and are famous for their purchasing power. If we are being waited on, the interest of the clerks usually shifts to any Japanese who enter the shop. In Kuching, Borneo, for example, we were buying postcards when two Japanese men walked in. The girl waiting on us walked away, without comment, and proceeded to sell $10,000 worth of samurai swords while we were standing there. She knew what she was doing!

`Women's lib' is slow to develop in Japan. There is an old saying that in her youth a woman must obey her father, in maturity her husband and in old age, her son. When a son is born large fish-shaped balloons fly in the breeze over blue tiled roofs in the countryside.

Japan's bullet trains are a miracle of efficiency. Trains of six to 10 cars often run two minutes apart and are so crammed with passengers that station attendants stand ready to shove the last ones in so the doors will close.

The world's first undersea railway tunnel and double-decker road tunnel connect the islands of Kyushu and Honshu. All driving is on the left-hand side of the road, in the British fashion. However, to say that someone is 'heavy on the left' does not mean he is driving too fast. It means he is a heavy drinker, since traditionally, saki wine was drunk using only the left hand.

The Ainu people of Hokkaido, the northernmost island, are an indigenous Caucasoid people, while the Japanese are classified as a branch of the Mongoloid race, akin to the peoples of eastern Asia.

The Ainus' Cult of the Bear offers a great deal of excitement at snow festivals during February, in Sapporo on the island of Hokkaido. Huge carved ice sculptures are featured. The 1972 Winter Olympics were held in Sapporo. In July many tame bears are used in the group's fire festivals. The head of the bear is used in shamanistic rituals.

Almost all Japanese performing arts originated from ancient magico-religious or shamanic seances, which developed into Shinto festivals and Buddhist rituals. The No Plays, Kabuki dancing and singing dramas, and Bunraku puppet shows developed from this background.

A final recollection of Japan is of leaving my red leather coat in a Tokyo taxi after a wild ride to Narita Airport to join the rest of our group on the first Chinese Boeing 747 to fly into Beijing. It is not without reason that these taxi drivers are called 'kamikazes,' according to our Air Force pilot friend who lives in Tokyo. He says that their suicidal driving maneuvers resemble those of Japanese pilots in WW II. We made the trip in two hours when it is often known to take five in traffic that must be seen to be believed. Knowing that it would be cold in Beijing, I just hoped that the woman in the driver's life needed that beautiful Turkish coat as much as I was going to need it.

Japanese Kimono

The *Encyclopedia Britannica*, not known for exaggeration, refers to the Japanese kimono as "the most beautiful garment in the world."

Kimonos are so expensive today that when they have been worn for awhile, many women sell theirs. This is a very fine old one. It was found in a handicraft shop in Kyoto, which is roughly 300 miles southwest of Tokyo. Once a capital of Japan and a residence of the imperial family, it is now a center of culture and costume shops.

This kimono is of a very pale gray-green pure silk, lined with a fine white silk, and has been dyed to fade into a pale apricot color at the edges. On the sleeves and from the hem, almost to the waist, are a background of clouds, mountains and a lake, hand painted in grays, greens and browns. On this background are flowers and leaves in colors of light and dark apricot, orange, blue and gold. The sharply pointed leaves of the lily are in green and gold. All of the designs are outlined either by paintbrush or by hand embroidery in gold. Some of the flowers are embroidered solidly in gold thread. A white silk slip and narrow silk scarf which lines the collar are worn. This lovely example of Japanese ethnic dress is the favorite of Japanese women who have modeled in museum costume shows.

An apricot obi, or large sash, is put on in a very special way, folded in half lengthwise, with the selvage edge uppermost, making a sash about a foot wide, which is wrapped tightly around the waist. The open edge forms a receptacle for a purse, handkerchief and cosmetics. The obi is tied in back in a complicated bow, with the insertion of a pillow in the knot. A silk cord passes through the bow and is fastened in front with either a knot or an 'abidome,' which is a jeweled brooch.

Two-toed socks, called 'tabi,' are worn with all of the kimonos. The shoes for dress wear are called 'zori' and made of ornamental fabric or leather. Two thongs pass between the first and second toe, holding the zori to the foot.

The left side of the kimono must be crossed over the right. We learned this the hard way in one of our first costume shows. A young non-Japanese girl wore the kimono crossed with the right side over the left. A Japanese woman in the audience informed us that our model was indeed an attractive corpse, since it is crossed that way only for burial.

Just as no Japanese girl is considered well educated until she has learned flower arranging, ikebana, and the intricacies of the tea ceremony, so must she learn the proper usage of her native dress. It must be appropriate to the age of the wearer, her marital status, her rank in society, the season of the year and the occasion.

The dainty fan has flower designs. It is from Nikko, which is an hour by bullet train from Tokyo. This is an important Buddhist center in beautiful Nikko National Park. Gorgeous red shrines in a setting of giant cedars, mountains, hot springs, lakes and waterfalls make this a popular holiday spot.

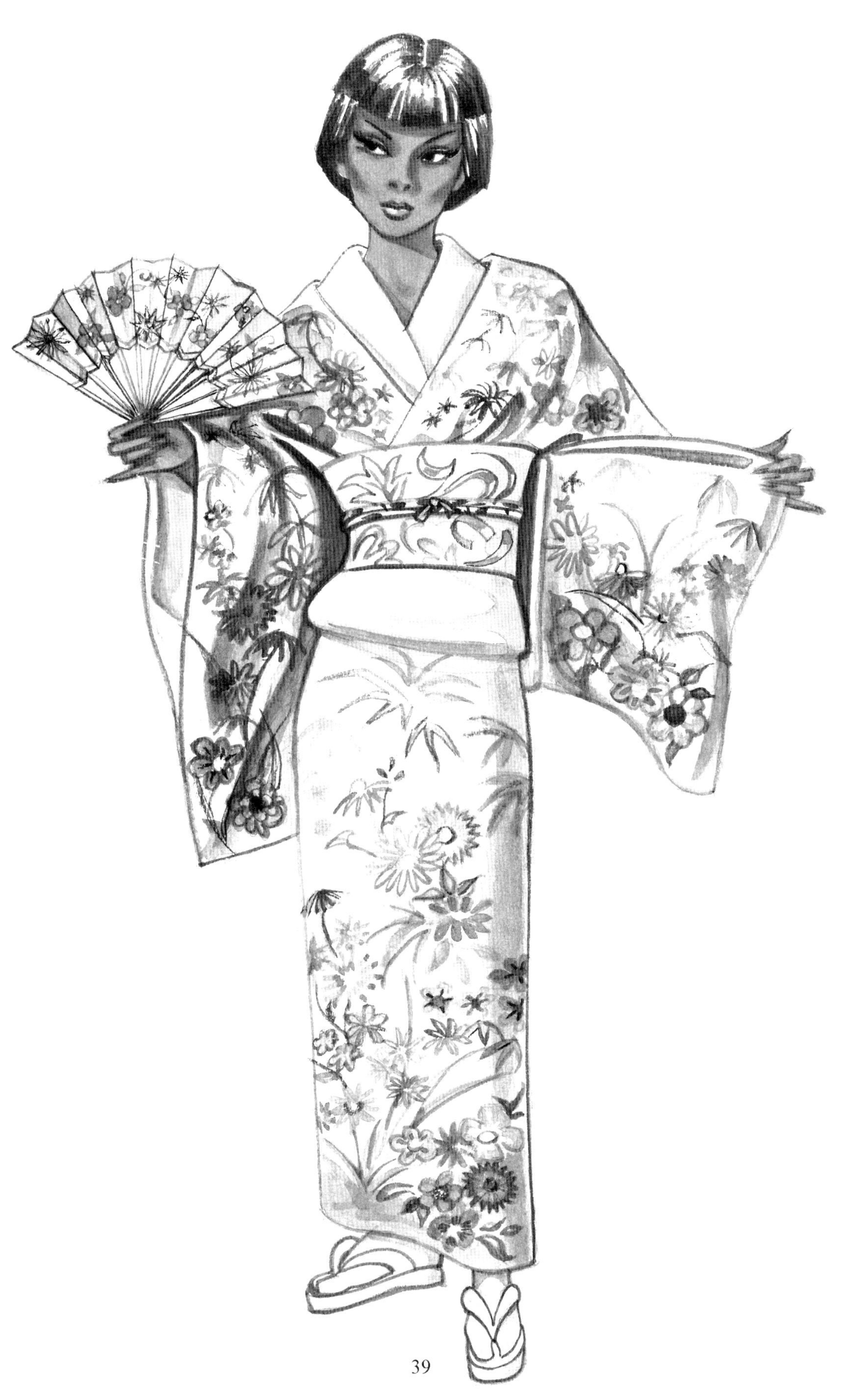

Japanese Wedding Robe

The goal of architecture in Japan, since the time of the shoguns, has been to achieve harmony with nature in order to enhance the lives of the people, their customs and their clothing. By tradition the kimono tries to show nature at its loveliest.

Robes like the wedding robe in the collection are now astronomically expensive. The average bride cannot possibly afford to buy one, so they are almost invariably rented. Most large hotels have shops where they can be found.

This robe is elegant, luxurious and highly decorative. It is of white satin, lined with an orange-red silk, which also covers the padded hem. It is six feet long and worn without an obi, hanging straight from the shoulders. Another kimono is worn beneath this robe, and it is worn with an obi. A narrow white silk scarf is worn at the neckline of both kimonos. Embroidery covers the entire robe. It was most likely done with an electric embroidery machine. The design is of flowers and leaves in various shapes, sizes and colors. Red, orange, shades of aqua, lavender and yellow flowers are plentiful, as well as large pink flowers with black centers. Gold and silver leaves with traces of green are part of the decoration. White tabi are worn with the zori, which are made of a white and gold silky fabric.

The bride's hairstyle is very ornate. There are wings on each side of her face and a large bun on the top of her head. She has been sleeping on a wooden pillow so that her hair will look perfect on her wedding day. Around her head is a loosely but carefully wrapped white silk double band about three inches wide. Tradition says that this hat covers the 'horns of jealousy' of the bride. Many glittery ornaments and flowers are worn in her hair above the hat.

This will be the most important and exciting day in the life of a woman, rivaled only by that of the birth of the couple's first child. The marriage ceremony will undoubtedly be conducted in the Shinto tradition.

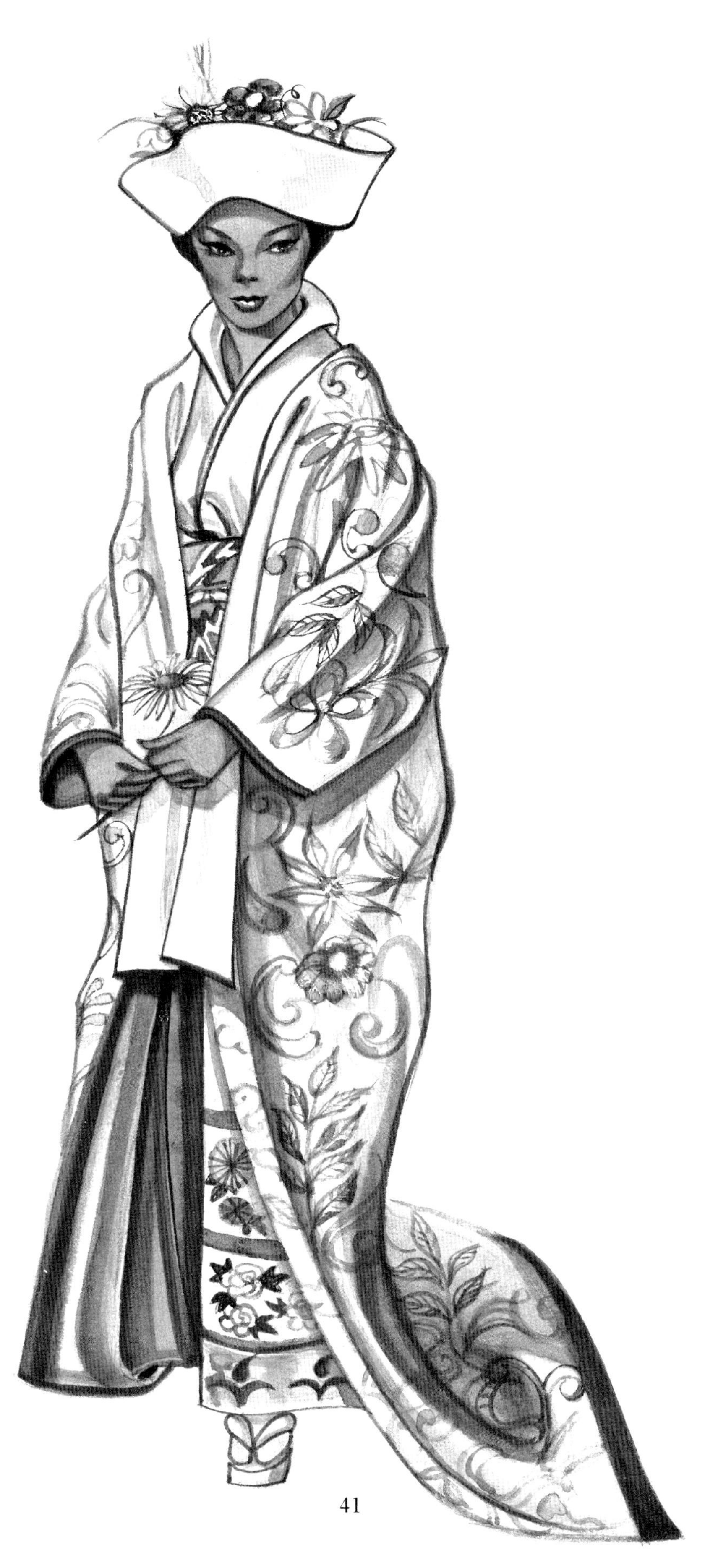

41

Tradition means giving votes to the most obscure of all classes -

our ancestors.

It is the democracy of the dead.

Tradition refuses to submit to the small and arrogant oligarchy

of those who merely happen to be walking around.

G.K. Chesterton

Republic of Korea . . . Land of the Morning Calm

South Korea is a peninsula thrusting from the northeast Asian mainland. It is slightly larger than the state of Indiana, with a population more than eight times that of Indiana, or about 45 million. The president lives in the 'Blue House,' reminiscent of our own White House.

The capital is Seoul, which was established before Columbus discovered Central America. It is the fourth largest city in the world, with two million more people than New York City. This city is a bustling, modern miracle that was rubble 50 years ago. The literacy of the people is 96 percent, and we have been assured by many Koreans that most of them can speak two languages. It is estimated that 49 percent of the population is Christian and 47 percent Buddhist. The currency is the won.

Korea has a recorded history since the first century B.C. In 668 A.D., the Silla Dynasty unified the country, forming the Koryo Kingdom, from which the present name is derived. During this period it began forming its own cultural traditions, distinct from the rest of Asia.

In 1392 the Yi Dynasty was established, which lasted until the Japanese annexed Korea in 1910, beginning 35 years of Japanese rule. Korean independence fighters fought with the Allies in China until the Japanese surrender in 1945. At the Potsdam Conference of that year the 38th Parallel, the site of Panmunjom, was a dividing line. It was agreed that north of the parallel the Japanese troops would surrender to the Soviets, and south of that line they would surrender to the U.S. When U.S. troops entered Korea in September of that year, they found that Soviet troops had entered a month earlier and had blocked all efforts to unite the country. There was now a North and South Korea.

North Korea invaded South Korea in June of 1950. Peace talks were begun in 1951 and lasted two years. The armistice was finally signed in July of 1953.

The 38th Parallel is only 35 miles from Seoul. When we were in South Korea in 1981 our guides told us that the North Koreans had built many tunnels under the border into South Korea, and the people lived in a daily state of apprehension. Security was of great concern.

Around South Korea

South Korea is one of our favorite countries, and we have visited three times. On the first trip my husband and I met, as planned, our good friends Tom and Sylvia who lived in Tokyo. They loved Seoul and wanted to see more of the country, so we planned an extensive trip by bus and train. We stayed in a suburb of Seoul in a large, pre-war mansion that once belonged to a Korean family and was sold to our Air Force during the Korean War. It was the best of both worlds...American comforts and food, and Korean surroundings. We felt very privileged.

We took an express bus from Seoul to Mt. Soraksen, a mountainous area on the Sea of Japan, about 250 miles across the peninsula. For the entire distance we were never out of view of yellow and purple flowers that bordered the highway. These were not wildflowers, but planted and well cared for. Everywhere were neat farmhouses with blue tiled roofs and not a scrap of paper or rubbish anywhere. The buses and restrooms on the express road were impeccably clean and modern.

Soraksen itself was a disappointment, as typhoon winds and rain pelted our hotel windows. We didn't see much of the vividly colored October leaves, but our hotel had three dining rooms to choose from, Chinese, Japanese and Korean, all of them nearly empty. Evidently other travelers had read the weather reports.

It took eight hours on local buses to reach Kyongju the next day. The scenery along the Sea of Japan was breathtaking. Since there was an excellent train from Seoul to Kyongju, the renowned 'Museum Without Walls,' in the south of the country, the bus was not the recommended way for tourists to travel to this area. The Korean women on the bus were used to the unisex restrooms along the way, and they even chatted with the men in the restrooms. I believe they were as surprised to see me there, as I was to be there.

Kyongju has been designated by UNESCO as one of the ten most important historic sites in the world. Its cultural heritage dates back 5,000 years. There are dozens of mounds that are royal graves and temples, magnificent gates, stone bridges, graceful pagodas and gilded Buddhist images, as well as a superb indoor museum. We took the train back to Seoul, enjoying sophisticated, modern travel with renewed appreciation.

The Folkloric Village near Seoul takes the visitor back 200 years in time to a Korean farming town. It is a living, functioning community, peopled by real artisans and craftsmen, doing what their ancestors did, dressed in the kind of clothing of that period and living in houses that are exact replicas of those in which their forefathers lived. There is even an old-style wedding ceremony.

Panmunjom

The men were anxious to go to Panmunjom. It is about 40 miles north of Seoul, at the 38th Parallel, in the demilitarized zone. Here, the armistice to end the Korean War was signed in July of 1953. We were told that South Koreans are not allowed in this area unless accompanied by military personnel. We took a tour.

A road into the town goes over Freedom Bridge and is the only road that enters North Korea from the south. We were allowed to go into a building which had a conference room with a large table in the exact center of the room. There was a yellow line drawn, dividing the table in half and continuing down the table to the wall on each side. No one needed to be told not to step across that line, since there were frozen-faced North Korean officers, well armed, zealously guarding their side. Through windows at the far wall the faces of other soldiers, equally somber, peered at the tourists. But they showed some curiosity, and some even took our pictures.

We could see, across the border, what appeared to be a small village. Our soldiers call it 'Propaganda Village' because, although there are a number of buildings, some even several stories high, it is a facade. It was difficult to find a purpose for this town, even for propaganda, since it obviously had no inhabitants. We were told that the largest of the structures was only 15 feet in width, but we never met anyone who had been in one. Apparently, information leaks are not a problem in North Korea.

There was no costume shopping this trip, so of course Korea was high on a 'must return' list. Meeting Sylvia again for a concentrated, delightful shopping trip was a 'must' also. Luckily we managed to make it all happen.

The Return

Jo and I like tours when traveling in foreign countries. Even with the best of planning there are details that need adjusting and expediting, often in a foreign language. Also, the local guides are nearly always dependable and knowledgeable about their own country. We've also traveled independently, but we prefer tours.

However, sometimes a tour is impossible, and that was true of this trip to South Korea. We were meeting Sylvia in Seoul. Our plane arrived after dark. It had been a tiring flight, and we took the first taxi driver that grabbed our bags. Relaxing in our seats for the long ride into town, we were anticipating with pleasure a great three-day shopping spree at 'It'aewon,' a bargain area for lovely clothes, eelskin bags and other wonderful things to fill the long Christmas and birthday gift lists we had brought with us. We had been saving up for this trip for a long time.

Seoul is a city approaching 17 million people. We knew the airport was far from town, but it seemed strange that after riding for quite a while, there was almost no traffic. We seemed to be on a country road. And horror...we were slowing down. Our driver, without a word, pulled over to the side of the road, got out of the car and disappeared. The headlights were still on, but all we could see were trees and bushes. There was not a single sign of habitation anywhere, just total blackness. We both admitted later that our first thoughts were that we should have called and waited for a hotel car. I also wondered, fearfully, if the bandits we expected to appear at any moment would be angered by our having only traveler's checks. Would they kill us? Neither of us uttered a sound. We were paralyzed, beyond speech.

In the stillness, through our partially open window, there were sounds from nearby bushes. Were the bandits congregating? Finally we realized that this was an open-air rest stop for our driver. He returned, got into the car and, without a word, drove to a busy highway and delivered us to our hotel. Our nerves were shattered. What a perfect setup we had presented for what could have been a real tragedy. Two older women, alone, arriving from the United States. How could we have been so careless, we who prided ourselves on knowing how to handle difficult situations anywhere?

The world is a wonderful place, but everyone in it does not think like we do, nor act as we think they will. Also, we do have a communication problem. Since we obviously do not know as much as we thought we did, in the future it would be tours for us, all the way!

Our hotel on this trip was hard to believe. Upon entering the Lotte Hotel, we were mesmerized by a natural waterfall cascading over huge rocks just outside the glass wall at one end of the lobby. The security in this hotel was very tight, and we learned that some high Philippine officials were meeting there. Metal detectors were used before entering an elevator, wielded by stunning young women in colorful satin hanboks. This was a wise move on the part of the management, since it seemed to keep the irritation of the delayed gentlemen at a minimum.

Under the Lotte Hotel is a large modern shopping mall. If there is better shopping anywhere in the world, these shoppers do not know where it is. We have heard many times that South Korea is the 'best-kept shopping secret' in the world of travel. We concur.

Hanbok Tailored to Tradition

From a Seoul newspaper article, 1994:

"The proprietor of a cloth and garment shop on Silk Street in Seoul refuses to make a traditional Korean costume in the modern style. He decries the new style of hanbok, claiming that it despoils the traditional garment of its beauty. Another store manager says, We do business our way. We aggressively exhort our customers to wear traditional clothes the traditional way. He is following an unwritten rule for the owners of shops on Silk Street, which is to convince customers to obey traditional dress codes. They say that the basics are being ignored, and that the contour of a hanbok should not be compromised. Also, when Koreans choose the color of their garment without expert advice, they are likely to depart sharply from the norm. The five elements that interact in the universe are arranged in the order of mutual benefit . . . blue (wood), red (fire), yellow (earth), white (metal) and black (water). The color red has a magical effect.

"There has been a gradual drop in master tailors. A trainee takes at least 10 years to become an expert. His training includes history, silk-making and the cultural and philosophical aspects of the garment."

The article adds that the long life-cycle of a traditional hanbok saves money. There are no strict measurements for adult hanboks. One size fits all, from slender ladies to pregnant women. Many people can share one garment.

Hanboks . . . the National Dress for Women

In the cities and towns in South Korea on Sundays and holidays, the parks, temple areas, museum and palace grounds are decorated with many bouquets of brightly colored flowers. The women and little girls in their bouffant hanboks show that South Korea's tradition of ethnic dress is still very much alive and in fashion.

This red satin hanbok has a short jacket called 'jhogori' and a very full long skirt, a 'chima.' Many half-slips are worn to make the chima as bouffant as possible. The jhogori has two long streamers that must be tied into a half-bow with a loop of the bow pointing toward the heart. Many white embroidered herons are in flight on the chima, and a golden sun rises over a silver cloud. Green fir leaves on boughs stretch along the hem. This dream of a hanbok was found at East Gate, one of South Korea's wonderful shopping areas.

A child's dress is made like the mother's. It is also red satin with gold trim, embroidered with circles of white herons. The long sleeves are of white satin with red cuffs and the long streamers on the jhogori must be tied exactly like the mother's. The striped rubber shoes, satin bag and tiny box-like hat with its pearl and flower trim are small versions of traditional wear.

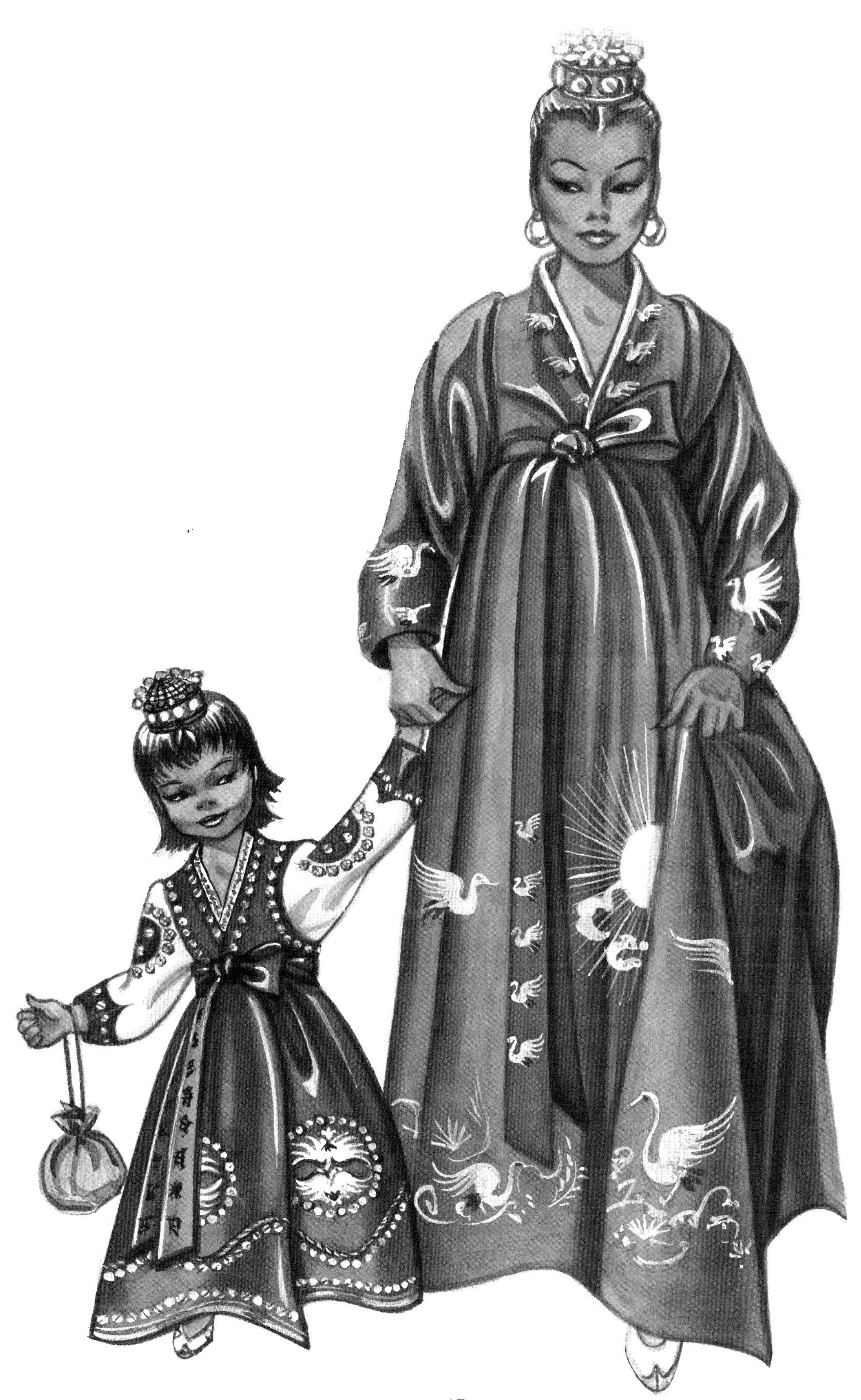

Korean Wedding Ducks

In Korea a family prepares for a daughter's wedding from her early childhood. The carving of traditional wedding ducks is a serious matter, because the man who carves them shares his spirit with the young couple. He must be honorable, and he may not accept money. His character traits are more important than his carving skill. He may carve only one pair of ducks in his lifetime, and he shares with the couple his FIVE FORTUNES, which are: He must be rich, have perfect health, never have been divorced (nor must there be divorce among his relatives), have a good wife and many sons.

The ducks are taken to the wedding. When the ceremony is over the bride and groom bow to the groom's mother, who throws the ducks toward the bride. If she catches them in her skirt she will have a boy as her first child. Next, the groom's mother throws jujubes. If caught this ensures a healthy future. Chestnuts are thrown, symbolizing the strong sons that will be born. The ducks are taken to the new home, and if the couple quarrels they point to the ducks to be reminded of their wedding vows. The bill of the hen is tied shut with a string that is finished off with a bow.

From an article on Korean customs from a folkloric center in Seoul.

Modern Hanbok

When the collector heard that the wife of President Ford had purchased two hanboks from a shop in the Chosun Hotel in Seoul, the temptation was too great to resist. The collection had to have one just like Betty Ford's. The result was a blue silk chiffon dress decorated with many white daisy-like flowers with pink centers.

The color-coordinated shoes are of solid rubber, low heeled with turned-up toes, and the bag matches the hanbok. Korean women are very color conscious.

A silk-tasseled jade ornament called a 'noreekay' is fastened at the neckline of the jhogori. These noreekays are handed down from mother to daughter, and some of them are very valuable. A nine-inch hairpin called a 'binyo' is made of a jade-like material and is worn pushed through the bun at the nape of the neck. This binyo has a flower-shaped head.

There are three pairs of fans in the collection. Any of the fans will transform an already beautiful hanbok into a dancing dress. One pair has red, white and green feathers. Another is made of a stiff, sheer material with large, hand-painted pink flowers. The third pair is all white feathers. Each fan is 18 inches long, opening to a width of three feet. The fans are very popular for home decoration as well as for dance performances. All of the accessories were found in Seoul.

My granddaughter Molly is modeling this hanbok.

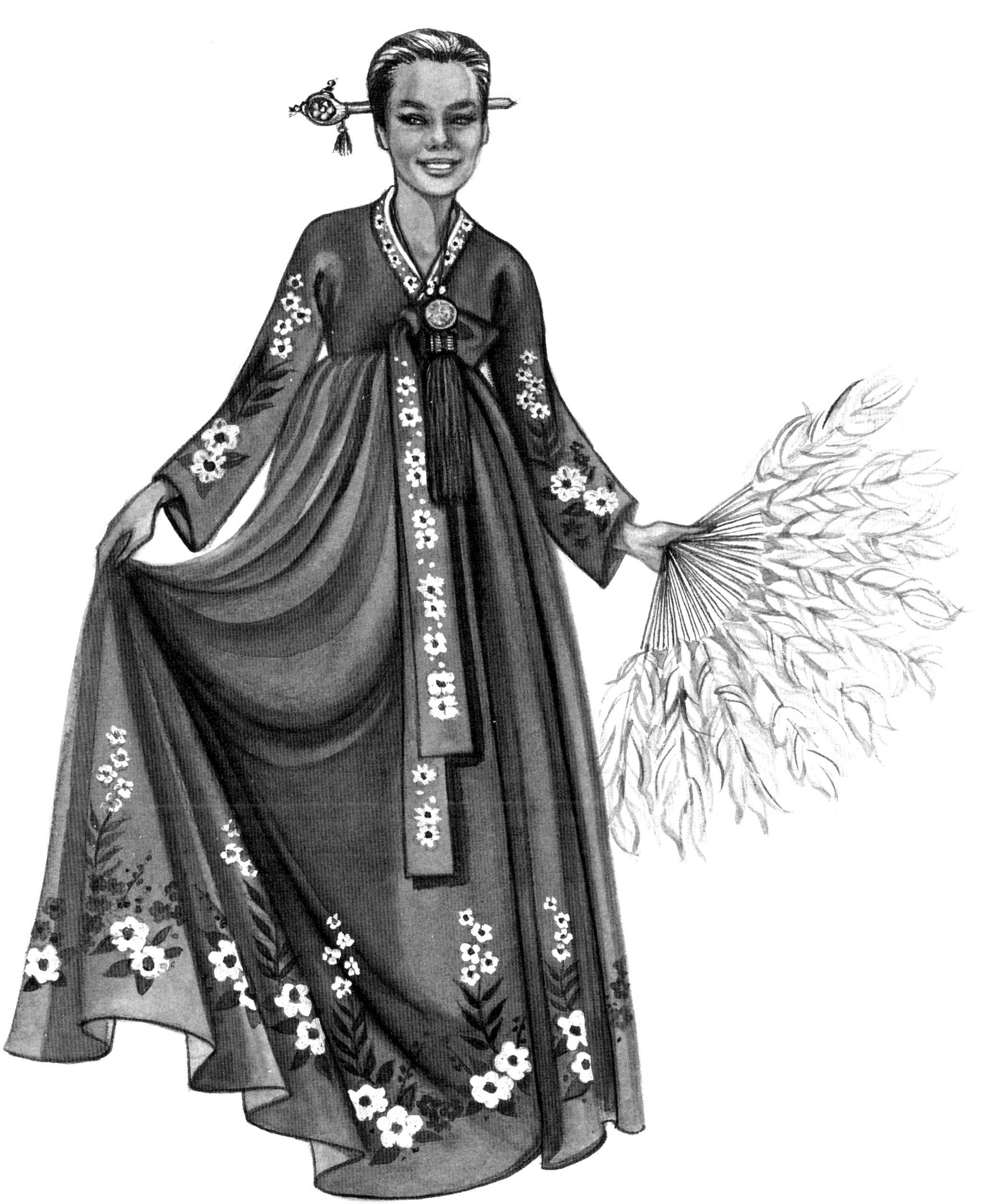

Ethnic Dress of Korean Man

The textile of this man's suit is a stiff, silky synthetic, similar to heavy organza, but more durable. A blue sleeveless vest is worn over a white shirt. The trousers, called 'bahji,' are white, wide at the waist and held up with a cloth belt. The ankle ties match the trousers.

A tall black hat called a 'gaht' is of horsehair. Black horsehair bands hold the hat on his head, keeping his long hair in place. There are two long ribbons that can be tied for extra security. In the National Folkloric Museum in Seoul there is a large case showing every step in making this distinctive traditional hat.

A blue satin handbag, larger than a woman's, but otherwise identical, is carried. The shoes, 'gomushin,' are the typical rubber shoes worn by men, women and children. They are all worn with heavy, white cotton, ankle-length socks. The pipe, a 'dahm bet dae,' is almost two feet long, and the three-foot cane, a 'jipang-yi,' is of wood with a curved handle.

Korean clothing is comfortable to wear. However, this particular costume is worn mostly by older men today, since younger men prefer Western dress.

The Lee Family Festival

We went to the Lee Family Festival in Seoul. It was held in a large park-like area near the city, and there were hundreds of Lees, as this is a very common name in Korea. The festivities included graceful dancers dressed in colorful hanboks with huge, feathery fans and long Korean speeches. A majority of the celebrants were elderly men wearing their ethnic dress, consisting of a blue vest, full trousers tied at the ankles, white rubber shoes and a tall, black horsehair hat. A short coat is often worn.

Many of the men had long gray beards and ponytails. However, it is most unusual to see gray-haired Korean women. They obviously dye it. It's too bad that wrinkles cannot be hidden so easily. Our nice young Korean guide even tactfully offered to get his mother's formula so I could do something about my unnecessary handicap. After having dyed my hair for many years and tiring of the process, I just pretended to be grateful for such useful information.

Jo and I were observing the festivities when a young man approached. He asked my age, pointing out the gentleman who wanted to know, who was smiling at us in a very friendly fashion. He wasn't very young-looking himself. All over the Orient it is obviously considered proper to inquire about a stranger's age. He could not have meant to be rude, after all, he was a Lee! At least I was getting attention. Jo's naturally brown hair was considered normal and they did not ask her age.

This incident brought back memories of a similar one in Bontoc, in the Philippines, when an old man in a breechcloth also wanted to know my age. A Muslim veil may have some advantages.

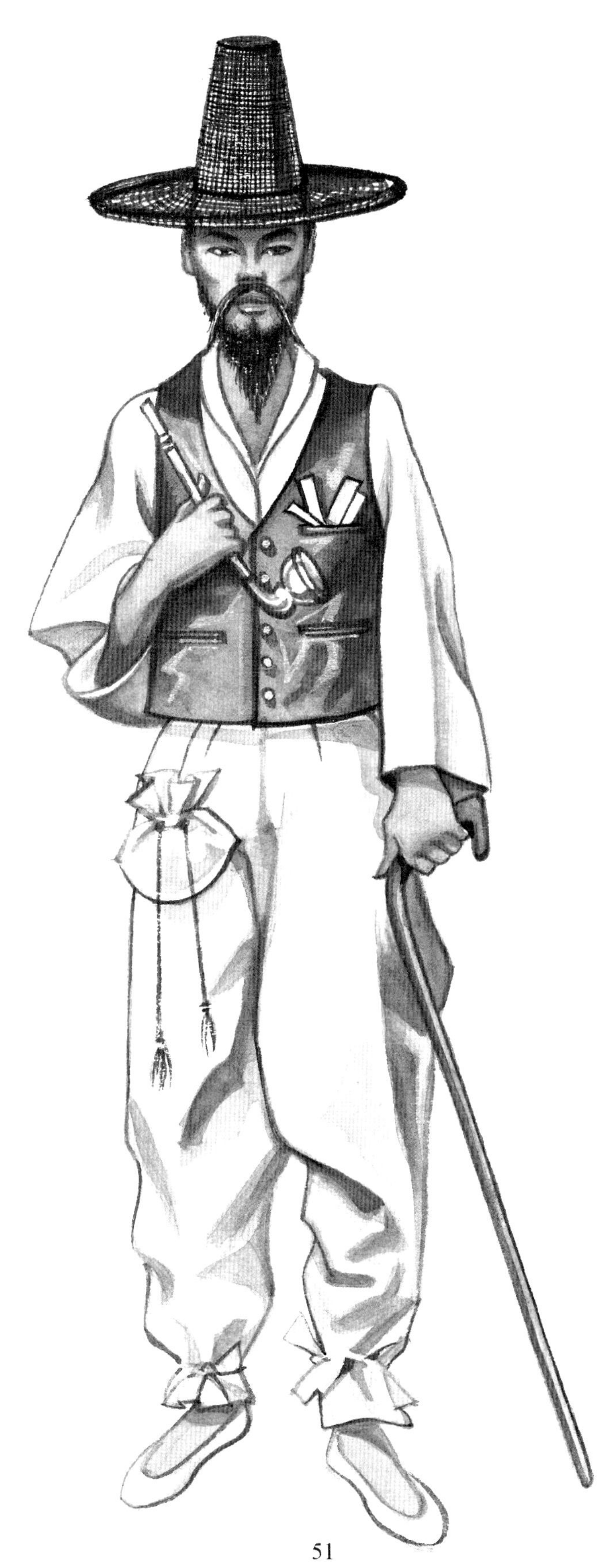

Hwarang-Do . . . A Military Martial Art

Hwarang-Do means 'The way of flowering manhood.' This military institution was developed in the ancient Korean state of Silla 2,000 years ago. It is a combination of both karate and kung fu. Karate movements are hard and linear, and kung fu stresses soft, circular movements. Hwarang-Do was the original system of hand-to-hand combat, and it developed into the most fierce fighting force in Asia. It was important in the formation of Korea. The groups, composed of Sillan young men of aristocratic birth, numbered in the thousands. The 'Hwarang' were the generals, statesmen and leaders of the kingdoms. Their civilian charges were called 'Rang-do.'

The spirit of chivalry resulted from their training. The guiding principles can be found in the five commandments: loyalty to one's country; loyalty to one's parents and teachers; trust and brotherhood among friends; courage in battle; never take a life without cause, as indiscriminate killing is evil.

One of the young men who participated in the Sun Cities Art Museum shows explained, "The ancient master believed that if one has the capacity to kill, then one should be able to heal as well. So when a student receives his first-degree black belt certification, he then studies acupuncture, acupressure, bone-setting, herbal medicine and inner strengthening, called the 'ki gong' technique."

Some of the results of this training were demonstrated in our show as students leaped at each other, flooring their adversary by well-placed kicks to the torso. A brick was broken in half with a single blow of a bare hand, and a young girl displayed the art of cooling the ardor of a man with evil intentions with the innocent swing of a handbag.

A humorous note came out of the invitation of the young men to the men in the audience to partake of this training for purposes of self-defense. Amid laughter, one elderly gentleman took the microphone to explain that just delivering one leap like the ones demonstrated would probably 'finish off' the majority of that audience of retirees.

Costume and Hwarang-Do information are courtesy of Master Instructor Tim Elliott of the Hwarang-Do Phoenix Academy.

The Hwarang-Do uniform has evolved through the ages. It consists of a knee-length, black, sleeveless cotton vest with a narrow orange stripe around the neck and down both sides of the front. It is open on each side and in the back nearly to the waist. There is a round, orange medallion embroidered on the right shoulder, with a wreath of green leaves. On the left shoulder there are two Korean characters which say 'Hwarang-Do.' The white cotton blouse, worn under the vest, is tucked into the trouser waist. The trousers are black. A long white cotton belt is tied into a bow at the left side of the waist, over the vest. It is tied with a single bow pointing toward the left, and long streamers at the right of the knot. The athletes perform barefoot.

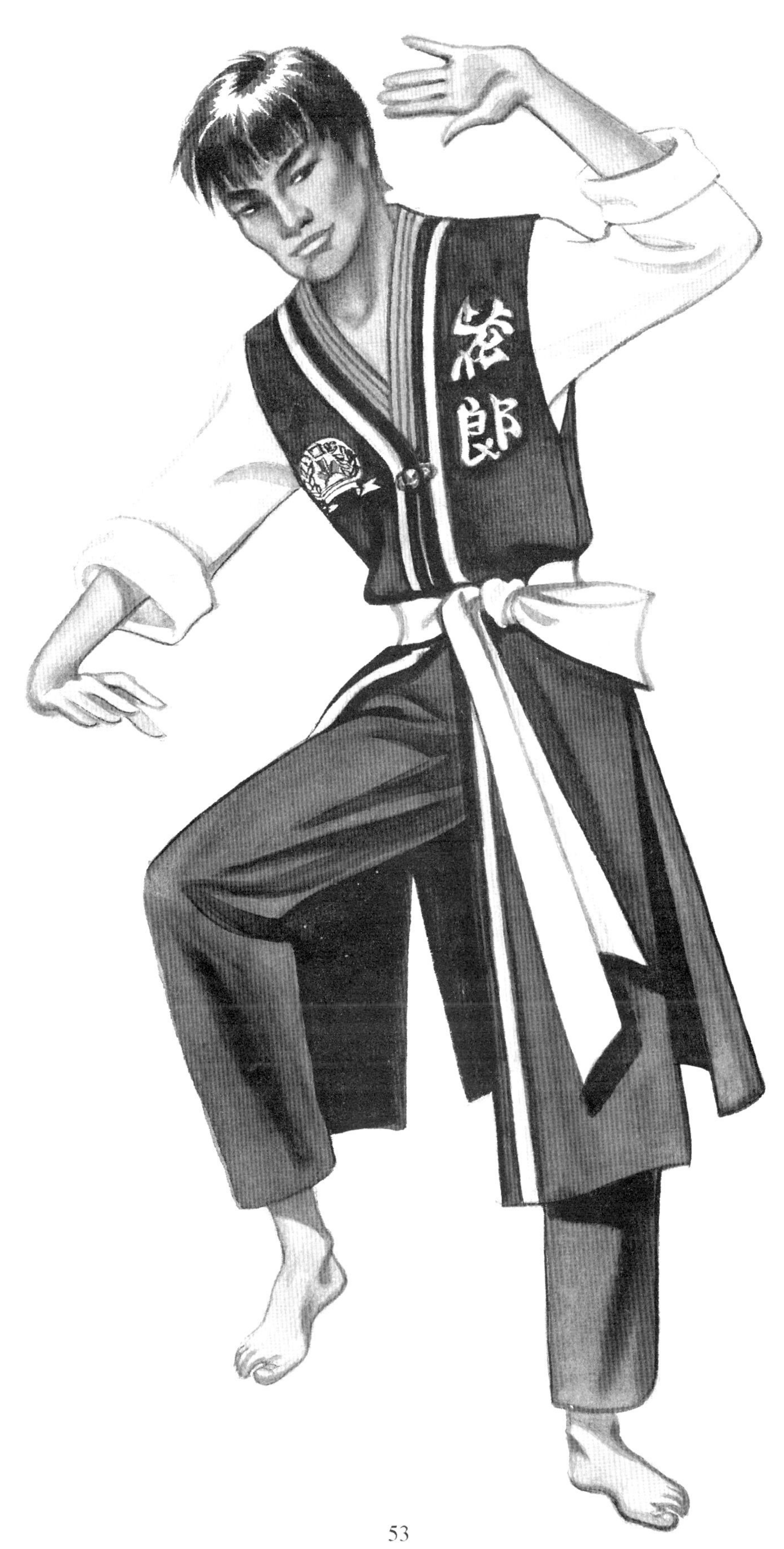
花郎

A market stall,

a fine Bokara rug,

a scrap of Chinese embroidery -

food for the eye is to be found almost everywhere.

Jocasta Innes

Hong Kong . . . Fragrant Harbor

Not too many years ago Pan American pilots voted Hong Kong the most glamorous stopover on earth! They should know, since they carved out the first regular flight routes around the world.

This city is a British Crown Colony at the mouth of the Canton River in China, 90 miles south of Canton. Its nucleus is Hong Kong Island, approximately 35 square miles, acquired from China in 1841. Victoria, the capital, is located on this island. Across the bay are the small areas of Kowloon Peninsula and Stonecutter's Island. An additional 355 square-mile area known as the New Territories was leased from China for 99 years in 1898. Britain and China signed an agreement in 1984 allowing Hong Kong to keep its capitalist system for 50 years after the lease expires in 1997.

Hong Kong's total area is 409 square miles, with a 1992 population estimate of 5.8 million, with less than 20,000 British. From 1949 until 1962 Hong Kong absorbed more than a million refugees from China. Hong Kong Harbor was long an important British naval station and one of the world's most important trans-shipment ports.

The fact that in 1997 China will again own the most important manufacturing region adjoining Kowloon hasn't dampened Hong Kong's progress as much as would seem probable. An editor of the *South China Morning Post,* one of the city's largest newspapers, said, "Grim forebodings are an exercise in futility, because it is hard enough to predict what will happen in so many days, much less so many years...Hong Kong has learned to live for today."

The Star Ferry still plies its way across Hong Kong Harbor, but less patient commuters prefer the subway under the bay. A few of the old red double-decker buses are to be found now on the freeways that twine around the island like a giant pretzel.

Hong Kong is still mysterious and romantic, and at night there is an air of excitement about the city that may be unrivaled by any other.

Hong Kong *Is* the Most Wonderful City in the World

To most world travelers Hong Kong is exciting, glamorous, a good place to shop and a place that must be seen at least once. But to me, it is the most wonderful city in the world. This is why.

We planned a trip around the world at an inauspicious time in history. It was at the height of the Vietnam War and our Marine son, Dave, was in Danang. He was a forward observer at the enemy line, directing the fire of our troops. We hadn't heard from him for several months, and the headlines were frightening. We had contacted Arizona's Barry Goldwater, who was having some success in reaching the fighting men with his short-wave radio, but he could not help us. We were not in a traveling mood; in fact, I resisted leaving our telephone. What if something happened to Dave and we couldn't be reached?

Our daughter Sally was flying for Pan American Airlines, and the company was making it possible for its employees to take their relatives around the world with them for a fraction of the normal cost. Knowing that we could do nothing for Dave, whether we went or not, we finally decided not to turn down the opportunity. It certainly would never happen again.

The itinerary consisted of Tokyo, Hong Kong, New Delhi, Istanbul, Beirut, with short round-trip flights to Jerusalem, Athens, Rome and Madrid. We would leave the flight at Nice and go by train to Amsterdam, with a flight from Frankfurt to Berlin sandwiched in. From Amsterdam we would fly to London and then home. Before leaving we would flood the mail with letters to Dave, hoping that at least one would get through, giving him our itinerary and names of hotels.

Tokyo had been interesting, but Hong Kong took our breath away. It was dusk when we landed at Kai Tak Airport. A fairyland of lights and colored streamers was spread out before us. Our hotel, the Mandarin, is still rated one of the top ten in the world.

We were escorted through the magnificent lobby to our rooms, where the phone was ringing. A man's voice said, "Welcome to Hong Kong! This is your son's captain. I left him in Danang this morning in good health and he says to tell you to have a wonderful trip and not to worry...he's fine." The captain then explained that he and his wife were staying in our hotel while he was on R and R (Rest and Recreation). He invited us to join them at the bar on the top floor of the hotel for a toast to Dave.

What a celebration! We laughed, we cried, from relief and happiness. It was a most memorable evening! Our son was well, and he was here with us in spirit. One of our letters had reached him in time to give his captain the name of our hotel. Hong Kong Harbor lay before us with its battleships, freighters, private cruisers, houseboats and junks spread out at anchor under a full moon. Without a doubt, we all agreed, Hong Kong was the most beautiful and wonderful city in the entire world.

Hong Kong Cheongsam

The Chinese cheongsam is a delightful version of Chinese costume, which has become very popular on Hong Kong Island and in Kowloon. A glamorous version of this dress can be seen in every elegant nightspot. It complements the beauty of an Asian woman in a way that cannot be matched by ordinary Western wear.

This cheongsam is of pure-white satin, with the high, stiff collar and right underarm closing which are important parts of Asian ethnic dress. The collar has a gold binding and the beads of the dragon down the front are gold, with an occasional red bead as a color accent. The opening on each side of the long skirt should not be more than four or five inches above the knee, although this rule is not always followed in today's Hong Kong. Bar girls often wear their skirts split on the sides nearly to the waist.

We found this stunning gown in Jonnie Ho's shop in the Hong Kong Hilton Hotel.

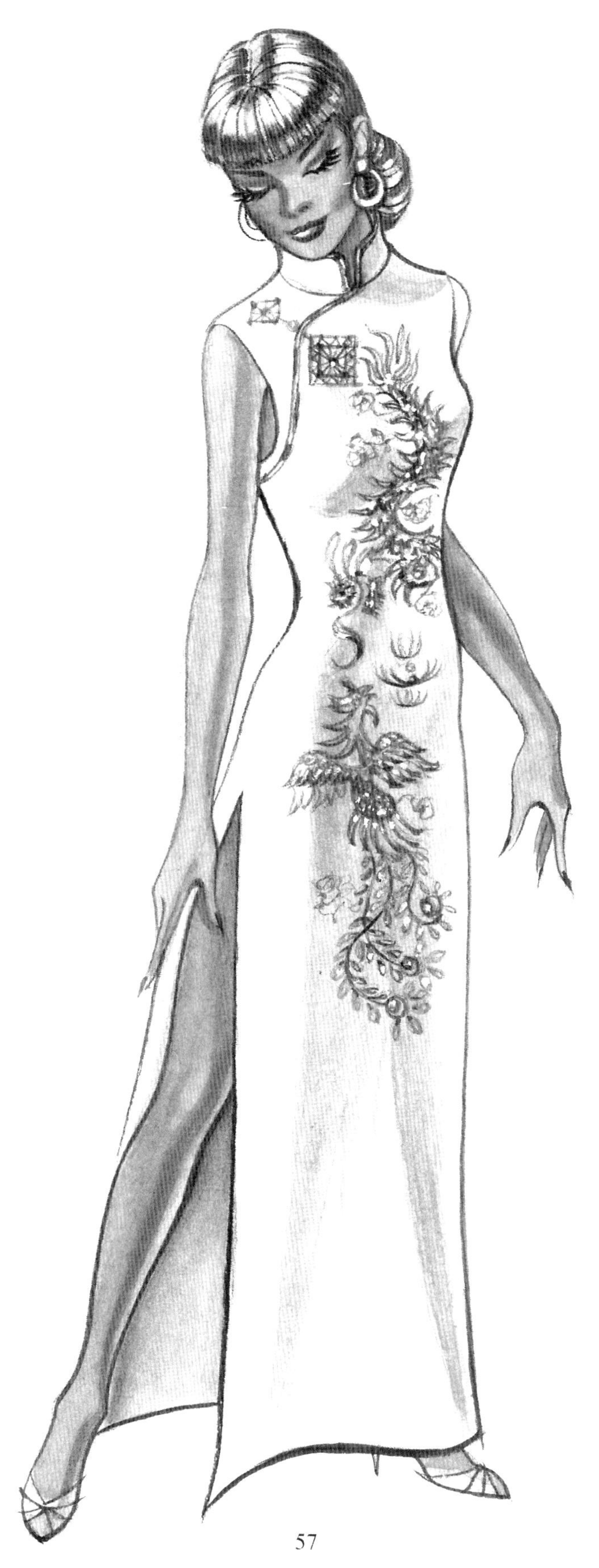

The world is a sure teacher, but it requires a fat fee.
Finnish Proverb

The world is a rose. Smell it and pass it to your friends.
Persian Proverb

What was hard to bear is sweet to remember.
Portuguese Proverb

Trust in Allah, but tie up your camel.
Turkish Proverb

When you go to buy, don't show your silver.
Chinese Proverb

One picture is worth a thousand words.
Chinese Proverb

Life is a book, and he who has not traveled has read only one page.
Anonymous

Chapter Four

Southeast Asian Odyssey

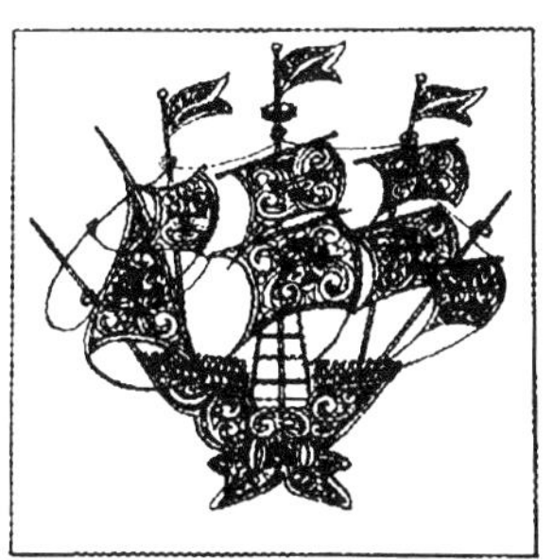

Vietnam
Thailand
Myanmar

The Socialist Republic of Vietnam

Vietnam is on the east coast of the Indochinese Peninsula in Southeast Asia. It is the size of New Mexico, with a population almost 48 times that of that state. The capital is Hanoi, the currency is the dong, and the literacy rate is estimated at 88 percent. The government is communist, with a president who is head of state and a prime minister who is head of government.

Vietnam's recorded history began in Tonkin, before the Christian era. Settled by Viets from central China, Vietnam was held by China from 111 B.C., until 939 A.D. In 1288 it defeated the armies of Kubla Khan. Conquest by France began in 1858 and lasted nearly 30 years. In 1940 the Japanese occupation began. The Independence League was formed, headed by Ho Chi Minh, a communist guerrilla leader. The French again sought to gain control and were finally defeated in 1954, and a cease-fire accord was signed in Geneva. Under the agreement the communists gained control of territory north of the 17th Parallel. Its capital was Hanoi and its president was Ho Chi Minh. South Vietnam consisted of 39 southern provinces, with Ngo Dinh Diem as president. Almost a million North Vietnamese fled to South Vietnam.

In 1954 North Vietnam tried to take over South Vietnam. The U.S. aided South Vietnam and the Soviets and Chinese gave arms assistance to North Vietnam. U.S. air strikes began in 1964, and troop strength reached a high of 543,400. Withdrawal of troops began in 1969, but air strikes resumed in 1972. A cease-fire agreement was signed in Paris in 1973 by the U.S., North and South Vietnam and the Vietcong, but it was never implemented.

Heavy fighting continued for two years throughout Indochina. The Saigon regime surrendered April 30, 1975. Reportedly, more than 58,000 Americans lost their lives in this conflict and displaced Vietnamese refugees and civilian dead numbered 6,500,000, in addition to a million Vietnamese killed in battle. We lost the war! What a sad era in American history!

Vietnamese and Chinese relations soured when ethnic Chinese charged discrimination. China cut off economic aid. Vietnamese reforms followed, and in 1994 the U.S. ended the 19-year trade embargo it had held on trade with that country.

Vietnam Visits

The Vietnam War played an important part in the lives of many Americans for many years.   With two of our children involved in that conflict, we had double worries. While son Dave was at Danang near the 17th Parallel, Sally, a `stew' for Pan-Am, decided she had to be part of the action and volunteered for Military Air Transport flights from San Francisco to Saigon. These flights (MATS) took troops to the combat areas and brought returnees to San Francisco, along with the remains of our soldiers killed in action.

A remarkable thing about these flights, she reported, was that the noise of the engines was the only sound to be heard. No alcohol was served, as our government and Pan-Am had an agreement on this issue. The men were engrossed in their own thoughts. Some were preparing themselves for what lay ahead and others were reliving their experiences. This quiet, contemplative bunch of young men were not in a mood for conversation.

Sally told of a 20-year-old Vietnamese girl who had lost her leg to an American truck and was being sent to the U.S. for a prosthesis. A touch of Vietnamese etiquette became evident on this flight. Although there were Vietnamese officers on the plane, none spoke to the girl on that long flight, as it would not have been appropriate without a proper introduction. But upon landing, when the time came to help her off the plane, they all leaped to offer assistance.

Both Dave and Sally have birthdays Christmas week, and Governor Love announced on television that a Colorado brother and sister were going to get together in Danang for a birthday party and that the celebration would be on T.V. We didn't turn off our set for the whole week, but got no further word. Weather interfered with the filming plans. A large birthday cake was picked up in Guam, decorated with palm trees and dancing dolls in grass skirts. After a five-hour delay, it was decided a landing could be made, and the pilot 'dive-bombed' the plane into Danang, in order to avoid snipers. A Pan-Am pilot had told us in Hong Kong that the sniper problem was the most dangerous part of being in Vietnam. Not a comforting thought for any parent!

The television crew did not arrive, but Dave had been waiting for hours. It was a good party, and the flight crew and others sang "Happy Birthday" and had some cake, and brother and sister had a good reunion.

Ethnic Dress of Vietnam

This Vietnamese 'au-dai' is correct in every detail. There are small differences between the au-dais of northern, central and southern Vietnam. This one is from Saigon, which is in the south. The long-sleeved tunic top is made of green embossed Chinese satin and the trousers are of a white synthetic fabric. The bodice is fitted, and the sides of the garment are open nearly to the waist. There are the soft, stand-up collar and a closing under the right arm, like many Oriental garments. In ancient times, when China controlled Vietnam, Chinese clothing and hairdress became obligatory. It is not surprising that this garment strongly resembles the Chinese cheongsam of Hong Kong. The pointed straw hat is typically Vietnamese.

My Marine son brought what I considered to be a lovely au-dai when he returned from his tour of duty in Vietnam. After proudly displaying this outfit in a show in Colorado, I was approached by a Vietnamese woman who asked, pointedly, how I happened to have the garment. When she heard it was a gift from a serviceman, she said, "That explains it. Enterprising Chinese were selling anything they could find to the American military personnel. Please let my husband make one for you that is like the ones worn in our country. He was a tailor in Saigon. We were fortunate in being able to leave South Vietnam just before it fell to the North. We appreciate being safely in your country and would like to have Americans see our native dress as it should be worn."

Her criticism and offer of help and advice were very welcome. It is difficult to keep from being misled when one has never been in a country and, after all, Marine training does not include details of ethnic dress. We learned that black trousers can be worn for work, white ones only for dress wear, and the blue top and green trousers of my costume were just not acceptable by Vietnamese standards.

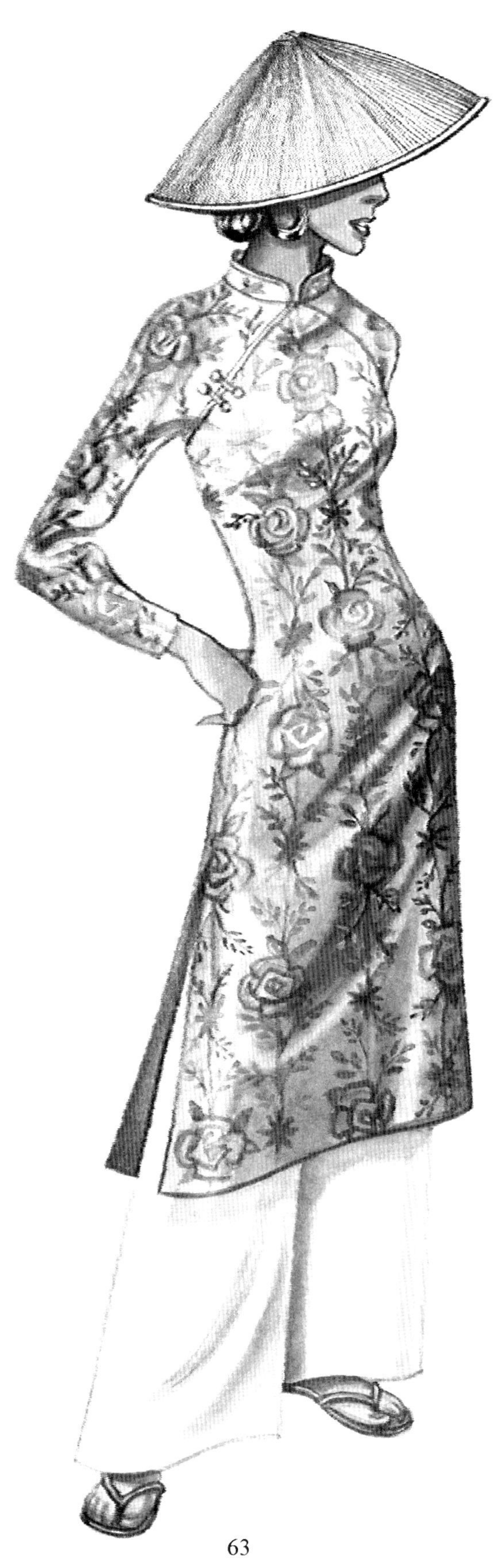

When the dancers dance badly,
they blame the musical accompaniment.

Don't sew your clothes while wearing them.

When walking behind an adult, the child will not be bitten by the dog.

Don't sing during meal time, because you'll get an old husband.

Contributed by Khacheenuj Chaovanapricha
A student at Seattle University, from Bangkok

Kingdom of Thailand . . . Formerly Siam

Thailand is a lovely little country on the Indochinese and Malayan Peninsula, in Southeast Asia. It is about the size of Texas, with more than three times the population of that state. The capital is Bangkok. The currency is the baht, and literacy is 89 percent. The government is a constitutional monarchy, and the king and queen have warm places in the hearts of their people. Many Thais believe that Queen Sirikit is one of the most beautiful women in the world. Nearly everyone visiting Thailand comments on the striking beauty of these dainty women.

Although surrounded by Burma, Laos and Cambodia, all of which have autocratic governments, the people of Thailand are determined to remain free. The word 'Thai' means 'free.' This is the only country in Southeast Asia that has never been taken over by a European power. Buddhism is the religion of 95 percent of the population, while four percent are Muslim.

Thais began migrating from China in the 11th century and the Thai nation emerged around the 13th century. King Mongkut and his son King Chulalongkorn ruled consecutively from 1851 to 1910 and signed trade treaties with Britain and France. They also developed a constitutional monarchy from an absolute monarchy. A popular musical, *The King and I,* was based on King Mongkut's reign and his supposed romance with a British schoolteacher.

Japan occupied the country in 1941. After World War II Thailand followed a pro-Western foreign policy and in 1969 was one of the participants in the Association of Southeast Asian Nations, which promoted economic, social and cultural cooperation and development.

Visiting this country is a delight. The 'klongs,' or waterways of Bangkok, are canals where flat-bottomed boats are loaded with every type of merchandise. Some of them are so covered with flowers that the boats look like huge floating bouquets. Many of the owners of the crafts live along the waterways, and some even live on the small boats. Life along these canals is a never-ending source of interest. The Rose Garden in Bangkok, where all things Thai are displayed, should not be missed. One should also see as many as possible of the 20,000 fabulous Siamese temples all over the country and the Emerald Buddha and the huge, golden reclining Buddha.

On our trip around the world during the Vietnam War, we stayed at the Siam Intercontinental Hotel in Bangkok. At that time Pan-Am owned these hotels. We had fun spotting important personages attending the airline's board of directors meeting. Colonel Charles Lindbergh was one we recognized.

A Bangkok Incident

While planning a trip to Burma and Thailand, a search was made for contacts that might lead to help in locating a man's traditional dancing dress. My Thai friend, Yuma, was from Chanthaburi, where *Bridge Over the River Kwai* was filmed. She had been a great help with the ethnic-dress shows given for charity in the Denver area. Her best friend in Bangkok owned a jewelry store near the National Theater, and her friend, Harold, had been a missionary in Thailand. Harold wrote immediately to Bangkok to contact an Italian businessman, a Mr. Minelli, whose wife was Thai. We were assured that with these contacts we would have no problem finding what we wanted.

Yuma's friend's jewelry shop was so tempting that both Jo and I found some pieces that we felt we could not do without. We then set out for the National Theater with Sapai, one of the shopgirls who was bilingual. The theater was old and impressive. The uniformed guard at the huge iron gate looked fierce and spoke no English. Without Sapai our search would have ended right there at the gate. We entered the lobby, and there it was! In a glass case in the center of a large expanse of marble floor was a spectacular, glistening dream of a man's traditional Thai dancing costume. All that remained now was to obtain this wonderful find at the right price.

Sapai spoke to the attendant on duty, and in a few minutes a slender young man appeared, bowed politely and spoke to Sapai. After a long conversation, Sapai finally explained that this man would come to our hotel the next morning to discuss the matter. Raising his hands in the formal Thai farewell gesture, we were dismissed. This gesture, known as the 'wai,' is made by placing one's palms together with the fingers pointed upward. The higher they are raised, the greater the respect shown.

The next morning the phone rang and a man's voice said, "This is Siripong, from the theater. We are in the lobby and have something to show you. We'll be right up." Seconds later the young man of the National Theater (whom I had thought did not speak English), accompanied by three lovely young girls, bounced into the room. They were casually dressed and were carrying, in all its splendid glory, the very dancing dress we had admired in the case in the theater lobby.

Siripong and I got down to business immediately, and soon had our purchase details completed. This was not difficult, because I was so excited by my overwhelming success that I neglected to bargain. For several hours we worked with the girls to learn how to put this extremely complicated outfit together properly.

We asked why he pretended not to understand or speak English, and he said that people were always trying to get free admissions to the theater, but our story was so different that they called him to check it out.

The girls danced every evening at a popular folkloric restaurant, and they studied dance during the day. Siripong was the choreographer for theater productions. They had all danced abroad and had just returned from Burma. Ladda put on the Burmese dancing dress that we had recently acquired and did a Burmese dance for us. It was full of slashing motions, in contrast to the rather gentle movements of the Thai dance. By this time we were all good friends. Jo and I treated the group to lunch in the hotel's garden, and they, in turn, invited us to that evening's performance. Of course we accepted eagerly.

We had invited the Minellis for cocktails, but calculated that surely they would leave for their dinner before it was time for the show. We miscalculated by just a few minutes, with nearly shattering results. Siripong and his lively crew, still in T-shirts and slacks, arrived at the hotel lobby while we were bidding farewell to our guests. Mr. Minelli looked as though he was about to have a heart attack. His face transfixed with horror, he shouted, "You do not know these people and you are going out in a car with them?"

"No, in a taxi," Siripong answered, although he had not been addressed.

"Are you taking a hotel taxi?" Mr. Minelli asked.

"No, they are too expensive; we'll pick up one at the street," countered Siripong.

Addressing Jo and me, Mr. Minelli queried, "Have you lost your senses?"

His concern was justified, for we had traveled enough to be aware of the danger of becoming friendly with strangers in a foreign country. There were many tales of robberies and even murders of tourists in the Bangkok papers every day. For a few moments we thought our chance at a magical evening was lost. Siripong looked very annoyed and the girls kept looking at their watches.

Our new self-appointed guardian decided against bringing in the police and asked what time we would be returned to our hotel. Eleven o'clock turned out to be the zero hour for this pair of grandmothers. The words, "I will call your room at exactly 11:10 and you had better be there," followed us as we ran out of the hotel lounge.

Six of us were squeezed into a tiny cab with the driver, and I didn't open my eyes once as we dashed wildly through Bangkok's crowded streets. Valuable time had been lost, and the girls had just two minutes, instead of the usual five, in which to get dressed in their intricate costumes.

In spite of its embarrassing beginning, that evening was the highlight of my entire costume-collecting experiences. How could we ever have dreamed of getting behind the scenes of a traditional dancing performance put on by Thailand's National Theater? The dinner was delicious. We were even introduced to the audience as the dancers' and Siripong's friends. We felt very important, and a part of the Thai world, as tourists rarely are.

The call came at exactly 11:10 p.m., and we were safely back in our room to receive it. Our caller was so relieved that he would not have to explain to his missionary friend about our demise, that we were truly sorry to have caused him an evening of so much anxiety.

Siripong called the next morning to say that his conscience bothered him because he had charged too much for the costume, so he would be over with another sarong. He gave us the most beautiful pure silk handloomed sarong we have ever seen. Thai visitors to the museum have declared it to be beyond price.

Traditional Thai Dancing Costumes

Man's

The man's role in this dance is performed by a woman. The costume is of gold satin, trimmed with red satin bands and embroidered all over with silver wire and sequins. The top is heavily embroidered in an all-over geometric design with solid silver flower-like discs. The short sleeves are trimmed with red satin and silver.

Yellow cotton trousers with wide decorated bands come to just below the knee. A sarong, three yards in length and a yard wide, is pleated and draped around the hips of the dancer. It is covered by three panels that hang from the waist. Another piece wraps around the waist.

The man's pointed, golden headgear is very much like that of the woman's, but it is not quite as ornate. This item could never have been found without the help of Sapai, the Thai shopgirl who was our guide to the National Museum. She shopped the huge Indian Market where everything anyone needs is said to be available . . . and was, for us.

This complicated costume can be put on by trained performers in five minutes, even with the necessary sewing to hold it in place. However, when it was shown at the museum, it became necessary to call in a Thai dancer from a temple in a nearby town for help.

In classical dances, body movements have great significance. The students must go through long periods of rigorous training to maintain disciplined and flexible bodies to perform and hold the 64 difficult positions which comprise the 'Alphabet of Dancing.' Each of these positions has a name, such as "The Bee Caressing the Flower," "Wedded Love," and "Walking Gracefully."

Orchestras accompanying the dance consist mostly of woodwinds and percussion instruments, with the melody provided by an instrument called the 'gong wong wai.' The musical scale has no halftones.

Woman's

We had been warned that finding the right skirt for the woman's dancing dress would be difficult. Fortunately, there was a dressmaking shop in our hotel that made designer clothing for the ethnic fashion shows which Queen Sirikit sponsored for charity. Miss Thailand, who had won a Miss Universe contest in the 1970's, was a model for these shows. She and her friends loved the type of skirt we needed. They wore them to court events, as well as modeling them, with embroidered and jeweled `sabais,' wide scarves wrapped around the upper part of the body with one end tucked into the skirt and the other end worn over one shoulder.

The textiles for these skirts were woven on order in only one factory, and that was several hundred miles from Bangkok. The shop proprietor had an extra length of the silk needed and promised to make exactly the right skirt for us and to have it ready when we returned from Chiang Mai. It was very elegantly made of cream-colored heavy silk, with an all-over design in red, green and gold thread. There is a box pleat down the front from waist to hem with pleats on both sides, finished with a flat, double bow at the waist and worn with gold mesh belts with large, ornate gold buckles. The dancers are barefoot.

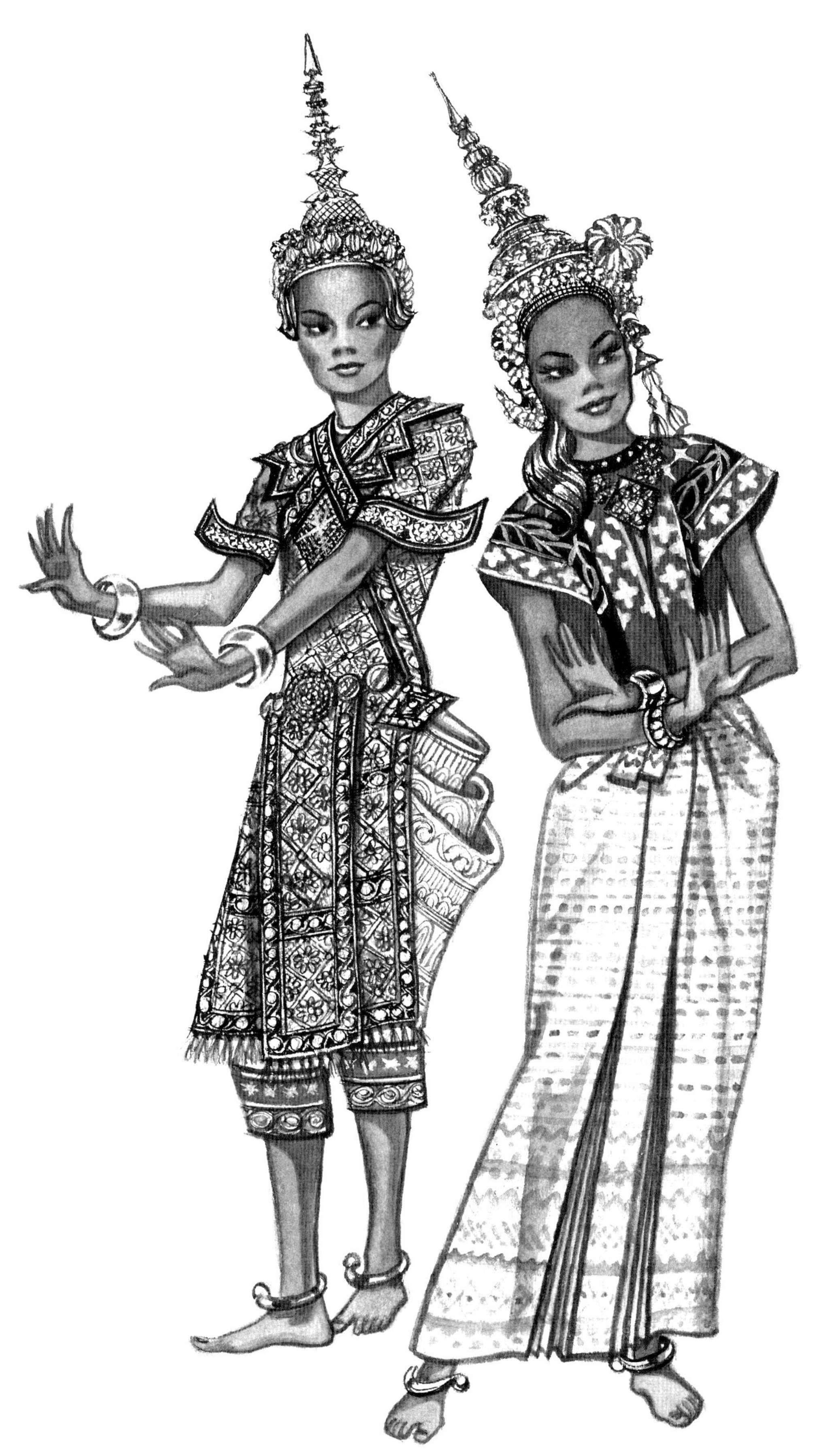

We visited the College of Dance in Chiang Mai in northern Thailand. The school's director was very kind in helping us put this outfit together. A green satin cape is worn over a sleeveless red cotton blouse, both of them tucking into the skirt. The cape and separate collar are heavily embroidered with silver wire, and synthetic gems are worked into the embroidery on the collar. Earrings, bracelets, anklets, a gold necklace and pendant and a gold mesh belt and buckle complete this outfit, except for the headgear. The director had the perfect gold-covered papier-mâché hat with its high, pointed top, made especially for this woman's dancing dress. An important finishing touch was the red flower with its strings of Persian jasmine that dangle from the left side of the headpiece. My Thai friend back home had provided the 'year-bra-bra,' or large imitation Thai blossom, but jasmine was needed, and the school had used all of theirs. In an incredible showing of a desire for perfection, the school's conscientious official arrived at the airport with a small bag of jasmine, just as our flight was being called. The wonderful people with whom we dealt in our costume searches made the project a series of stimulating and gratifying experiences.

It should be noticed in the drawings of the dancers that their fingers are bent backwards in an exaggerated position. Little girls practice bending their fingers in this way so that they can become dancers when they grow up. Long fingernails exaggerate this graceful, curved effect, and sometimes metallic nails several inches long are worn for dancing. However, artificial nails are not used in this particular traditional performance.

Travel Trials

Broad-brimmed, flat-topped Thai straw hats, with lacy straw pieces securing them to the head, are seen everywhere in Thailand. They are light, and provide much needed shade. Nearly every boatman and woman on the klongs and most field workers wear them. Two of these hats were stacked together and I wore them on the plane back to the United States. Except for carrying an extra large package, there was no other way to assure their safe arrival. Getting complicated and fragile hats to their ultimate destination was perhaps the most difficult single job of costume collecting. It took insistence, pleading, defiance and a great deal of nerve in handling airline personnel, who are accustomed to dealing with overloaded people on international flights. It is with pride that I state that at least 16 extremely fragile pieces of headgear were transported safely without a harmful scratch. However, the most difficult pieces were the Thai golden dancing hats. The only way I was able to keep the airline from putting them in with the rest of the luggage was to create such a furor that the pilot picked the boxes up and allowed them to ride with him in the cockpit.

As to the question of how anyone could carry, in an already full suitcase, all of those costumes without sending any of them by mail, there is a simple answer. Some people give their old clothes to charity. Mine end up in hotel rubbish baskets, with a note attached to be sure that they do not arrive at my home months later, sent by a conscientious hotel manager. With an almost empty suitcase, the costumes themselves are not a problem. But, oh, those unmanageable ornamental hats!

The Meo of Thailand

Originating in China, the Meos have been known as a distinct nation in Chinese history for 4,000 years. They are proud of their history and culture. Their costume will never be allowed to be forgotten, as wherever the tribe finds itself, its ethnic dress remains a symbol of home. The method of agriculture is slash and burn, which is very destructive to the land, so they move an average of every three years. A Burmese guide took us from Chiang Mai into the mountains to a Meo village. They like to settle on the highest spot, and their compound is built around the tallest tree. A hen is sacrificed every year to this tree, and a gun is never fired in its direction. The village was a group of houses with dirt floors and a place for a fire in the center of the room, with a hole in the roof to allow the smoke to escape.

There are White, Blue, Black, Red and Flowered Meo tribes, each named by the color of the dress of its women. The dress in the collection is that of a Blue Meo. There were no shops in the village, nor did we see any tribal clothing for sale in Chiang Mai. A treasured possession of every household is its sewing machine, and we saw a woman completing a dress in her home. It was meant for a neighbor, but the idea that their beloved traditional costume would be shown in a museum in the U.S. proved irresistable. We were allowed to purchase it. While waiting for it to be completed our Burmese guide translated additional information about Meo customs. It is the differences in culture that make the world so interesting.

The head villager, a 'pookang,' is elected by the people and is held responsible for their welfare. If anything goes wrong, he is fined. The religious leader is a shaman who exorcises evil spirits. Most of the people are animists. Justice is harsh. In the case of a murder, the guilty person is buried with the victim. In this tribe the women are as strong as the men, and rape is unknown. Although polygamy is accepted if the husband can afford more than one wife, if his behavior causes the wife to commit suicide, he is punished by tying his arms and legs to two bulls and turning them loose. Punishment is severe, swift and final.

In the mountains near Meo villages there are large teak forests where elephants provide the heavy labor for harvesting the timber.

Ethnic Dress of a Meo Woman

Blue and White Meos are seen more than any other tribes in northern Thailand today. This dress has a blouse of black sateen, embroidered in front with a collar decorated in back with 25 silver coins. The skirt is blue, accordion-pleated cotton, with bands of cross-stitching in yellow, blue and red. A foot-wide panel hangs from the waist in front to the bottom of the skirt. It is embroidered with petit point, and it is believed that by dipping this cloth into warm water and bathing the face and brow of her husband, a woman can cure him of many illnesses.

There is a red sash about nine yards long and over a foot wide that has 14-inch-long red wool fringe on each side. It takes some time and effort to adjust this waistband properly, since the wearer must wind it several times around the body to get it tight enough.

A small bag of black handwoven fabric has a petit point insertion and fluffy red balls at each of its four corners, with a handle made of braided red wool. A silver neck ring completes the costume, and a decorated headband keeps the complicated hairdo in place. Women fashion large buns to wear in their hair by collecting clippings of their own hair and that of women relatives.

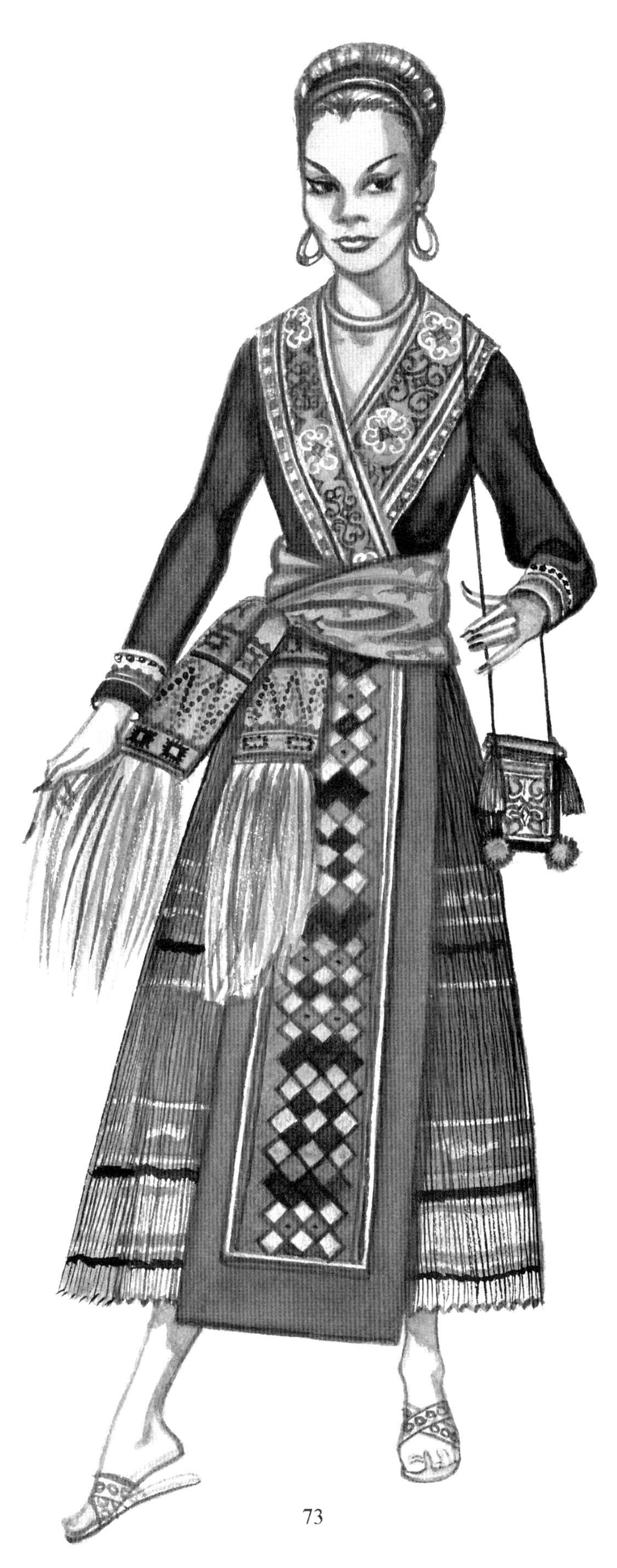

A man with little learning

is like the frog

who thinks its puddle is a great sea.

Burmese proverb

Union of Myanmar . . . Formerly Burma

Burma was once the richest nation in Southeast Asia and was known as the Golden Land. However, in 1987 it was given 'Less Developed' status by the United Nations.

Myanmar, located on the Bay of Bengal, is nearly as large as Texas, with a population more than two and one-half times that of Texas. The capital is Yangon, formerly known as Rangoon. The currency is the kyat, and literacy is 81 percent.

Mountains rise to a height of 20,000 feet on three sides of the country, which is covered with tropical forests. The sources of three of the world's greatest rivers are in these mountains, the Mekong, the Yangtze and the Irrawaddy, which is navigable for 900 miles. These rivers flow through deep gorges within a few miles of each other. The climate of this wild and forbidding land is tropical monsoon.

It was across this land that the ancestors of the present-day Burmese people traveled from Tibet in the late 8th century. By the 11th century a Buddhist monarchy was established. Since 1824 Burma was more or less under British control until Japan gained nearly complete authority over the country from 1942 until 1945, when the last Japanese forces surrendered in World War II. In 1948 Britain agreed to Burma's independence, and since then it has been ruled by military leaders. When the first free multiparty elections in 30 years took place in 1990 the main opposition party won, but the military rulers refused to relinquish power. Aung San Suu Kyi, the chief leader of the opposition, was put under house arrest before these elections. In 1991 she was awarded the Nobel Peace Prize, and in July of 1995 she was finally unconditionally released.

General Than Shwe is head of state and head of government, and what the people call V.I.P.'s (Very Important Persons) run the country. These are military personnel with broad powers. People will go to great lengths to keep from offending a V.I.P. We never heard anyone use a Burmese word for V.I.P., so we assume that everyone uses the English form.

There does not appear to be any restriction on religion. Buddhism is practiced by 89 percent of the population. It has been suggested that this religion has been allowed to exist because its doctrine of peace would not encourage rebellion against the government.

Every Burmese with whom we spoke expressed the dream of being able to someday leave Burma and travel to another country. Only people related to V.I.P.'s are allowed to leave, we were told. Burma remains, in today's world, a country that time left behind. It is secluded, insular and remote.

Myanmar Memories

Rangoon (Yangon):

Htroi-Ra met us at the airport. She said to call her Tryra, which was a relief. She took us to the Inya Lake Hotel, which was like many Burmese hotels, not so bad on the outside, but disintegrating inside. It was built by Russians, whose plumbing skills left something to be desired. The first floor was nice, but the upstairs was disappointing, to say the least. We were upstairs.

Rangoon has a population of two and one-half million. The Shwe Dagon Pagoda stands on a hill, dominating the city. It is over 300 feet in height and is covered with 90 million dollars' worth of gold leaf. This magnificent temple was built, according to Buddhist doctrine, to house eight hairs of the head of Gautama Buddha. Rudyard Kipling called this temple "golden mystery, a beautiful, winking wonder." We were a little surprised that none of our guides in Burma had ever heard of Kipling, since he was a source of much of our interest in Burma.

Tryra was a Kachin, from a hill tribe in northern Burma, which has given the government a lot of trouble. Tryra herself was a rebel. When asked how Burma was under British rule, she replied, "Much better, my parents tell me." She also told us that Yangon means 'End of Strife,' but that the tranquility which permeates Burmese life is a product of Buddhism, not good government. She was a Christian, not a Buddhist.

We were not allowed on the train which runs along the Irrawaddy River to Pagan and Mandalay. Canadians and Australians could ride it, but Americans were banned. We never discovered the reason for this ban, but arranged to fly on Union of Burma Airways, although they were not a member of the International Air Transport Association. It was the only way we could travel the 400 miles to Pagan.

Pagan:

This city is a national treasure. It is said that there are as many temples as people in Pagan. In the 11th and 12th centuries wealthy people competed by building imposing pagodas as memorials to themselves. The armies of Kubla Khan put an end to this in 1287, but over 1,200 Buddhist temples in various stages of restoration still rise from the site of this famous city.

Our guide's name was Lwyn Aye. He was 26 years old and had a bachelor's degree in marine biology, but he could not leave the country to work. His father, a teacher, did not know an important enough V.I.P. to help. Fourteen members of his family live together, two grandparents, two brothers, seven sisters and his mother and father. Lwyn told us that most of the tourists were French and Italian, and that Japan and Germany were providing technical aid in joint ventures. Buddhist priests were everywhere, hoping for rice to be put in their begging bowls.

The floors of the temples were covered with gravel, and no one could go inside wearing shoes, so it didn't take much temple sightseeing to bruise our feet and bring this particular activity to an end. Although Lwyn considered Pagan a modern city, there were only two washing machines in the entire town, and both of them belonged to the hotel. Jo had brought dozens of balloons to give to the children, and we were soon so surrounded that she threw them all at the crowd, and we ran. We heard calls of "chocolate, chocolate!" from the children. They were putting in their order for the next time.

Mandalay:

Mandalay is the second largest city in Burma. It has about one-half million people, all dressed in their longyis and pasogs and on bicycle, or so it seemed. Our guide, Maymi, was lively and chatty. We learned more from her than from anyone in Burma. It was Maymi who told us that a women's liberation movement was not needed in her country, as women enjoy an equality with men that is rare in Asia. Upon marrying the woman retains her name and property rights. She does not wear a wedding ring, and either party can instigate divorce. Maymi was an ardent Buddhist, explaining, "We care little about getting rich. We just want enough to keep our families from need and as we grow old to have something to give to the temple." She also told us that another name for Burma is "Happy Land." But Maymi seemed very nervous, and with a reason. When she knew us better she told of her problem: "An idiot of a newspaper man from Italy hired me to take him around. When he went back home he wrote in his column that Maymi, in Mandalay, could get anything you wanted, under the counter. If the V.I.P.'s learn of this I could be in real trouble." She was even afraid to ask for a pass to go to Rangoon to see her sister for fear it would trigger an investigation. We wondered if the writer's action was due to deliberation or ignorance.

The less said about Mandalay's best hotel the better. The small town of Pagan had decent beds and air conditioning in its hotel, but Mandalay had neither. There was a thin layer of bedding over what felt like a slab of cement on which to sleep. We didn't see any other Americans there.

As we drove along the Irrawaddy River to the `Buffalo Rest,' we saw colonies of houses on stilts in the riverbed, which was nearly dry at that time of year. When the water is high the inhabitants can fish from their doorways, and when it is low they can get two harvests of rice a year. We were "On the road to Mandalay, where flying fishes play." They weren't out playing that day, although there were lots of nets around.

The Buffalo Rest is what we called a coffee break for water buffalo. It was in a protected bay of the river, where teak logs were floated from the forests of northern Burma to be loaded onto trucks. Trailers were backed into the water. The trucks pull, and teams of four buffalo push the trailers onto land. When a rest period is due the animals are allowed in water deep enough to float their heavy yokes. Although their eyes and noses are almost under water, they sleep peacefully until the next loading.

Our last morning in Mandalay we had to get up early because our plane was due at 7:30 a.m., and we knew we mustn't be late. As though we could sleep on those beds! On our way out of the hotel we saw a boy cleaning the floor of the lobby by pushing one-half of a coconut around with his foot. We couldn't tell if he was asleep or awake by his motions.

We were on time for the plane . . . it left at 3 p.m., because a V.I.P. (a BIG one) was late. Maymi cried while saying goodbye, wishing she could go somewhere too. Without her it would have been impossible to be as successful as we were in the costume search. We have often wondered how Maymi has fared in that far-off land.

When we finally boarded, the crew rushed around frantically in a great show of efficiency. But the stewardess forgot to check the overhead railing where the hand luggage was kept. A package that looked like a wrapped parasol stuck out into the aisle, over the low railing that was supposed to keep the hand luggage in place. As the jet rose into the air, the package turned slowly and headed for Jo, who was in an aisle seat in front of me. I saw it coming and yelled at her. As she turned her head the object slid across her forehead and one eyebrow, down her shoulder and across the hand I had instinctively put out. It bumped into the back of her seat and fell to the floor with a clank everyone around us could hear, above the noise of the engines. It turned out to be a piece of metal pipe.

The woman in the next seat screamed. I was paralyzed, and Jo didn't move. We thought she was dead. It seemed hours before the stewardess came, although it was probably minutes. She said with a touch of hysteria in her voice, "That idiot of a German salesman should have known better. We have a V.I.P on board and didn't have time to check the overhead."

Jo asked for ice, so we knew she was still alive. From then on everything that happened was part of a scheme to keep the V.I.P. from knowing that such an inexcusable accident had occurred. We always carry insurance, and I asked for a note from the pilot to verify that the accident had happened on the plane. In a little while he came out and assured us that everything would be taken care of at the airport. The minute we were on the ground in Bangkok, everyone connected with that plane disappeared. No one even helped Jo down the steps with her heavy bag. We were the only Americans on that plane, and we know why, now.

Rangoon, Again:

Tryra met us at the airport. She was horrified at our story and found the airport manager and insisted he find the pilot. She was told that the pilot had left and had no telephone at home. (A pilot on a scheduled airline with no telephone?) Tryra then called the American Embassy and made an appointment for the next morning.

Jo awoke with a black eye, but not even a headache. A fraction of an inch difference in that pipe and the story would have had a different ending. This was not the kind of excitement we were looking for. Tryra was thrilled to go to the American Embassy. She said she had always wanted to go, so we invited her to stay with us while we talked to the consul. He was a very nice young man who had graduated from a college near our home and had visited a good friend who lived across the street from us. We felt like old friends and were soon on first-name terms. He said that Burma is considered a 'plum' job for embassy people because they have no responsibilities of any consequence. The V.I.P.'s make every important decision. Household help was very inexpensive, and the wives loved it. There were lots of parties and 'fun' places to go (as long as one traveled in embassy cars and stayed away from Union of Burma Airways). He signed an insurance claim, which, fortunately, Jo did not need. She recovered without so much as a headache, and her eyesight was undamaged.

This was the worst experience, and yet the luckiest, that we have had on any trip. Tryra wept when we left. All those tears in such a 'Happy Land?'

By the old Moulmein Pagoda, lookin' eastward to the sea,

There's a Burma girl a-settin', and I know she thinks o' me;

For the wind is in the palm-trees, and the temple-bells they say:

"Come you back, you British soldier; come you back to Mandalay!"

Come you back to Mandalay,

Where the old Flotilla lay:

Can't you 'ear their paddles chunkin' from Rangoon to Mandalay?

On the road to Mandalay,

Where the flyin' fishes play,

An' the dawn comes up like thunder outer China 'crost the Bay!

Rudyard Kipling

Woman's Longyi

The 'longyi' is the national dress of Burma. The man's skirt is almost the same as the woman's, except that it is called a 'pasog' and is tied in a different manner. In the less industrialized cities, nearly every man, woman and child still wear their longyis everywhere. Westernized dress has slowly been gaining ground, but with the exception of Bhutan, nowhere has traditional dress been more in evidence than in Burma.

This longyi was made in Mandalay by a local seamstress. It took her just 12 hours to have it ready. The fabric was found at a government store and came from under the counter. Our enterprising guide, Maymi, had the nicest colors and patterns put away for her. She told us that very few good textiles are available to the average Burmese woman. This one is salmon colored, with a beige and brown overall conventional design. A two-inch border runs along one side of the fabric.

The tops can have sleeves of any length. This one is sleeveless, for a hot tropical country. There is a round neck and an opening down the left side. The top is tucked into the longyi, which is made into a wide tube with a black band at the waist and the border design around the bottom of the hem. It is ankle length and tied on the left side. There is a special way of tying this skirt. A wide pleat is made, with the fold toward the left hip. Two pieces of the top of the skirt are grasped at the left hip and tied, with the ends tucked into the black band. The wide cotton band, always in black, is a feature of nearly every woman's fashionable longyi.

Women wear flowers in their hair whenever possible. Brilliantly-colored blossoms encircle a large bun on the top of the head or at the nape of the neck. Ponytails are popular too, and there are usually flowers in them somewhere.

'Ton-a-kan,' a paste made of sandalwood, is worn on the faces of men, women and children. It is said to protect the skin from the sun and to be good for the complexion. Women and children paint designs on their faces with this paste.

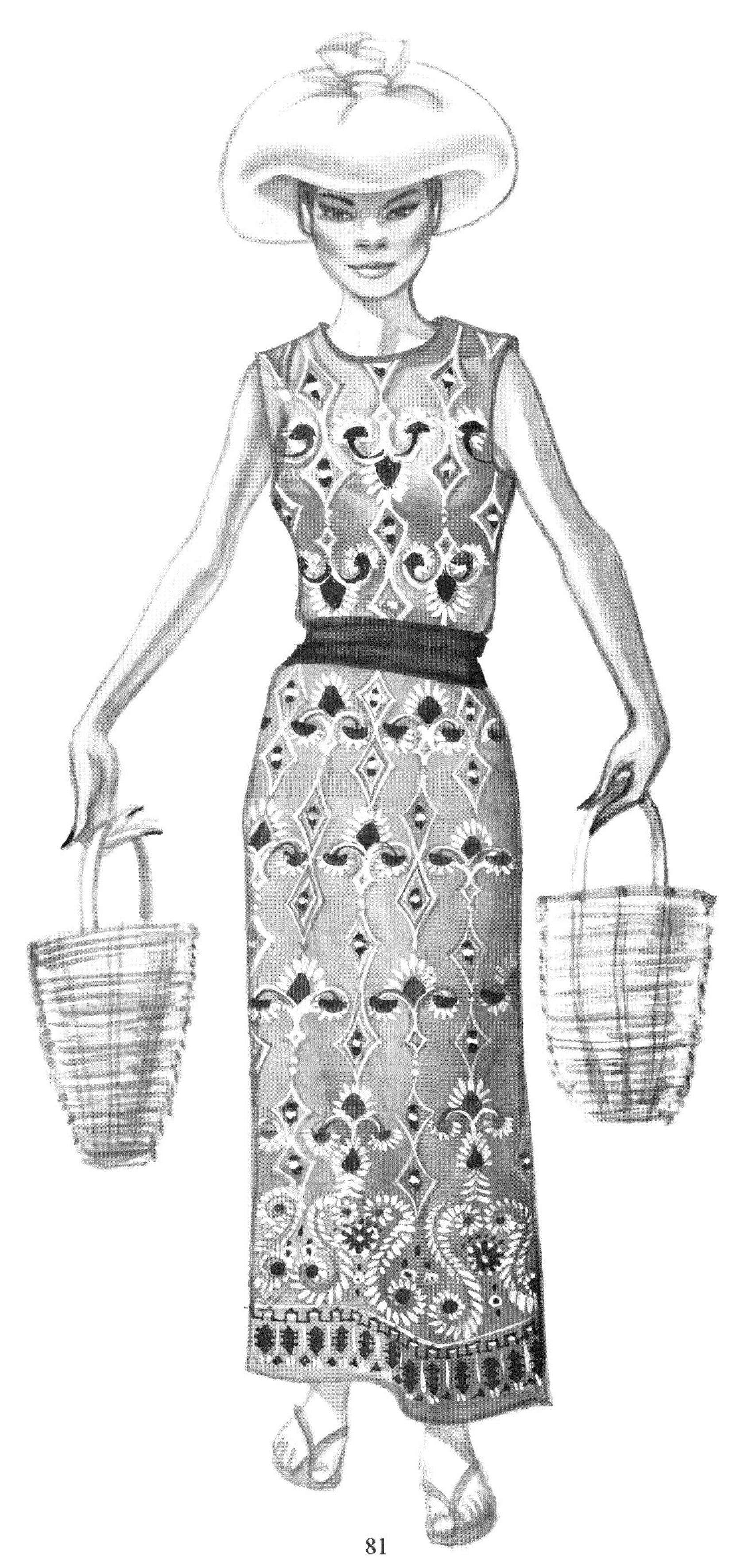

Burmese Dancing Dress

Although Burma is now 89 percent Buddhist, this dance has come down through the centuries from ancient Hindu culture. The dancing costume reflects sculptures seen on ancient Hindu temples. Dancers, according to a travel brochure describing Burmese dance techniques, "swirl with litheness that seems beyond the capacity of human joints." We saw the veracity of this description when Ladda performed a Burmese dance for us in Bangkok. Television and movie theaters are slow in coming to Burma, and traveling dance groups provide welcome entertainment.

Maymi took us to a shop in a private home where costumes are made-to-order for entertainers. There, hanging on a rack among other beautiful costumes, was this dream of a lavender silk chiffon dress decorated with hundreds, perhaps thousands, of sequins in pink, fuschia and lavender, with splashes of green, gold and silver. The search was over! Another 'no bargaining' dress. Maymi said later that she was ashamed of me. This simply is not done in Burma. I believe she was embarrassed by such stupid behavior. She inferred that in the future she would take over and I was to remain quiet. In my own defense, I felt the dress seemed very reasonably priced and worth settling before anyone changed their mind.

The top of the costume is wired at the hipline to create bird-like wings. The wire is covered with lavender lace. The sleeves are long. The entire sheer, jacket-like top is embroidered with deeper lavender sequins. A vestee covers the front neck opening, and a small, stiff collar covered with sequins in the designs and colors of the skirt goes around the neck and down nearly to the waist, in two points.

The long skirt has the customary black cotton band around the waist and a wide white cotton band around the hem. It is wrapped around the body and decorated with flower and leaf sequins patterns in all of the colors mentioned above. A large, lavender net shawl is draped around the shoulders.

Fuschia and gold-colored sequins decorate the close-fitting headgear. It is made of papier-mâché and covered with gold cloth, comprising the background for the tiny flowers made of sequins. An S-shaped ornament on top has white beads dangling from it and from the rim. Purple velvet sandals were acquired in a shop in a Buddhist temple, completing a dazzling creation for a traditional Burmese dance. Maymi handled the purchase of the sandals.

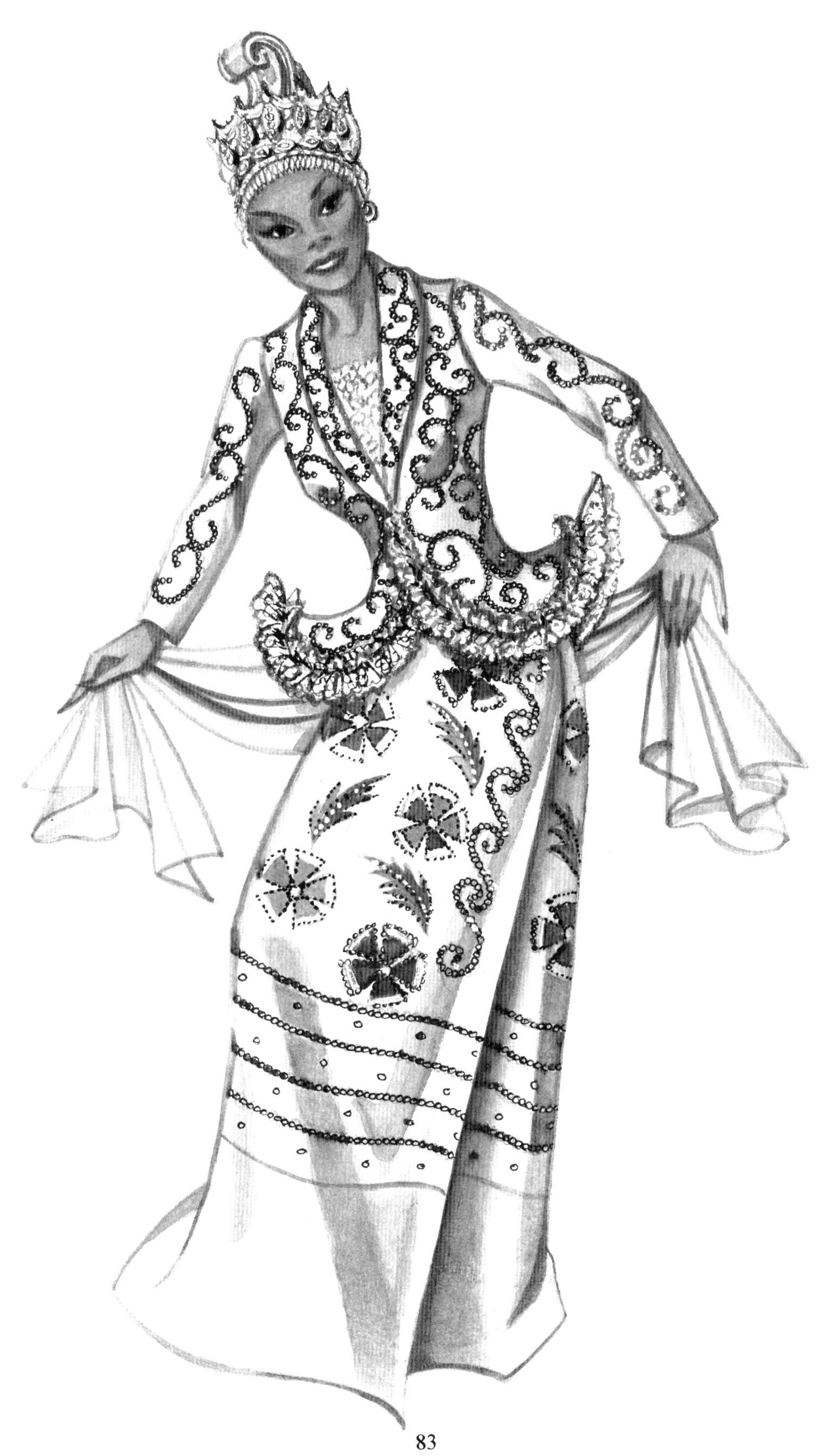

The cares that infest the day

Shall fold their tents like the Arabs

And silently steal away.

Henry Wadsworth Longfellow

Chapter Five

Lands of Muhammad

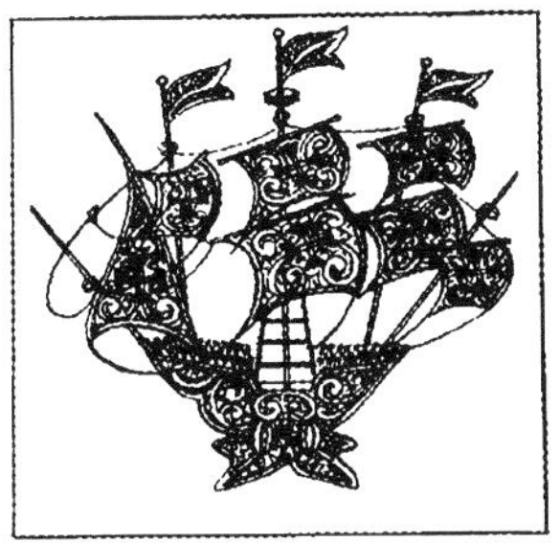

Egypt
Saudi Arabia
Afghanistan
Pakistan

Islam and Ethnic Dress

Throughout history, religion has affected the dress of its followers, and the religion of Islam is commonly believed to have influenced the attire of its women. Since in the collection there are 13 costumes from nine countries whose populations are almost 100 percent Muslim, a limited discussion of this religion and some opinions of its followers should result in a better understanding of the extent of this influence.

Islam is the religion of the Muslims. It was founded in the seventh century by the prophet Muhammad, who was born in 570 A.D., in Mecca, now Saudi Arabia. He was also the founder of the Arab empire and the initiator of religious, social and cultural development. The Kur'an, or Koran, is the holy book of Islam, as revealed to Muhammad.

It is estimated that there are over one billion Muslims in the world today. They are called either Muslims or Moslems, and their prophet is properly called either Muhammad or Mohammed. There are many sects, the largest of which are the Sunnis and Shi'ites. Muslims are bound together by faith and a sense of belonging to a common community. Uncompromising monotheism is mandatory. The word Islam means 'surrender to the will of Allah.'

Wherever Islam has become dominant, the veiling and secluding of women in homes and harems has followed, with varying degrees of restriction.

We were told in Egypt that the veil had been banished in 1925, but that since the late 1970's there has been a movement by women toward more conservative dress, which includes veiling their faces. We were also given to understand that this trend is becoming popular in other countries with large Muslim populations.

In Kashmir, older women may prefer the veil, but young women customarily wear long scarves.

Although nomadic Muslim women travel through countries with strict dress codes, their lifestyle necessitates more freedom than is allowed women with sedentary habits. Large shawls are customary.

Muslim society in Indonesia is matrilineal, with inheritance descending through the female line. There is little veiling on these islands. Also, literacy rates are much higher in Indonesia than in other predominantly Muslim countries, since education for their girls is considered as important as it is for their boys.

Saudi Arabia demands that women conform to rigid dress codes when in public. The hair, face and body must be covered.

In 1991 Albert Hourani wrote in *A History of the Arab Peoples* that not only was the veil less common in Morocco, but that other forms of segregation of men and women were disappearing.

Linda Donley, on loan to the Lamu Museum from the Smithsonian, wrote in a letter enclosed with the costume she sent from Lamu, "Before 1900 women either stayed indoors all their lives or went out in groups of ten or more under a tent-like veil called a 'sharr.' Then the bui-bui was introduced from Persia. Women believe in covering themselves so as to not show their shape and thus tempt men into sinful ways."

Our guide at the Khyber Pass told us that the clothing of the peasant woman of Afghanistan today is exactly like it has been for hundreds of years. Since we were unable to go to that country, but are in possession of an example of their ethnic dress, the Afghan Embassy in the U.S. assisted us in finding a source of information on their present-day dress. Mr. Ghulam Kosham, secretary of the Afghanistan Cultural Society of Hayward, California, was recommended. In a letter he explained that changes are taking place in Afghanistan. He wrote, "Our Holy Kur'an has not imposed the veil for Muslim women . . . Our veil is tradition, sometimes even a tradition copied from the West, but a large scarf to cover the hair and neck is advisable . . . It is allowable to leave the hands and feet uncovered . . . Islamic teaching never, never said to cover the face."

A Pakistani government official who spoke to our group in Pakistan said, "Our tradition holds that women are the honor of our families. To safeguard their honor, a family keeps a woman in 'purdah' (the veiling of the face), behind four walls and behind the veil." He also told us that the Koran allows four wives, but that the husband must treat them equally.

Our guides in predominantly Muslim countries have mentioned this, adding with a smile that few men take advantage of this opportunity today, because one wife is about all they can handle. The inability of a woman to bear a child is the usual reason for acquiring another wife.

Benazir Bhutto, the current prime minister of Pakistan, is the first woman ever to lead a Muslim nation. She graduated from Harvard University and attended Oxford University in London. When in public she wears a silk scarf draped over her hair and around her face, but her lovely face is not covered. In her 1989 autobiography, *Daughter of Destiny,* she wrote:

> *"My father was determined to bring his country - and his children - into the 20th century. 'Will the children marry into the family?' I overheard my mother ask my father one day. I held my breath for his answer. 'I don't want the boys to marry their cousins and leave them behind our compound walls any more than I want my daughters buried alive behind some other relative's compound walls,' he said to my great relief. 'Let them finish their educations first. Then they can decide what to do with their lives.'*

> *"His reaction was just as welcome the day my mother covered me in a 'burqa' for the first time. We had been on the train from Karachi to Larkana when my mother took a black, gauzy cloth out of her pocketbook and draped it over me. 'You are no longer a child,' she told me with a tinge of regret. As she performed this age-old rite of passage for the daughters of conservative land-owning families, I passed from childhood into the world of the adult. But what a disappointing world it turned out to be. The colors of the sky, the grass, the flowers were gone, muted and grayish. Everything was blurred by the pattern over my eyes. As I got off the train, the fabric which covered me from head to toe made it difficult to walk. Shut off from whatever breeze there might be, the sweat began to pour down my face.*

> *"'Pinkie wore her burqa for the first time today,' my mother told my father when we reached Al-Murtaza. There was a long pause. 'She doesn't need to wear it,' my father finally said. 'The Prophet himself said that the best veil is the veil behind the eyes. Let her be judged by her character and her mind, not her clothing.' And I became the first Bhutto woman to be released from a life spent in perpetual twilight."*

It is evident that the veiling and secluding of women in Muslim countries is due to governmental and family authority and in adherence to local custom. It is not the result of religious doctrine, either as taught by Muhammad or found in the Koran. However, some cultures in which men have had complete domination over women for centuries are resistant to change.

I met a traveler from an antique land
Who said: "Two vast and trunkless legs of stone
Stand in the desert . . . Near them, on the sand,
Half sunk, a shattered visage lies, whose frown,
And wrinkled lip, and sneer of cold command,
Tell that its sculptor well those passions read."

"My name is Ozymandias, king of kings:
Look on my works, yet Mighty, and despair!"
Nothing beside remains. Round the decay
Of that colossal wreck, boundless and bare,
The lone and level sands stretch far away.

Percy Bysshe Shelley

The Arab Republic of Egypt

Egypt is located in the northeast corner of Africa, and is about the size of Texas, Oklahoma and Arkansas combined, with a population of two and one-half times that of all three of those states. The capital city is Cairo, the currency is the Egyptian pound, the literacy rate is 44 percent and the people are 94 percent Sunni Muslim.

Most of the people live in the Nile River Valley, which stretches for 550 miles. The rest of the area is barren and desolate. Egyptians call their country the 'Mother of the World.' Archeological records of Egypt date back to 4000 B.C. Around 3200 B.C., there was a unified kingdom in which rulers and priests built a culture based on fertile soil, serfdom and the annual flooding of the Nile. In 341 B.C., the Persians won control of the country, as did the Greeks, Romans, Byzantines, Arabs and British in turn.

Cairo is the largest city in Africa, with more than 10 million people. Traffic is such that the first part of a car to wear out is the horn. It is needed to get through the goats, camels, donkeys and carts, taxis, buses, trucks, British right-hand and American left-hand drivers. The housing shortage is so acute that if the family of someone who died has been able to build a tomb of any size, it may be necessary to live in it. We saw many families living in cemeteries.

We stayed in a beautiful hotel in Giza, originally called al-Jizah, southwest of Cairo, within walking distance of the pyramids of Khufu, Khafre and Mankaure. Khufu is still considered one of the largest buildings ever built. There are many other pyramids, especially along a 50-mile stretch of the west bank of the Nile just south of Cairo. The consensus of most scholars is that the pyramids were built as burial places for Egyptian rulers in order to bring about a closer union between the ruler and the afterworld. Of the original Seven Wonders of the World, only the pyramids are still in a recognizable state. If the Arabs had not stripped them of their hard polished casing stones they would look new. It is believed that they will last for a hundred thousand years.

Near the pyramids is the Great Sphinx, an imposing figure of a creature with the facial features of King Khafre and the body of a lion. It was carved out of a single block of stone. We attended a dramatic light and sound show one evening in the shadow of the pyramids, and enjoyed it immensely. It was wise to have a sweater along, as the desert can be very cold when the sun goes down.

One afternoon I set out alone to look for some shoes to match a costume. A group of five pre-teen boys followed me, trying to sell some uninteresting artifacts. We bantered a bit. It was fun for a while, until they started pushing to make a sale and were informed that I had no money with me. I knew better than to carry a purse. Several of them tried to lift my blouse, looking for a money belt, and that is exactly where my air tickets, passport and credit cards were. Before there was time to become annoyed enough to call for help, a man wearing a long, loose 'galabia' and a headscarf (kaffiyeh), held in place with a cord (agal), appeared suddenly. "Are these children bothering you?" he asked. I told him that they were beginning to, but that it was my fault as I was encouraging them by teasing. He let them go with a lecture in Arabic, bowed politely to me and left. After finding the shoes I wanted to purchase and returning to the hotel, I saw the same man at the lobby door. Again, he bowed and walked away. At dinner our tour guide explained that these men are hired to keep an eye on tourists, in order to avoid unpleasant incidents. That was why not one of those brazen camel drivers came near . . . I was off limits!

The Nile

Called the 'Father of Rivers,' the Nile is the longest river in the world. The White Nile, whose source is in Lake Albert, forms part of the border between Uganda and Zaire and joins the Blue Nile in Khartoum, flowing jointly over 4,000 miles to the Mediterranean Sea. It flows from south to north, which is unusual for great rivers. The early Egyptians and Greeks found this unexplainable. Also, not understanding the location of the Nile's source, they developed a belief that the waters rushing down in summer were the tears of the goddess Isis weeping for Osiris, the god of fertility, her dead love. Great feasting and rejoicing took place in the fall when the waters sank into the rich fields that appeared. Each year an elaborately dressed young virgin was thrown into the waters to be the bride of the river god.

Egyptian life centers on this river, and the economy of the country depends on its annual floods, which provide life support for over 50 million people. The treasures of the world also came up this waterway on ships from faraway lands.

We sailed down the Nile on a riverboat, or more correctly, we sailed up the Nile about 300 miles to Luxor. This was like a trip into past centuries. Luxor occupies the southern half of what used to be Thebes. Karnak occupies the other half, where we visited magnificent ruins dating back to 2000 B.C. In the temple of Karnak is a hall of pillars in which enormous 78-foot columns raise the central nave above the 140 slightly lower pillars which form several lateral aisles. The opening is placed so that the sun's rays shine into the temple from wherever the sun is in the sky.

Luxor is a favorite city for travelers, who can also visit the fabled Valleys of the Tombs of the Kings and the Queens and the tomb of Tutankhamen, across the river.

Bedouin Woman's Ethnic Dress

The Bedouins are Arabic-speaking nomadic tribes, who roam the deserts of the Middle East in search of water and pasture for their herds. Although these people constitute only 10 percent of the population, they utilize almost nine-tenths of the land area of the Middle East.

There are cattle, sheep, horse and goat nomads, but the camel tribes rate highest on the Bedouin social scale. No member of a camel tribe would ever demean herself or himself by marrying into a tribe of lesser rank. Bedouins live in long, low, black tents made of goat hair. Men and women live in separate sides of the tents, and the male side is always away from the wind. When a girl marries she goes to live with her husband's family.

This dress was found in Luxor and purchased from a Bedouin. Although it is carelessly made, the cross-stitching embroidery is lavish and beautiful. The fabric is a heavy black cotton and the garment is long with three-quarter-length sleeves. Bands of cross-stitching in red, yellow and white decorate the neck, and there is a wide band across the bodice, down each sleeve and covering the skirt below the waistline. A three-yard-long black shawl has a long silky fringe. It is draped across the face to show that our Bedouin lady is modest and not seeking the glances of men. It also provides protection from the sandstorms of the desert.

With a herd of gold-colored camels crossing the front panel of the skirt, there can be little doubt that the original owner of this dress was a member of that loftiest of social classes, a camel tribe.

Two Bedouin adages may aid understanding of the culture of these tribes:

"A man must do three things quickly . . . bury the dead, serve a guest and marry off a daughter, the sooner the better."

"Pampering a girl will disgrace thee, pampering a boy will make thee rich."

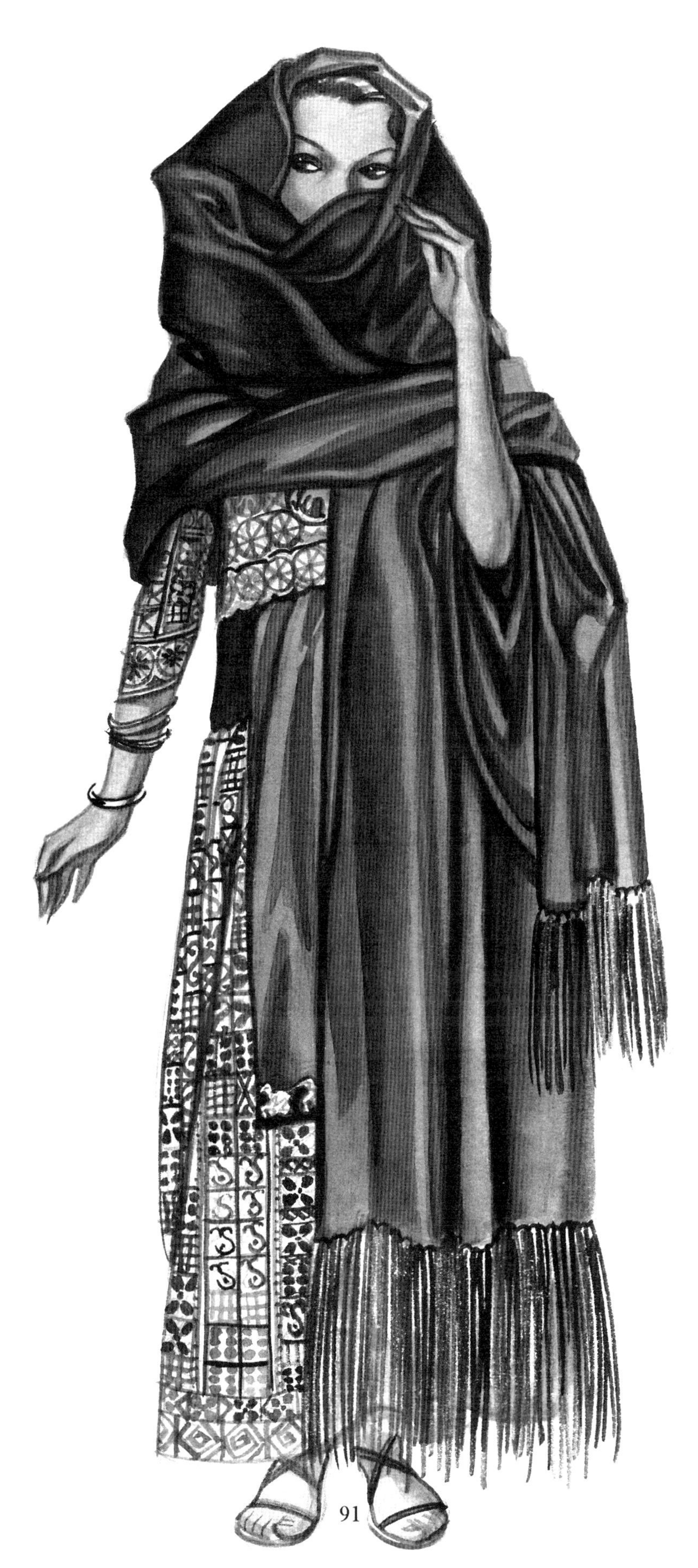

Saad Al-Ali

The Arab name for the Aswan High Dam is Saad Al-Ali. It is a rock-fill dam across the Nile River, four miles south of Aswan. This dam, including the moving of the complex of temples of Abu Simbel to higher ground, was one of the world's great engineering feats. It was completed in 1970, impounding Lake Nasser for 200 miles in Egypt and 100 miles in Sudan. As the waters rose, the temples as well as 90,000 fellahin (peasants) and Sudanese nubian nomads were relocated. Fifty thousand Egyptians were transported to the Kawn Umbu Valley, 30 miles north of Aswan, to form a new agricultural zone. Egypt received funds from 30 countries to engineer this awesome project. The city of Aswan is the capital of the governate of Aswan. It is now a popular resort area and commercial center.

A flight across Lake Nasser brings one to the new location of the sandstone cliffs of the temples of Ramses II. Four massive statues, two on each side, are placed at the entrance of the main temple. Two of the statues have small figures of Ramses' queen, Nefetari, and their children, at their feet.

Graffiti is not usually considered to be valuable to historical data, but that of Greek mercenaries in the sixth century B.C., carved on these statues, provided significant evidence of the beginnings of the alphabet.

It is believed by many scholars that the temples of Abu Simbel were built in the time of Moses, who delivered his people from Egyptian slavery. This coincides with the time in Biblical history when Egypt ordered death to all newborn Hebrew males. Moses' parents set their baby afloat in a basket woven from papyrus reeds strengthened with pitch. He was found by the daughter of the Pharaoh and raised in the court of Egypt.

Woman's Galabia

This woman's costume is an example of the movement by young women toward more traditional, religious-oriented dress. The galabia is black, has long sleeves and is floor length. The fabric is cotton with black embroidery decorating the front panel of the dress. A white wool knit cap is worn under a shawl, which comes down over the shoulders. The cap and shawl are knit in an attractive loose stitch. The galabia was found in Aswan and the cap and shawl are from Luxor.

The flat, green leather shoes have a painting on the toes of a horse and chariot with a driver aiming a drawn bow and arrow. The necklace has a large gold head of Tutankhamen on green enamel bordered with silver. Both the shoes and the necklace came from shops near the pyramids at Giza.

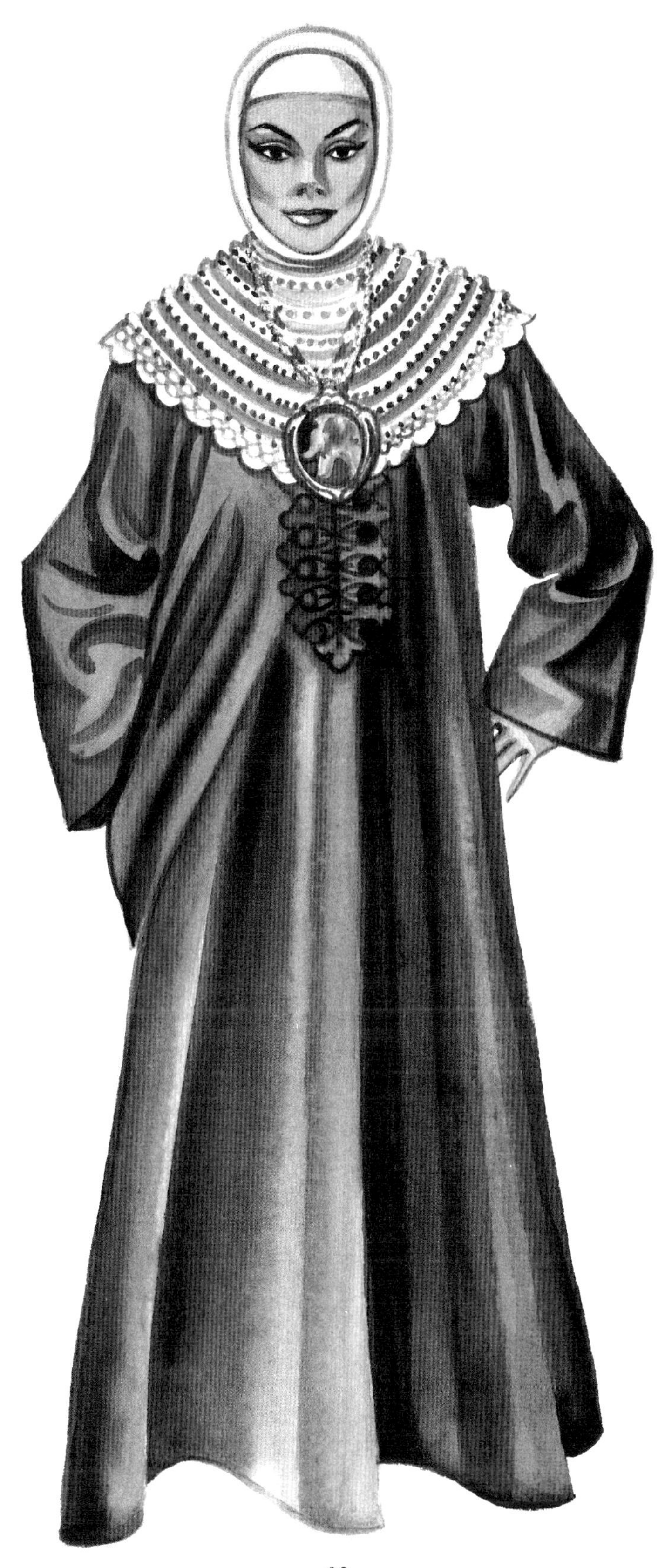

Then at a wave of her sunny hand
The dancing-girls of Samarcand
Glide in like shapes from fairy-land,
Making a sudden mist in air
Of fleecy veils and floating hair
And white arms lifted. Orient blood
Runs in their veins, shines in their eyes.
And there is this Eastern Paradise,
Filled with the breath of sandal-wood,
And Khoten musk, and aloes and myrrh,
Sits Rose-in-Bloom on a silk divan,
Sipping the wines of Astrakhan;
And her Arab lover sits with her.
That's when the Sultan Shah-Zaman
Goes to the city of Ispahan.

Thomas Bailey Aldrich

Kingdom of Saudi Arabia

Saudi Arabia is approximately one-third the size of the U.S., with a population of around 18 million. It occupies most of the Arabian Peninsula in the Middle East. The highlands in the west reach 9,000 feet in altitude, and are a barren, arid desert, sloping to the Persian Gulf. The capital is Riyadh, and the monetary unit the riyal. The language is Arabic, the religion is 100 percent Muslim, and literacy is 62 percent. The government is a monarchy, with a council of ministers. There is no constitution and no parliament and the law of the land is the Islamic code.

Arabia was united in the early seventh century by Muhammad. His successors conquered the entire Near East and North Africa, bringing Islam and the Arabic language, but Arabia itself soon returned to its former status, a country of Bedouin tribes.

Ibn Saud was born around 1880 to a family who controlled much of central Arabia. While he was still an infant his family was driven out by rivals and forced to live as penniless exiles in Kuwait. At the age of 21 he set out with a small fighting force and in two years reconquered half of Central Arabia. He fought the Turks for nearly 12 years, vanquishing them and gaining territory. In 1932 he created the Kingdom of Saudi Arabia and became king.

The Saudi family runs the country. By 1992 there were 4,000 male members of the ruling house of Saud. This is the only country ever named for a family. The official title of the king is 'Custodian of Holy Places.' The two holy cities are Mecca, the birthplace of Muhammad, and Medina, the site of his tomb. Mecca is the foremost sacred city of the Muslim world. Every Muslim is encouraged to make a pilgrimage to Mecca once in his lifetime. This pilgrimage is the fifth in the Five Pillars of Islam, and must begin on the seventh day and end on the tenth day of the last month of the Muslim year. Until 1930, when oil was discovered, a large source of the country's income was from these pilgrimages. The country was transformed by the sudden, enormous wealth.

During our travels we have often seen pilgrims traveling to their holy cities. They were always recognizable because of the dress of the women. The largest group we observed was gathered in the airport in Johannesburg, South Africa. The evening paper verified that 10,000 Muslims of East Indian descent were making a pilgrimage to Mecca.

Dancing Dress of Saudi Arabia

It is very difficult for women to obtain visas to visit Saudi Arabia, unless accompanied by a man. Four of us, including two travel agent friends, tried for months to get visas, and finally gave up. Jo and Grace were widows, Claudia was unmarried, and my husband absolutely refused to go on a shopping trip with four women.

When Pam Franklin of International Media Services of Colorado Springs said she would find an example of Saudi ethnic dress while she was in that country on business, we were delighted. The company had contracted to film the Saudi Arabian Navy. Pam was a photographer and would be accompanied by men. When she discovered that she could not go shopping by herself, probably because she was not veiled, an obliging friend located this 'thoob,' or dancing dress. The thoob is worn on the stage for performances at private social events, and also by women dancing privately for their husbands. Tradition has it that the wife will then conceive, hopefully a son!

This long, flowing silk chiffon gown is a deep royal blue, lavishly trimmed with gold braid and sequins. There is a wide band with two narrow bands of gold braid hand-stitched down the front of the gown to a large gold medallion just above the hem. On the back there are two bands of braid from the shoulder to the hem. Gold medallion circles, two inches in diameter, surrounded by gold sequins, are hand-sewn all over the thoob. The neckline, hem and full, flowing sleeves are all edged with gold braid. The hair is worn loose, and the dancer may or may not be barefoot.

We are very grateful to Pam of IMS for making it possible to add this glamorous Saudi dancing dress to the collection. Customs papers required to get this costume out of the country seemed excessive. No other country, with the exception of Lamu, has required even one document for this purpose. Saudi regulations are very rigid, and this rigidity extends to the out-of-doors dress of the women. Her hair, face and body must be completely covered when she can be seen by men other than those in her own family.

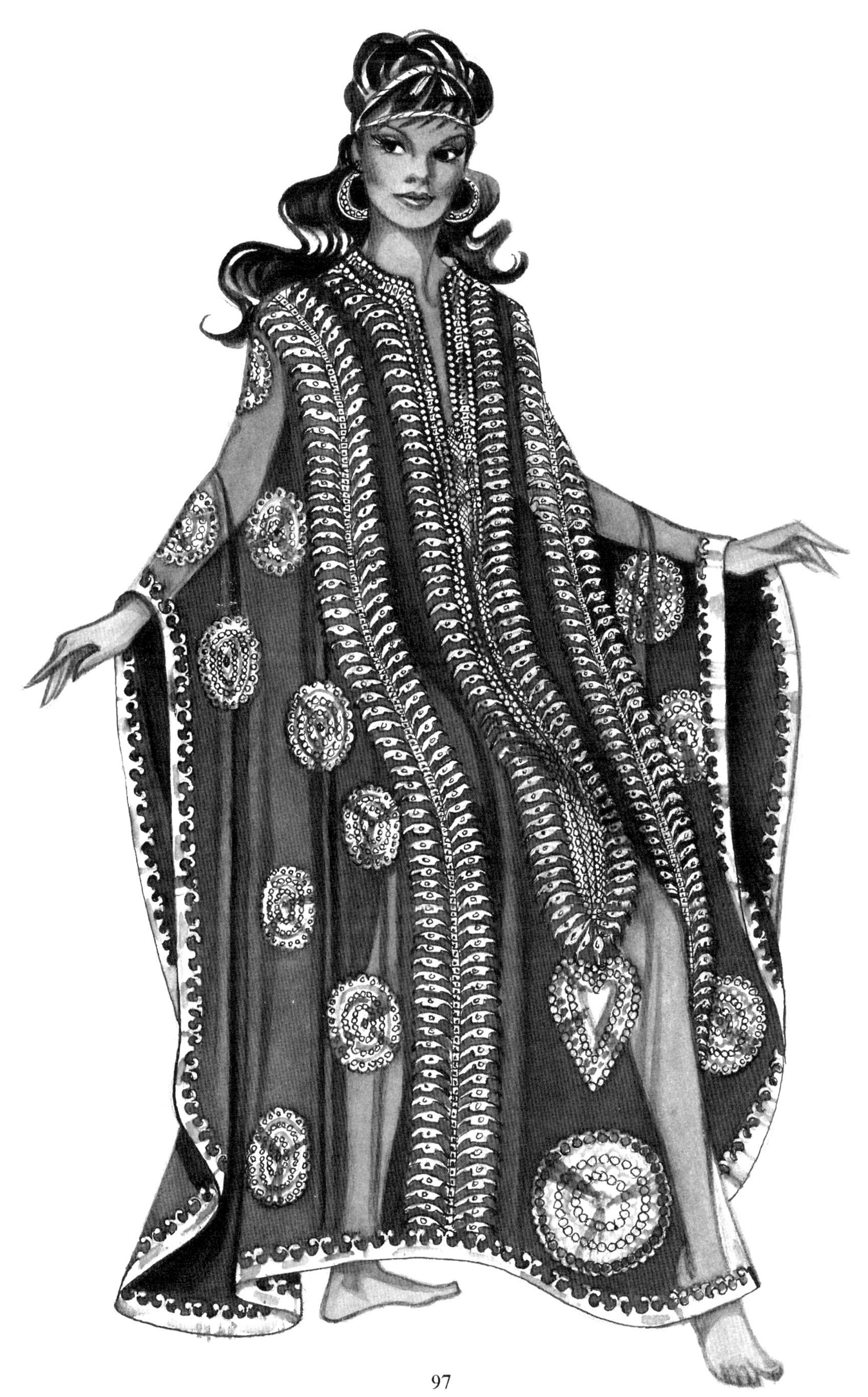

Republic of Afghanistan

Afghanistan is a landlocked, mountainous country between Soviet Central Asia, Iran and Pakistan. It is about the size of Texas, with almost the same population. The capital is Kabul, and the currency is the afghani. The religion is Muslim, and literacy is 29 percent. Approximately 88 percent of the adults have had no formal education.

The government, which is now in transition, was backed by Soviet force until very recently. There is now a president, who is head of state. Historically, foreign empires alternated rule with local emirs until the 18th century, when a unified kingdom was established. In 1973 a military coup ushered in a republic. Then in 1979 the Soviets began an airlift into Kabul, resulting in a coup that brought in a pro-Soviet leader. There was fighting for nine years, when as many as 100,000 Soviet troops fought Afghan rebels. A United Nations agreement was signed in 1988 that provided for Soviet withdrawal, with the U.S. and USSR pledged as guarantors, but this agreement was rejected by the rebels. In 1992 the Soviet-backed regime withdrew, but Islamic fundamentalists and moderates have continued to clash, with fierce fighting around Kabul.

The Chadri of Afghanistan

The 'chadri' was introduced by the Muslims in Afghanistan. When we were in Pakistan we saw this same costume being worn in the area of Peshawar and the Khyber Pass, where it is called a 'burqa.' Webbed face-covering is a distinctive feature of both the chadri and the burqa. It is possible for a woman to see out through the webbing, but impossible for anyone to see her face. Her hair is completely covered, as is the rest of her body, except for her feet.

This chadri is made of a synthetic navy fabric, decorated on a front panel with eyelet embroidery in the same dark blue color. The sides and back are accordion pleated and it is hip-length in front and floor-length in the back. It can be worn several ways, as shown.

A friend who lived in Kabul while her husband worked as an attorney for the Dupont Corporation in Afghanistan donated the costume in the drawing on the right. Under this chadri a Western-style dress is often worn, but the legs are covered. The pants are made of an off-white Chinese silk and trimmed with ivory-colored handmade lace. The high-heeled sandals are typical of those worn by well-dressed women in Kabul.

When we were invited to do a costume show benefit for the library of the University of Colorado, we recruited our models from the International Club. An attractive young Afghan student wore the chadri, showing the skirt of her dress which was worn over her trousers when she was out-of-doors. She told us that in her country, before the communist invasion, this type of chadri was often worn in Kabul over beautiful designer dresses from Paris.

Our lovely model was fascinated with the Bedouin costume and its huge shawl, and wore them with a flair. She regaled us with stories of how her brother escaped the country by joining a group of Bedouin nomads.

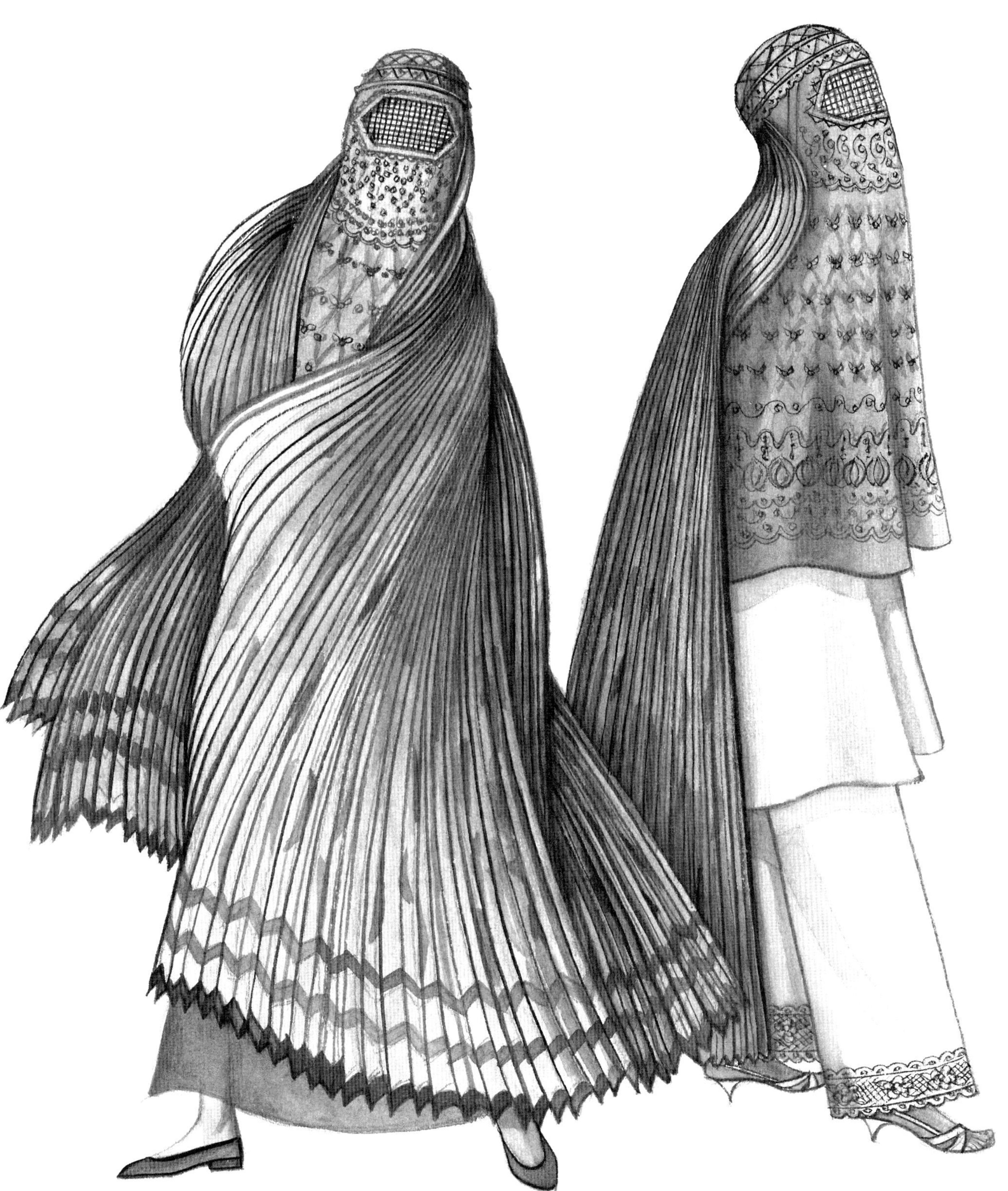

The Ballad of East and West

Oh East is East, and West is West,

and never the twain shall meet,

Till Earth and Sky stand presently

at God's great Judgment Seat;

But there is neither East nor West,

Border, nor Breed, nor Birth,

When two strong men stand face to face,

tho' they come from the ends of earth!

Rudyard Kipling

Islamic Republic of Pakistan

Pakistan lies in the western part of South Asia. It is about the size of Texas and Washington together, with a population over five times that of those two states. The capital is Islamabad, the currency is the rupee and literacy is 35 percent. The religion is 97 percent Muslim, and Islamic law has been adopted over the secular code. It is a parliamentary democracy with a president and prime minister.

The Indus River rises in the Hindu Kush and Himalayan Mountains and flows 1,000 miles through fertile valleys, emptying into the Arabian Sea. The highest mountain in Pakistan is K2, the second highest in the world, at 28,250 feet.

Present day Pakistan shares the 5,000-year history of the India-Pakistan subcontinent. From around 1500 B.C., a Hindu civilization dominated both Pakistan and India for 2,000 years.

Beginning with the Persians in the sixth century B.C., and continuing with Alexander the Great, Pakistan has been influenced by nations to the west, separating it from Indian culture. The first Arab invasion, in 712 A.D., introduced Islam. Muslims ruled most of India, yielding to British rule and a Hindu resurgence. When the British withdrew in 1947, Pakistan was divided into two sections, West Pakistan and East Pakistan. These sections were on either side of India, nearly 1,000 miles apart. India helped the Easterners gain independence as the nation of Bangladesh. After full scale war between India and Pakistan, a pact was signed in 1972. Troops were withdrawn and an agreement was made to seek peaceful solutions to their problems.

Zulfikar ali Bhutto became president, but was convicted of complicity in a political murder and executed in 1979. Bhutto's daughter, Benazir, returned from exile in Europe in 1986 and was elected prime minister, after President Zia was killed in a plane explosion. She is the first woman to lead a Muslim nation. However, she, too, was accused of corruption by the president and dismissed, but was again elected to power in 1993.

People and Places of Pakistan

Our introduction to Pakistan was a very intimate relationship with the Lahore Airport. The plane from Nepal was late, very late. The rest of our group was elephant-riding in Nepal, and we were meeting them at this airport to fly to Islamabad. Everyone in that group was a member of the Denver Botanical Gardens, except us. We were there because my husband and I had met the travel agent and guide on a Greek cruise, enjoyed his company and kept in touch. My husband decided against this trip and Jo agreed to go in his place. To us, even the name Pakistan, which in the Urdu language means 'Land of the Pure,' was exciting. We waited, and waited. Every half hour, for eight hours, we were told the plane was due. This is a bad habit lots of airlines have.

When the plane arrived it discharged 26 exhausted-looking passengers, most of whom were having trouble getting around because of too much use of unused muscles. When the announcement was made that the plane was overbooked and three people were needed to be 'kind enough' to ride to Islamabad by car, a distance of 200 miles, we decided to be kind enough. We weren't as tired as that bunch looked, so Jo and I, and a younger woman who had survived the elephant safari in good shape, volunteered. It was a good decision.

Lahore at dusk was a dream city, clean, with streets shining as the lights came on, outlining ornate monuments, tombs, Mughal-style buildings and mosques of Oriental architecture. All were seen through the flowering trees of April that lined the roads. Lahore seemed like a Persian fantasy. We hadn't been to Persia (Iran) except for the Teheran airport, where we weren't allowed off the plane, but we had read *A Thousand and One Nights,* and this was it! All of the trucks passing us were gaily decorated in bright colors and intricate designs. Every truck driver in Pakistan must have at least one artist in his family. The prospect of spending three days in Lahore before leaving Pakistan at tour's end delighted us, especially when we would visit, with botanically knowledgeable companions, that magnificent garden of all gardens, the Shalimar.

As we left the city, we were amused by road signs in Urdu and English, such as "No Overtaking" and "Squeeze Left," and they meant it! Our Pakistani driver gave us a language lesson. A multi-purpose greeting is "Al Salaam Alikomm," meaning 'Peace be with you.' If that doesn't fit, and one is in a spot that requires an answer, just a smile, a shrug and "Inshallah," meaning 'God willing,' will probably do the job. And with "Khuda Hafiz" for 'goodbye,' we felt prepared for any event and slept the rest of the way to Islamabad.

Islamabad to the Khyber Pass

Poppies, poppies, poppies, miles of them, are beautiful to look at, but deadly. These are opium poppies, used to make heroin and that useful painkiller, morphine.

Few passes have had the strategic importance and historic associations of the Khyber Pass that links Peshawar, Pakistan and Kabul, Afghanistan. Through it have passed Persians, Greeks, Mughals and Afghans. It was crucial to British control of the Afghan border. The summit of the pass is almost 3,600 feet in altitude, and there are three roads: the top one is the Mughal road, built in the 14th century; the middle road is the ancient one, built in 327 B.C.; and the bottom road is the one the British built in 1929.

The Landi Kotal, at the high point of the pass, is an important market center. Much of the merchandise is brought in by camels and mules. This was where we saw some of the women of Pakistan, wearing pastel-colored burqas, and webbed face-screens, buying fashionable Italian shoes at an outdoor shop.

At a compound near the pass we were introduced to all the men who lived there, but the only female we saw was a three-year-old girl, who was evidently the favorite of someone important. She was even allowed to have her picture taken with the men. We knew women lived in the compound, because we were shown their dining room. We were told that the women of western Pakistan are very traditional and shy.

Getting into Gilgit was not easy, and getting out turned out to be even more difficult. The weather had to be just right, so that a small plane could wend its way around high mountain peaks.

The very first game of polo was played here, imported by the British, we were told. The game we saw was the most exciting game of any kind that we had ever witnessed. A Scottish marching bagpipe band piped the players onto the field, but that was the end of ceremony and civility. The contestants aimed not just at the ball, but at each other, and often connected. It was rough and bloody. We had seen bullfights in Mexico and

Valencia, Spain, and had to admit that these horses had almost as bad a time as those bulls. However, an article in *The Wall Street Journal* of September 7, 1984, "Remote Pakistan is Land of . . . Pure Polo," convinced us that Gilgit polo was a mild version of the real sport.

In that article a prince of Hunza, the Rajah Ali Ahmed Jan, was quoted: "Polo is the traditional sport of these people and particularly of their mirs and rajahs. Our polo is pure polo. Polo without rules. We play 30 minutes with no stops and no change of horses. You change horses only if yours dies. In our polo, the purpose is to crash each other. In our polo, killing is not a crime. Half of my family has died playing polo . . . The British added rules. They tried to spoil our polo."

The mountain valley of Hunza is just 30 miles south of the China border. It is a tiny principality that, until 10 years ago, was ruled by mirs, hereditary monarchs that were ancestors of Rajah Ali. In the 13th and 14th centuries it was the meeting place of all trans-Asiatic caravan routes linking it to Europe via Iran and Turkey. The 'caravanserais,' or resting places, provided water, lodging, space and protection, not only for the travelers, but for 300 to 400 camels as well.

On a cold morning in spring, we rode in jeeps to Hunza. Flowering apricot trees transformed the valley into scenery worthy of an artist's brush. The wobbling passage across the river on a wooden suspension bridge was a thing of wonder, once we were safely across and opened our eyes. The inscription on the swinging bridge, stating it was built in 1927 by Bengal miners of the Indian army, certainly didn't add to our confidence.

Hunza is famed for the longevity of its people. Two reasons are given for this phenomenon, gold dust in the drinking water and a diet with lots of apricots and their powdered seeds. However, our consensus of opinion was that our male relatives of the same age back home looked younger. The old women were invisible, except for those we saw from the road, playing with their grandchildren on the flat roofs of their houses.

The time came to say farewell to Gilgit, but we couldn't leave! All airports were closed! A rock slide had blocked the single road leading to the outside world, and President Zia had caused Zulfikar Ali Bhutto to be hanged, and riots were anticipated. These things happening on the same day were not only a troubling coincidence, but we were trapped, and all supplies were cut off.

The hospitality of the hotel staff was remarkable, and they were in far better humor than we were. Every day we could not leave cut a day from our stay in Lahore. Our diet was limited, but we were served lots of delicious chocolate-covered custard, a specialty of the house.

On the third day, our plane came just in time to make it to Lahore to meet our ride to Amritsar, India. Looking back, except for our disappointment at missing having 26 botanists take us around the famed Shalimar Gardens, our only discomfort had been the ice-cold showers we had to endure. We had plenty of excitement in Pakistan and were treated superbly, and Jo and I still love chocolate-covered custard.

Our entire party agreed that this small Pakistani town of Gilgit, with its backdrop of 25,500-foot snowcapped Mt. Rakaposhi, would never be forgotten.

Khameez, Shalwar and Duppata of Pakistan

In western Pakistan and Afghanistan the 'khameez,' or tunic, and 'shalwar,' wide-topped trousers with a drawstring at the waist, are usually worn under burqas with webbed face coverings. In East Pakistan they are often worn with the 'dupatta,' or large shawl, draped around the head and neck.

This khameez and shalwar are of a medium blue, silky synthetic fabric. The front of the khameez, the bands around the wrists and the bottoms of the legs of the shalwar are embroidered in gold thread, which holds tiny mirrors in place. The dupatta is red chiffon and is worn around the hat, or 'gooshiiski farczin,' and across the lower part of the woman's face and neck. The skull-cap type of hat is solidly cross-stitched by hand in red, green and yellow yarn.

Typical jewelry for this costume consists of two necklaces with plastic and thread beads, the latter wrapped with gold thread. A tassel hangs from the center of each necklace.

We followed the Asian Highway that stretches from London to Singapore, through the Malakand Pass of the Hindu Kush Mountains in the Northwest Frontier Province. There, on a precarious turn, our bus narrowly missed a collision with a truck that would have hurled us hundreds of feet down a mountainside. When we reached a safe spot the driver pulled over, calming himself for the remainder of the journey. We were lucky, and happy, to arrive in Saidu Shariff, the capital of Swat, in one piece.

And there, not far from Churchill's Pickett, where Winston Churchill was based as a young captain in Britain's army, we found a shop in the upper story of a home that was the fulfillment of this costume-searcher's dream. It was there we found this modern version of a khameez and shalwar. The colorful gooshiiski farczin and dupatta are from Gilgit.

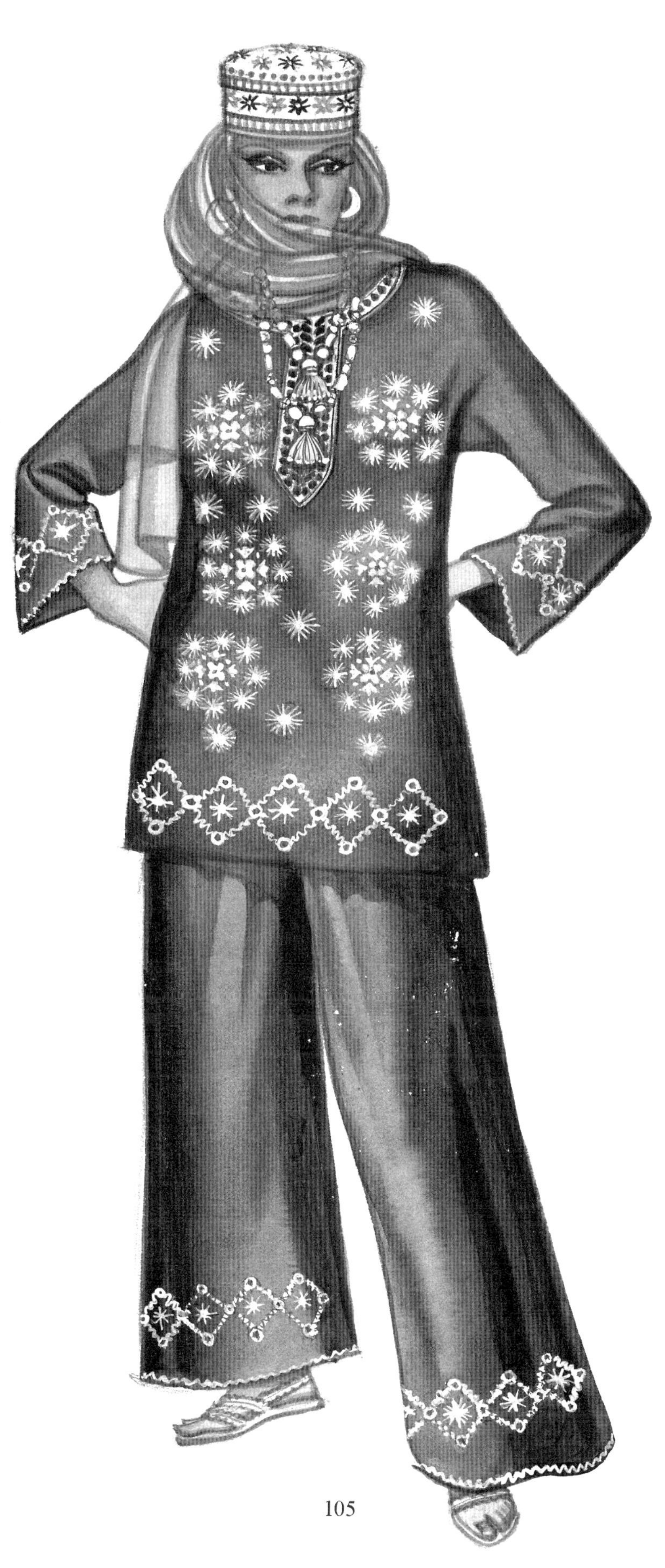

In Xanadu did Kubla Khan
A stately pleasure-dome decree:
Where Alph, the sacred river, ran
Through caverns measureless to man
Down to the sunless sea.
So twice five miles of fertile ground
With walls and towers were girdled round:
And there were gardens bright with sinuous rills,
Where blossomed many an incense-bearing tree;
And here were forests ancient as the hills,
Enfolding sunny spots of greenery.

Samuel Taylor Coleridge

Chapter Six

Developing Giants

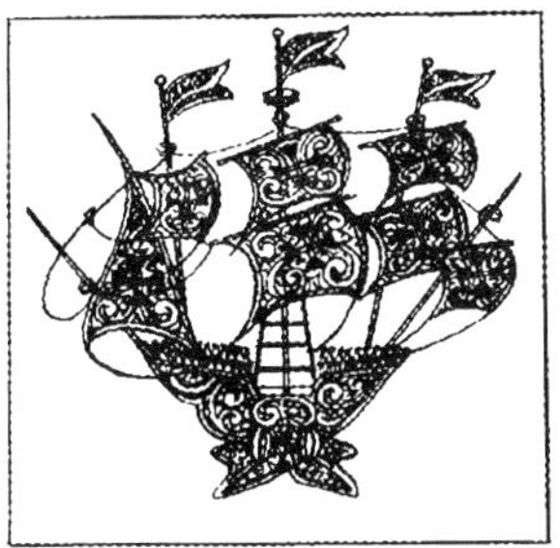

India
China

Be cautious about the man who sets himself as an expert on India.

It is too vast geographically,

its history is too complex,

its regional variations too many,

and all of the rules are riddled with exceptions.

India's Department of Tourism

Republic of India

India is one-third the size of the United States, with as many people as live in all of South America, Central America, North America and Canada combined. It occupies most of the Indian subcontinent in southern Asia. The capital is New Delhi, the monetary unit is the rupee and literacy is 48 percent. The government is a federal republic.

The civilization of India spans at least 5,000 years. Richly carved temples, the Taj Mahal and the famous Ajanta Caves are among the relics of the past. The caves are famous for their wall paintings, in temples hollowed out of granite cliffs. Work on these caves began in the first century B.C., depicting stories of Buddhist legends and gods.

Muslim invaders made inroads in the eighth century, and from 1526 to 1857 Mughal emperors ruled large parts of India. Britain, through the East India Company, gained control of most of India, and the British parliament assumed political guidance. The rule of rajahs was discouraged after 1828. Under Mahatma Gandhi, self-rule, non-violence and the abolition of untouchability were advocated. He worked for the emancipation of women. He is considered to be the father of his country. Nationalism grew, and in 1950 India became a democratic republic.

India is not just a country. It is the result of thousands of years of history. Its modern life is deeply embedded in its ancient past, showing an amazing continuity. A visitor to this country feels that he is living in several centuries at once. A computer technician on his way to work may have to wait for a camel or water buffalo to cross the road. He may find himself behind a broken-down jeep being pulled by a team of oxen, and he may pass barefoot women carrying their shoes in a bundle on their heads as they wend their way toward the modern factories where they are employed.

Untouchability in any form is now a penal offense. Divorce provisions have been added to the laws of Hindu society, and women no longer throw themselves on their husband's funeral pyres. Child marriages have been banned.

Mystery, excitement, color, poverty and grandeur . . . whatever emotion one feels about India, it is never indifference. This country has fired the imagination of many adventurers throughout history. The whole of Southeast Asia received much of its cultural tradition from India. Three thousand years ago Indian artifacts traveled the Old Silk Road to China and Central Asia. Exquisite ivories, muslins, dyed cottons and carved wooden beams were carried by Indian ships to the court of Israel's King Solomon.

By the time of Christ, Indian art had reached a high level. The premier craft is handloom weaving, and the sari is the main product. A fine cotton cloth known as madras became famous because an entire sari could be drawn through a wedding ring. This weaving was so skilled that traders came from all over the world for these products, especially silk and Bengal muslin. Handlooms are still important in the manufacture of Indian textiles which, as a commercial product, ranks second in importance only to agriculture.

Jewelry-making profits from the fact that Indian women love to wear it. Heavy tribal jewelry from Gumarat, Rajastan and Orissa is famous, and elegant costume jewelry in modern designs is made in Delhi, Bombay and Jaipur.

A Complicated Crossing

India and Pakistan comprise a large area south of the Himalayas. The division of India into two countries was due to centuries of Mughal and British rule and friction between Muslim and Hindu factions. By the time Britain withdrew after World War II, India had been partitioned into dominions of Hindu India and Muslim Pakistan. After a war in 1971 between the two countries, the assassinations of two Indian prime ministers and many riots, an uneasy peace was achieved. In addition to these problems, Mrs. Indira Gandhi had become prime minister for the second time but was killed by her Sikh bodyguards in 1984. The assassination was in retaliation for a government siege of the Golden Temple, the Holy Shrine of the Sikhs.

When we crossed the Pakistan border into Amritsar, India, we were made to feel like criminals. No one except our group was crossing at this time, so the Sikh border guards had plenty of time to work us over. We filled out so many forms that the process took five hours.

Our costume collecting was progressing satisfactorily, with one exception. A turban purchased in New Delhi along with the snake charmer's outfit had come apart. We later learned that the best way to preserve the complicated wrapping was to pin it in place and then spray it heavily with starch. But it was too late, as the damage was done.

Sikhs are very impressive people, with their fierce-looking black beards and magnificently wrapped turbans, into which they fold their long hair. Sikhs never cut their hair. I determined to learn to wrap my wilted turban into one like the Sikhs wore. This might be the last chance for such a lesson.

The wondrous Golden Temple, shining in its covering of tons of gold foil, should be an excellent place to find an expert turban-wrapper. After all, this temple was the very center of the Sikh religion. We saw no women, and the serious demeanor of the men was intimidating. The security guard at our hotel, though, looked friendly, and his turban was absolutely beautiful. He told us, in quite good English, that his wife wrapped his turbans. He said she was known to be more skilled in that art than anyone in Amritsar, and he offered to take me to his home so she could give me a lesson. What a thrilling development! This was a little-known craft outside of India. I would be the best turban wrapper in my state. Although Jo wasn't really into this art, it sounded like fun, even though we would probably miss the only dinner seating our small hotel offered.

We waited at the appointed place and time for our driver and car to arrive. He came . . . on a bicycle, and not even a very large one. It had only one seat. He assured me he was a good driver and would return me to the hotel safely after the lesson. Where would I put my legs? And where would Jo sit? I turned to her for help in explaining to the driver why this wasn't a good idea and found her with her back turned to us and her face in her hands, her shoulders shaking with laughter.

Oh well, we made it to dinner, and since we weren't leaving India yet, there could still be time for a lesson . . . somewhere.

Jo gave in to the temptation of fulfilling her son's wish for a sitar from India, although she could get it home only by carrying it over her shoulder. She proclaimed herself the oldest hippy to ever go through customs in the New York airport.

Of Tigers and Classes

We went to Khajuraho, in central India. The name Khajuraho derives from the prevalence of date palms in the area. This is an historic village in the Chhatarpur district of Madhya Pradesh state. Eighty-five temples were built here between 950 and 1050 A.D. Twenty of these have survived. Built of sandstone, they are richly carved with erotic sculptures, both on the outside and inside.

After spending the morning going through the temples, a group of tourists decided to rent a small bus and drive to an old monastery which had been turned into a fort. We were told that this fort was abandoned because of the man-eating tigers in the area. It was now unused and had fallen into disrepair. Of course we didn't want to miss such an exciting chance for adventure. What a story this would make when we got home. We might even see a tiger!

We passed through dense forests of palm trees and flowering bushes. For the entire 30 miles of our drive the only inhabitants of the area that we could see were small monkeys swinging through the trees. There was no sign of human life. We knew we were in the very heart of uncivilized India.

The monastery-fort was nearly hidden by a heavy growth of bushes and was covered with climbing vines. Our bus driver was our guide, and he told us stories of the man-eating tigers who had attacked the soldiers. He was very graphic, explaining how the tigers had caught the men when they were alone and away from the fort, killing and devouring those unfortunate souls. Eventually the fort was closed and the dauntless fighting men driven away, he told us sadly.

His inference seemed to be that if we lingered in this dangerous place too long we might be inviting a similar fate. Hastening back to our bus, we found a group of eight small children waiting for us. They were clean and quite well dressed and seemed out of place in such remote, dangerous surroundings. One small boy, perhaps 12 years old, approached me and in English asked, "Are you Swedish?" That question is often asked me in Asian countries. It must be because my hair is so white. He then asked, "What classes do you have in America?"

Here was the question I had been waiting for all the time I was in India. I would answer carefully, teaching a small lesson in democracy to this 'underprivileged' little boy. Launching into a mini-lecture, I informed him that America is a democracy and that we have no classes. The child listened politely and then asked again, "You have no classes in America?" I assured him that in our country everyone was equal and that we do not have a class system. He looked at us as if we were from another planet and said, "That is too bad. I have English, Hindi, Biology and Algebra in my class." Shaking his head, he slowly joined his friends and they walked away, undoubtedly discussing America's strange educational system.

Sorting out our impressions on the bus as we returned to Khajuraho, we were forced to conclude that as an ambassadress for my country and democracy, I had not earned a very good grade. We also decided that our guide's concern for the dauntless fighting men could have been equaled by his desire for some extra rupees, as a reward for having provided an exciting tour.

Punjabi Suit of Kashmir

The Vale of Kashmir is a scenic, fertile valley 85 miles long and 20 miles wide, lying between the Himalayan and Pir Panjal Ranges of northwest India. The "Happy Valley" is popular with prosperous Indian families and an increasing number of tourists.

Srinagar, the capital, is on the shores of Lake Dal and was a favorite spot of Mughal emperors. We wandered in the still-beautiful gardens built by a 17th century emperor for his empress and rode through the ancient city in a horse-drawn carriage. Across the lake we could see our temporary homes, gaily decorated houseboats floating in beds of waterlilies.

This region is predominantly Muslim, while most of India is Hindu. Some older women still follow religious tradition and shield their faces from public view, but young girls wear their scarves around their neck, letting the two ends hang down their backs and leaving their faces unveiled.

An Arab tailor was making this Punjabi suit for his wife. I ordered an exact copy to my measurements. It consists of a 'khameez,' a long-sleeved tunic that nearly reaches the knees, and the 'shalwar,' or trousers, which are very full at the waist and are held by a drawstring. They are made of shiny synthetic fabric with a beige and red print on a brown background. A plain brown cotton sleeveless coat is worn under a cape, with an attached veil of layered brown chiffon. The veil is impenetrable from the outside and almost so from the inside.

This type of khameez and shalwar is now the favorite traveling costume of many Indian women, who find the sari too cumbersome. It is also comfortable in the squatting position so commonly assumed for long periods of time by both men and women in this part of the world. It could be called a Far Eastern version of the Western pants suit.

Heavily embossed shoes have gold braid and low heels. The jewelry chosen to wear with this costume is a very fine agate necklace of 50 beads, graduated in size, with a gold bead between each agate. The necklace was acquired in Gulmarg, Kashmir, a town in the mountains where agate is found.

A Plot to Deceive Goes Awry

A planned joke turned into my most embarrassing travel experience ever! One of our group invited us to a party on his houseboat. My Kashmiri Muslim costume had arrived from the tailor. Our young local Indian guide would introduce me as his mother, and we would join the party. He warned me not to say a word and to keep my hands hidden. We met on the dock after dark, and if I do say so, my disguise was perfect. Even the guide was surprised. Veiling has some advantages . . . one can be anonymous if desired.

Unfortunately, our tour director answered our knock and refused admittance, shutting the door in our faces. My young guide disappeared, and for the rest of the evening I had trouble concealing my dismay from our rude leader. So did Jo, who had helped perfect the disguise. When I 'unveiled,' the rest of the guests thought it had been a great idea, and our director was embarrassed. This plot turned out to be bad judgment on my part, but now I had a small sampling of what it was like to be an untouchable - degrading! I never saw the local guide again to apologize, but what was there to say?

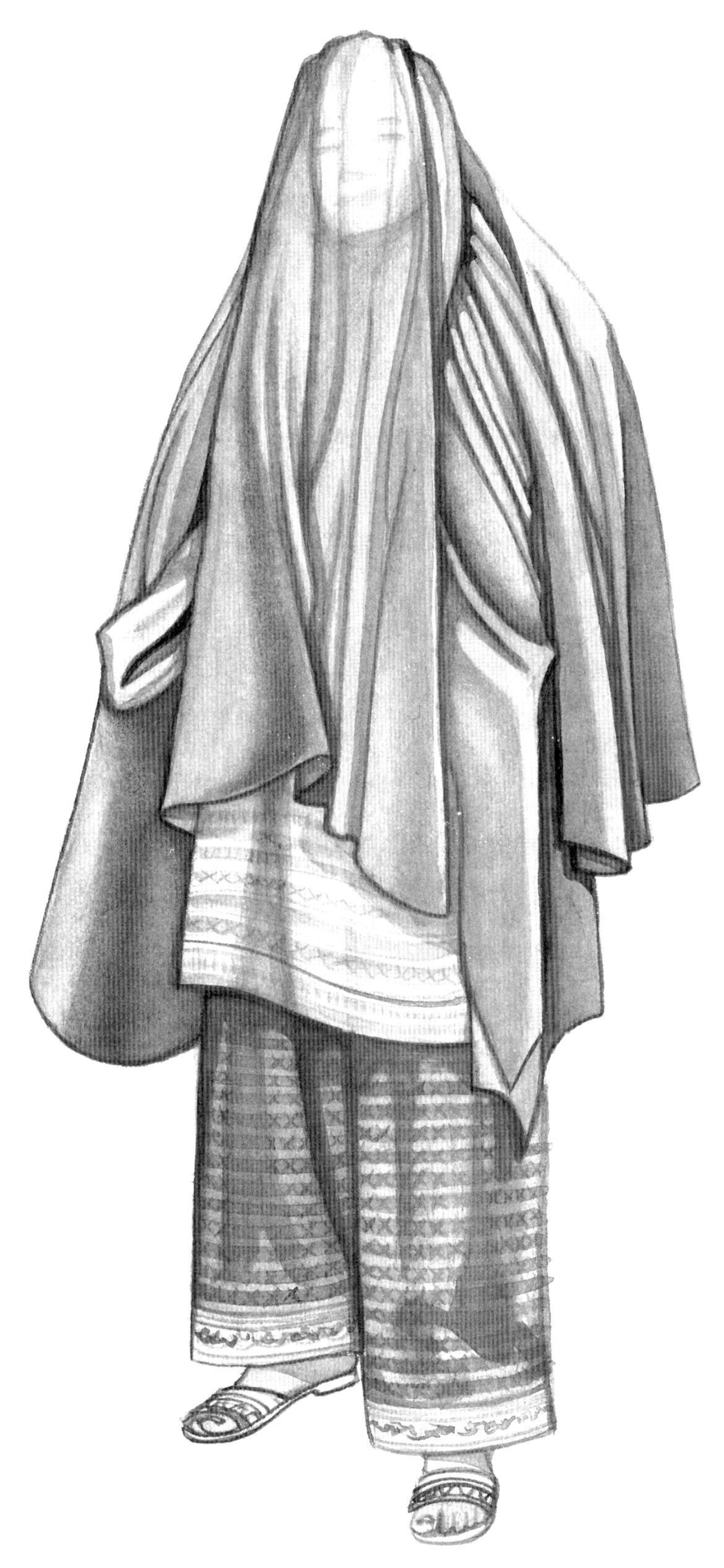

The Charmer and His Snake

India's serpent worship goes far back into time and into the culture of the land. The cobra is well suited for the type of ritual used by snake charmers. It is large, undeniably exciting and dangerous, and it responds to movement, striking with a slow, sweeping movement, minimizing danger to the native handlers.

It is not the music of the 'pungi,' or pipe, that causes the snake to sway in his act, as all cobras are deaf to high frequencies. He is hypnotized by the movement of his master waving the pungi, which usually has pieces of glass or mirror fastened to the tip.

This pungi was found in Bangalore, India. It belonged to a genuine snake handler, who was reluctant to part with it until persuaded by quite a few rupees.

The shirt or tunic, called a 'jubba,' and the sarong, were found in New Delhi. They are in the traditional shades of red and gold, favored by these handlers. The fabric of the jubba is a silky synthetic, gold in color, with white embroidery on the high collar and around the sleeves. The cotton sarong has a red background, with a design in gold and white. The shiny 'genie' hat was a real find in Khajuraho not only because it suits this dramatic act so well, but also because it was the answer to our 'disintegrated turban' problem. We hadn't done very well solving that problem in Amritsar, and no one since then with a really well-wrapped turban had looked approachable enough for us to ask for a lesson.

Since 1973, it has not been possible to bring a stuffed cobra into the United States because the stuffing was often opium. My Thai friend found the snake for us in a shop in Colorado, but she was unable to find a basket. (The snake's master usually weaves his own.) We saw many bread baskets in our search all over India before we finally found a suitable home for Naja-Naja. . . snake in Hindi. We hope that it was designed for him, not Indian bread. There has been discussion as to whether some handlers defang their snakes, but we can rest assured that our cobra poses no harm to museum observers.

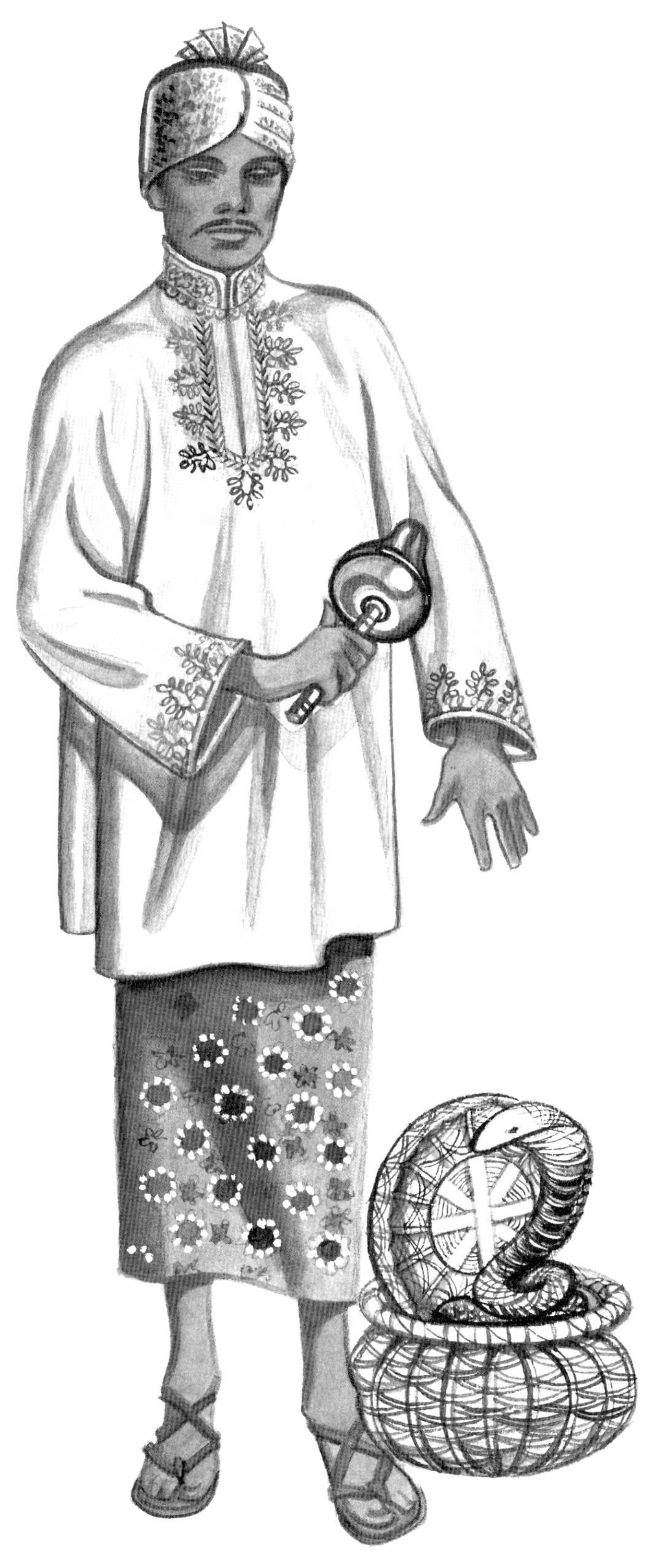

Madame Tendu-Fla in Darjeeling

Darjeeling, the Place of the Thunderbolt, is across a deep-forested valley from Mt. Kachenjunga, which towers into the sky for 28,208 feet. This magnificent snow-capped mountain is part of the Himalayan Range and is the third highest mountain in the world. Hindus believe its crest is in the shape of Lord Siva, in a prone position. To get to Darjeeling one must fly from Calcutta's Dum-Dum Airport to Siliguri and then travel by car or narrow-gauge railroad through breathtaking scenery with many tea plantations.

When Tibet came under Chinese control, Mary Tendu-Fla and her husband fled to Darjeeling and became owners and operators of the small but elegant Windamere Hotel. For many years Darjeeling was an escape for British families seeking relief from the steamy Calcutta summers and the Windamere, at an altitude of 7,000 feet, became a very pleasant summer home for many of them. Frequent guests were famed traveler Lowell Thomas and Sir Edmund Hillary, the first man to scale the world's highest mountain, Mt. Everest. Other well-known guests were a member of the British royal family and Hope Cooke, the American woman who became the Queen of Sikkim, which is practically next door to Darjeeling and is now a Protectorate of India. Hope Cooke became friends with 'Madame' Tendu-Fla, as she prefers to be called, and was initiated into the custom of the Tibetan baku for daily wear. The baku in this collection was donated by Madame Tendu-Fla.

A day at the Windamere may begin with coffee and croissants served in one's room before a log fire.   Then a drive to Tiger Hill to view the spectacular sunrise over the Himalayas, with Mt. Everest towering above all the other mountain peaks. Shopping in the town of Darjeeling for Tibetan crafts and mixing with Tibetan lamas, Burkhas of eastern Nepal, Gurungs of southern Nepal, the Bhutia Lepchas of northern Sikkim and Drukpas of Bhutan is an unforgettable experience. Adding to the color and glamour of the scene are the Tibetan women in their striped aprons and Indian women in their colorful, graceful saris. Then back to the hotel for Darjeeling tea with tiny cucumber and tomato sandwiches, served on the hotel terrace. The mesa on which the hotel is perched drops hundreds of feet into a heavily forested ravine. Beyond the ravine glow the plains of Bengal, over which the 'King of the Mountain's' snowy crest is beginning to reflect the pinks, lavenders, blues, golds and greens of the sunset. A delicious dinner is replete with stimulating conversation from globe-trotting guests. Among the guests we found particularly interesting was a handsome boy of perhaps six years, dressed in the reddish-colored robe of a student monk. He was dining with a lovely young American woman and an adult Buddhist monk. After becoming acquainted with this group of diners, we learned that the boy was with his mother and his teacher. The child, at this tender age, spoke four languages fluently. The monk was his constant companion. His mother, we were told, is the daughter of a star of the New York theatrical world. The boy will become a monk when he reaches the proper age.

And now to bed, snuggled under goose-down comforters, lulled to sleep by the crackling, flickering fire. As Shah Jahan inscribed in gold on the Red Fort at Delhi:
> *"If on earth there is a Paradise, then this is it, this is it, this is it."*

Madame Tendu-Fla is still, in 1995, managing the Windamere Hotel. She has visited the United States twice since we were in Darjeeling, and we were delighted to see her.

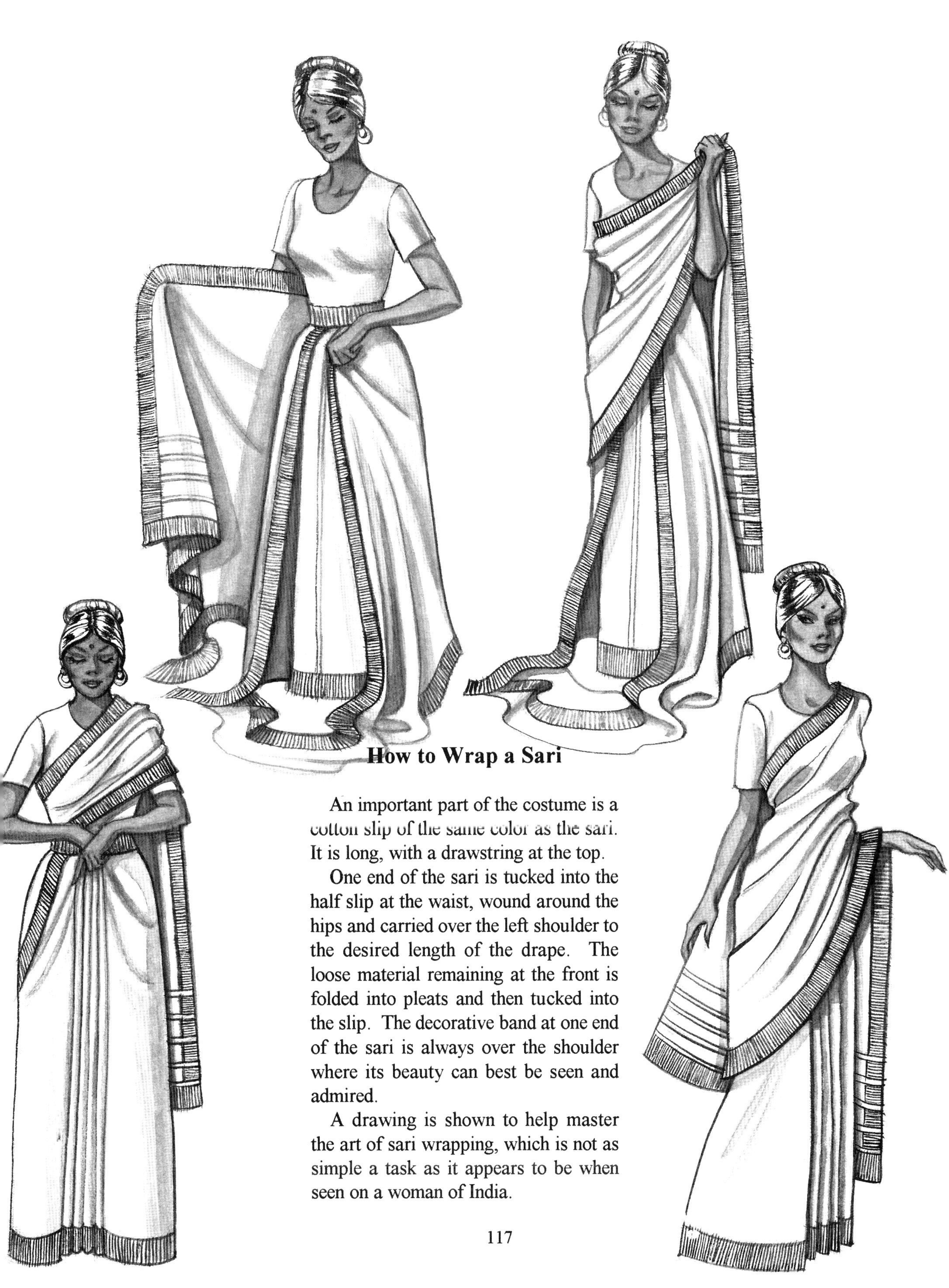

How to Wrap a Sari

An important part of the costume is a cotton slip of the same color as the sari. It is long, with a drawstring at the top.

One end of the sari is tucked into the half slip at the waist, wound around the hips and carried over the left shoulder to the desired length of the drape. The loose material remaining at the front is folded into pleats and then tucked into the slip. The decorative band at one end of the sari is always over the shoulder where its beauty can best be seen and admired.

A drawing is shown to help master the art of sari wrapping, which is not as simple a task as it appears to be when seen on a woman of India.

117

The Indian Sari...an Example of Grace and Beauty

India's sari is one of the world's best known examples of ethnic dress. It is the woman's garment of India, Bangladesh, East Pakistan, Sri Lanka, Nepal and Assam. It can be seen in all the large cities of the world, wherever there is an Asian population of any size. The grace and beauty of the sari are justly admired. It has been said that this is the most feminine of dresses. Exquisite fabrics are draped on the body in a variety of ways, almost always according to the regional customs of a country. It is possible for a knowledgeable observer to discern the part of India from which the wearer of a distinctively wrapped sari originates. Although Indian men have adopted western dress to a great degree, the women have clung to tradition. A woman may still be expected to bring enough saris to her marriage to last her a lifetime.

The finest saris are believed to be those woven in Benares, called Varanasi, that holy city on the Ganges River. The silk thread of these saris is from cultivated silkworms, which are fed the leaves of mulberry trees. The gold and silver designs are made by beating metal bars until they are flat, and then drawing strips through holes in a steel plate until they become fine wire. The design is then woven into the fabric by using a small, needle-like spool, carried in and out of the threads to develop the pattern.

Saris are all worn with a 'cholee' or 'choli,' a short jacket-type covering for the upper part of the body. It can be sleeveless or short-sleeved and is made of the same silk as the sari, but is undecorated. The jacket can be fastened either in the back or front, and the wearer has the option of covering the midriff or leaving it bare. The choli must always fit very snugly.

While Muslims prefer to cover the faces of their women in order to hide their beauty from the world, Hindus prefer to 'gild the lily.' Dark eyes are often made to appear larger with the use of kohl, and there is the 'bindi,' a small round dot worn on the woman's forehead. It originally meant that the wearer was married, but it is now worn as a colorful decoration by women in general, except for widows. Widows have a difficult time in India because their active lives are considered over when their husbands die. At least 'suttee,' the compelling of a woman to share her husband's funeral pyre, is now outlawed.

The wearing of jewelry is not only to enhance the beauty of the wearer, it helps establish her social status. A woman may wear her fortune in gold, silver and gems on her person. These include rings on her fingers and toes, many bracelets jingling on arms and ankles, elaborate necklaces and ornaments for her hair. A valuable gemstone, preferably a diamond, is often worn in a pierced nostril. This nose decoration is called a 'kalimpong.' The piercing of nostrils is as common in India as is the piercing of ears in America.

The fabric of this breathtaking blue silk sari from Benares was made with cultivated silkworm thread. Its extensive gold decoration makes it very valuable. The sari is about eight yards in length and 45 inches wide, with a six-inch border around the bottom in a golden pattern of hearts, leaves and stylized flowers. There are also bands of gold woven diagonally across the full length of the sari. On the bottom of the end that goes over the left shoulder there is an area of nearly solid gold embroidery measuring 12 by 45 inches. When no longer wearable this quality of sari is melted down to retrieve the precious metal.

Leather, hand-decorated, flat-soled, red and gold sandals are worn with this sari.

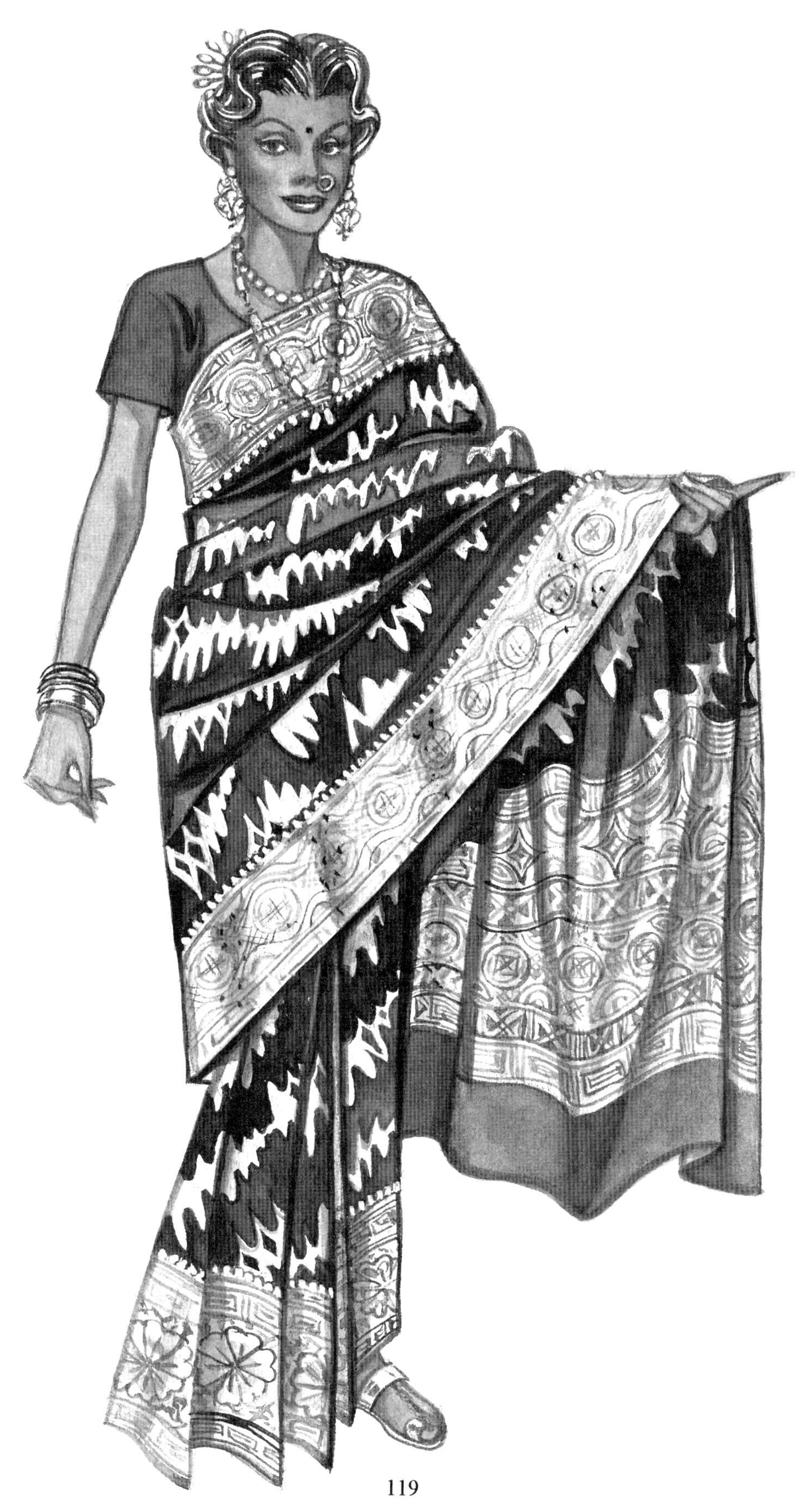

"Flowers open in the hands of the dancer
And birds fly from the tips of the fingers.
The body sways now in pride and now in devotion,
Even as the whole face expresses all the
Variegated splendour of forms and moods."

Source unknown

Bharata Natya Dancer and Dress

For many centuries religion has been communicated in India through dance. Hinduism, a major religion of India, has three main deities: Brahma, the Creator; Vishnu, Protector of the Universe; and Shiva, Destroyer and Restorer and Protector of the Dance. There is a myth that says when Lord Shiva shook a hand drum, the world heard its first rhythm. As he moved his body in time with the beat, the universe came into being.

Bharata Natya is not only the most important of all Hindu religious dance dramas, it is also the most popular form of traditional Indian dance today. It is a dance technique of the south of India and was the dance of the 'Devadasis,' or temple dancers, centuries ago.

The dancers' costumes worn today resemble those of the temple dancers in remarkable detail. These costumes consist of a sari stitched to sheath the legs from hip to ankle. Pleats in front unfold like a fan when the knees are bent, in a basic stance. A brief choli is worn, sometimes with a sheer veil. The palms of the hands and the soles of the feet are dyed red, the eyes of the dancer are lined heavily with kohl, and the hair is decorated with flowers. There is jewelry in profusion: a head pendant, necklaces, arm bracelets, ear pendants, nose rings, finger rings and ankle bells. On each ankle bracelet there may be 50 to 100 tiny bells, which are used to articulate the rhythm of the orchestra as the dancer stomps her feet. The orchestra consists of drums, drone (played on the tambura) and a singer.

Every feature of the dancer's face becomes the register of many emotions in response to the music, while the positions of the arms, hands and fingers tell stories and indicate moods. In a dance of the purest tradition there are just 11 hand poses.

Asha is a renowned Indian dancer from Bangalore, who won an Indian government scholarship and has studied and traveled in India, Canada and Europe. She has danced for many dignitaries, including Indira Gandhi, and represented India at world's fairs.

This dancing dress was worn by Asha at some of her important events, and later acquired by the collector. It is of heavy garnet-colored silk, trimmed with green silk bands that are decorated with a floral design in gold thread.

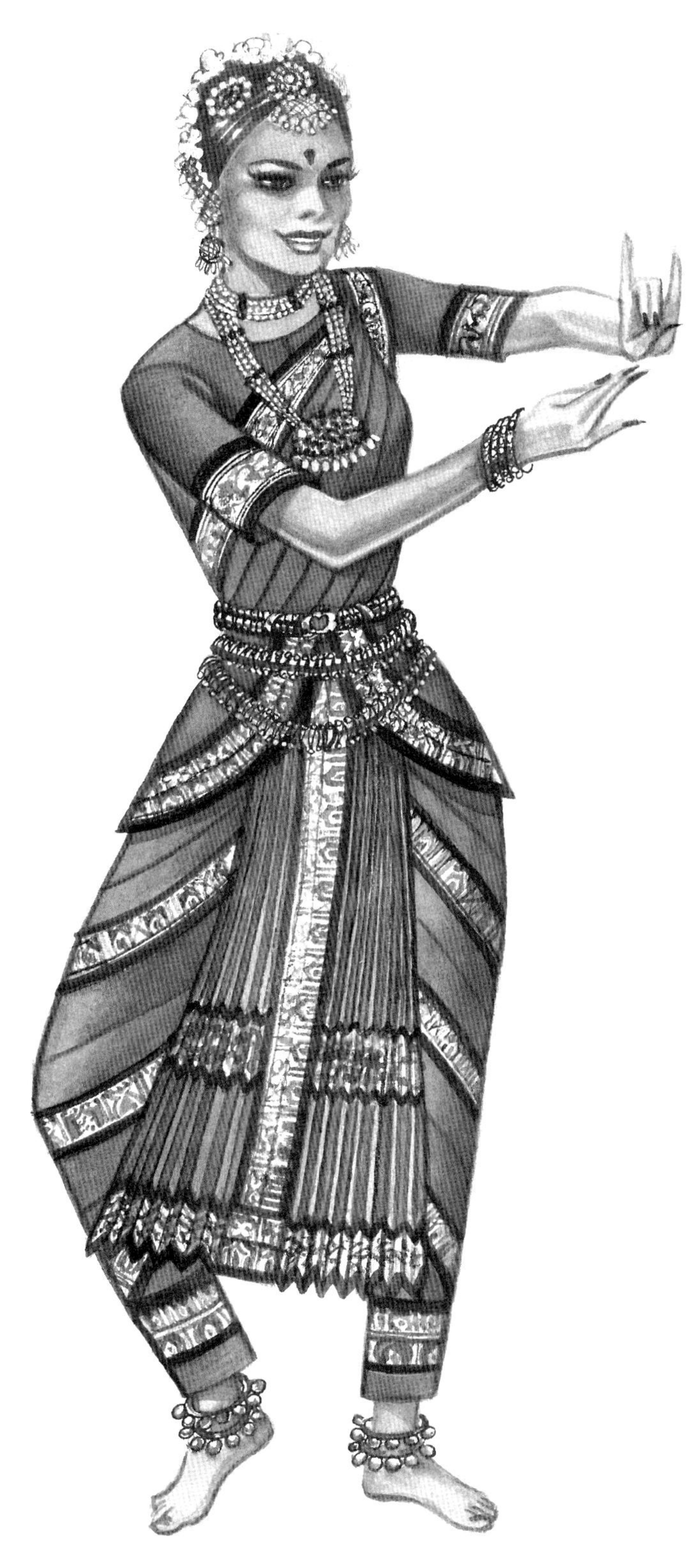

The People's Republic of China

China occupies most of the habitable land of East Asia. It is slightly larger in land mass than the United States, with a population of over one billion, which is more than four times that of the U.S. Ninety-two percent of the people are Han Chinese. The religions are traditionally Buddhism and Taoism, but the country is now officially atheist. The currency is the yuan and literacy is 70 percent. The government is that of a Communist Party-led state.

Remains of various man-like creatures who lived several hundred-thousand years ago have been found in China. Neolithic agricultural settlements dotted the Huanghe basin from about 5000 B.C. Chinese civilization was built on the language, religion and art of these people.

The Shang Dynasty ruled much of north China for 500 years, and the next 3,000 years were a succession of dynasties and interdynastic rule by warring kingdoms. A brilliant society, technologically and culturally, was developed. Russia, Japan, Britain and other powers exercised political and economic control in large parts of the country. China became a republic in 1912. In 1949 China came under the domination of communist armies, and the Kuomintang government, led by General Chiang Kai-shek, was forced to move to Taiwan. The People's Republic of China was proclaimed in Beijing under Mao Zedong. China and the USSR signed a 30-year treaty of "friendship, alliance and mutual assistance." Forcible relocations to the countryside were launched. Millions of teenagers were relocated and massive purges took place. After Mao and Chou En-Lai died, Mao's widow and three other leaders were arrested. In 1972 President Nixon visited China, and the two countries opened liaison offices in each other's capitals. In 1978 the U.S. formally recognized the People's Republic of China.

In 1989 sweeping reforms were demanded. More than 100,000 students staged a march, and a million people gathered, demanding democracy and the ousting of Deng and other leaders. Marshal law was ignored and protesters were crushed and arrested by Chinese troops. China maintained its totalitarianism, but with a more market-oriented economy.

Beijing

Six of us were traveling together, Grace and Claudia, who were mother and daughter travel agents, Sue, (our son's wife,) my friend Jo, my husband and I.

We flew out of Japan's Narita International Airport on the first Chinese 747 to land in Beijing. Even the stewardesses were excited. We were meeting the rest of our tour later. The country had just opened to tourism the year before, in 1979, and the Chinese people examined us with great interest wherever we went.

It was snowing . . . ridiculous weather for May, and I missed the coat left in that Japanese taxi! My trusted long underwear and borrowed sweaters were not enough. I bought a Mao suit and cap at a 'Friendship Store' near the hotel. No gloves were available, so I borrowed my husband's woolen socks. At least they matched the outfit, and now I could enjoy sightseeing. Keeping notes up-to-date with frozen fingers, or in socks with no fingers, wasn't easy.

While writing this chapter I called Sue. She was the youngest of the group and should have the best memory. She said that what she remembered most was how funny I looked in my Mao outfit and the faces of the Chinese when they saw me. Just the memory caused her to dissolve into laughter, and when she mentioned the 'gloves' it set her off again. A lot of help she was!

Beijing was teeming with building projects. There were bamboo scaffolding and piles of bricks everywhere, but we didn't see many workers. We went to the Peking Duck Restaurant, the same one that entertained President Nixon. Sue had been told by some students at the Capital Medical School nearby that they called it the 'Sick Duck.' We hoped this was a joke. We also had our usual language lesson: 'Neehow' is hello, 'Shy-Shy' is both thank you and goodbye. Since nearly everyone with whom we came in contact spoke English, we agreed that that was all the Chinese we needed.

The Forbidden City

A first glimpse of the Forbidden City, in the center of Beijing, comes from the incredible 98-acre public square. This famous Tien-an-Men Square easily holds several hundred-thousand people.

An entire inner city, containing hundreds of buildings, is surrounded by a 35-foot wall, with 17 gates. The gates, halls, gardens and palaces within the Forbidden City have names such as Gate of Correct Deportment, Hall of Perfect Harmony, Garden of Earthly Tranquility, and Palace of Peace and Longevity. The structure was built by the third Ming emperor after moving the capital of China to Beijing in 1421. Careful consideration of the principles of 'yin and yang' was taken.

The concept of yin and yang permeates every aspect of Chinese thought. It has influenced art, medicine, architecture, astrology, government and the daily lives of the people. As early as the third century B.C., there was an entire school of cosmology formed on the basis of yin and yang.

Yin is earth, female, dark, passive and absorbing. It is present in even numbers, valleys and streams and is represented by the tiger.

Yang is heaven, male, light, active and penetrating. It is present in odd numbers and mountains and is represented by the dragon. The two are shown as light and dark halves of a circle. Both are said to come from T`ai Chi, the Supreme Ultimate, with their interplay on one another being a part of the process of the universe and everything in it.

Since the emperor's role was central to this theme, his residence was a place where heaven, earth and man can meet. Thus, his responsibility was for the harmony and prosperity of his empire, seeing that the cosmological order of the universe was obeyed.

Mao Suits

This example of the dress of China from 1945 until the mid-1980's consists of jacket and trousers in navy blue, and a cap with a small bill. The red star on the cap denotes status. This all-occasion outfit was worn by both men and women for work, sightseeing, entertaining, housework and attending the opera.

The jacket, trousers, cap and shoes were purchased in Shanghai in 1981, at the Friendship Store. Even at that time, in warmer climates, one could see the occasional colorful jacket or slacks. But the love of color inherent in the Chinese nature came out in their art, their opera and the dress of their children. We saw babies bundled up in red, purple or orange quilted jackets, with little pink bottoms peaking through the `convenience' opening in the seat of the trousers (a simplified type of toilet training).

It was difficult to believe that a people who once named their public buildings "The lodge of fresh fragrance," "The pavilion of floating green," "Listening to the orioles among the willows," would be content to dress in drab grays and blues forever. As recent history has shown, they were not.

In the early 1980's, when the museum was giving costume shows as fund-raisers, it was impossible to find a Chinese refugee female or male to wear these coats and trousers. The Taiwanese were insulted when asked. Now, except for the military and government officials, there is not much of this uniform-style dress left on the streets, unless it is being worn as old clothing to save their new Western-style fashions.

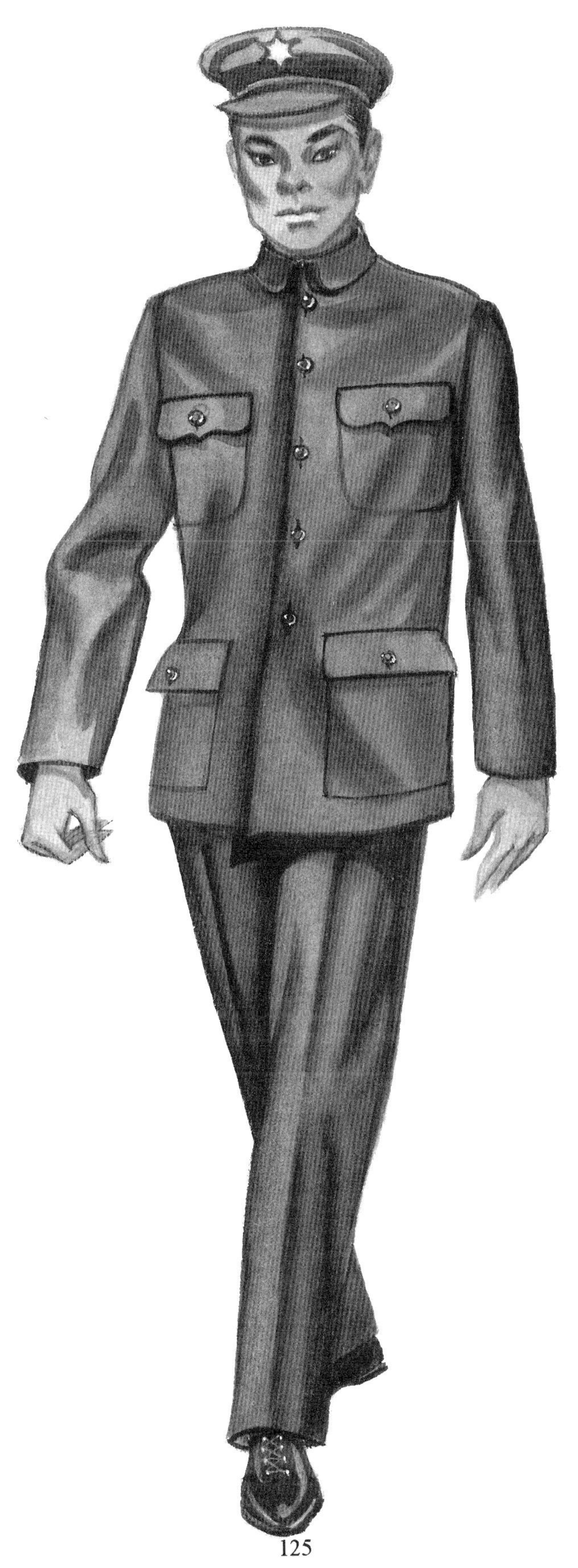

The Great Wall

The Great Wall of China has long been known as one of the wonders of the world and is one of the last sights visible to the astronauts as they leave the earth on a space mission. It is estimated that the bricks and rocks used for all of the Great Wall building projects would stretch 40 times around the equator.

Walls were built in many parts of China, but the one in the north of the country is by far the largest. It is 1,500 miles in length, running from west to east, like a huge dragon, winding through deserts, pastures and towering mountains to the Yellow Sea, where a barely distinguishable dragon's head looks over the Gulf of Chihli.   The first brick of the wall was laid in the seventh century B.C., and the construction continued for more than 20 centuries. It is difficult for us to understand the tremendous amount of work involved in building these massive barriers. Bricks, hewn stones and mortar were brought to the site either by hand or by cable.

The forts were built at such strategic spots that one soldier of the garrison could block the inroad of thousands of an invading army. The beacon towers were on peaks or mounds and were a means of communication. Smoke during daytime and fire at night were used as alarms. A mixture of wolf dung, sulfur and nitrate was used for these alarms. One column of smoke, with a single gunshot, meant that there was an enemy force of about 100, two columns with two shots meant 500, three columns and three shots meant 1,000, and five columns and five shots signified a 5,000-man army.

At certain periods of history the Great Wall was superior to any other kind of defense anywhere in the world. One wall protected the Silk Road with its precious cargo of silks for the west and its equally valuable cargo of woolens, melons and fruits for east Asia.

A story is told of a woman whose husband was conscripted in the early third century B.C. into the Great Wall project. She walked thousands of kilometers to take her husband winter clothing she had made for him, only to find that he had died of hard labor and miserable living conditions. As she walked along the newly-built Great Wall, she mourned so intensely that a part of the wall burst open to expose the body of her husband. Although a legend, it is an expression of the people's hatred of oppression and tyranny. There is even a special rock to mark the legendary tomb of the widow Mengjiang.

Shanghai, On the Sea

Shanghai, which means 'on the sea,' has the most Western look of any Chinese city. It was the first port opened to Western trade. There are 1.1 million bicycles in Shanghai, a city of seven million people.

Medical schools there specialize in teaching 'barefoot doctors,' who are sent to the communes. One hospital just teaches acupuncture.

We visited a commune within driving distance of Shanghai. Sue sat next to our guide. He was a college professor and spoke excellent English, but he answered her questions in the Chinese way.

Since he had said he had a wife and children, Sue asked him where they were. He answered, "Back in the country." When asked if he could see them on vacations, he replied, "Yes." However, when asked how long his vacations were, he responded, "We don't get vacations, just a few holidays." On further questioning he revealed that it had been two years since he had seen them, and the only possibility of their coming to live with him would be when the population of Shanghai goes down. He also said that the workers in the countryside are called peasants, no matter what their background.

The commune we visited was enveloped in an unpleasant odor that permeated the entire environment. It was because of the use of 'nightsoil' as fertilizer. A young Alabama farm girl in our group remarked, "Our cows back home live better than these people do." We had a little trouble managing to eat lunch, but that gave the commune managers more to eat. The food in China was certainly not like 'Chinese chop suey' in our country.

Sue loved talking to the natives, and was often surrounded by a large group of young people, many of them college students. Their comprehension of English was remarkable. The interest of those she talked with centered on economics and money. The usual salary of college graduates in 1980 was $30 a month, and after graduation it often took them two years to find a job.

Children are very precious in China. The family's first child is subsidized by the government. With the second one, there is half the subsidization, and when the third child arrives, there is a salary deduction. One would assume that anything less than a wage of $30 a month would be a very good incentive for birth control.

Dress of Chinese Peasant of Shanghai Before 1945

Jonny Ho was making me a beautiful, long, elegant, red and black Chinese satin dress. This was strictly a tourist acquisition, not for the museum. It was just for parties, made to my own specifications.

When Jonny, who owned a tailoring shop in a Hong Kong hotel, learned that his customer collected native costumes from all over the world, he told his mother, who insisted on presenting a gift to the museum. It was still in its original package. When Jonny, his mother and their family fled Shanghai in 1945, she brought with her enough traditional clothing to last for many years.

Mrs. Ho's gift was very welcome as it was exactly what I was searching for. It consists of a long-sleeved, high-necked top with the Oriental right-shoulder closing, and calf-length trousers with the usual voluminous drawstring waist. The fabric is a gray synthetic material. The pointed hat and basket are of woven straw and were found in the Red Chinese shop in Kowloon, which is across the harbor from Hong Kong. The soft, felt shoes also came from this store. Even today Hong Kong's elderly citizens enjoy wearing these comfortable shoes.

This fine example of a costume of old China was made during a time when an individual's social and economic status were obvious in his or her dress. Jonny's own success was mirrored in his Westernized suit and tie, but his ethnic interests were strong. His mother's outfit was of the peasant, or serving class, and she was proud of it, as was her son.

Such situations are not unusual. In countries where national states impose upon their subjects a goal of one nation, one people, one government, one religious belief (or lack of belief), they also encourage one type of dress. These states resent the folk order, and fleeing refugees are prone to treasure their unique clothing and to make great effort to preserve it. Jonny's mother wanted the world to know about her life and that of her ancestors. Knowing that her ethnicity would be recognized in a museum in the United States helped fulfill her strong desire to keep a part of her cultural heritage from being lost to future generations.

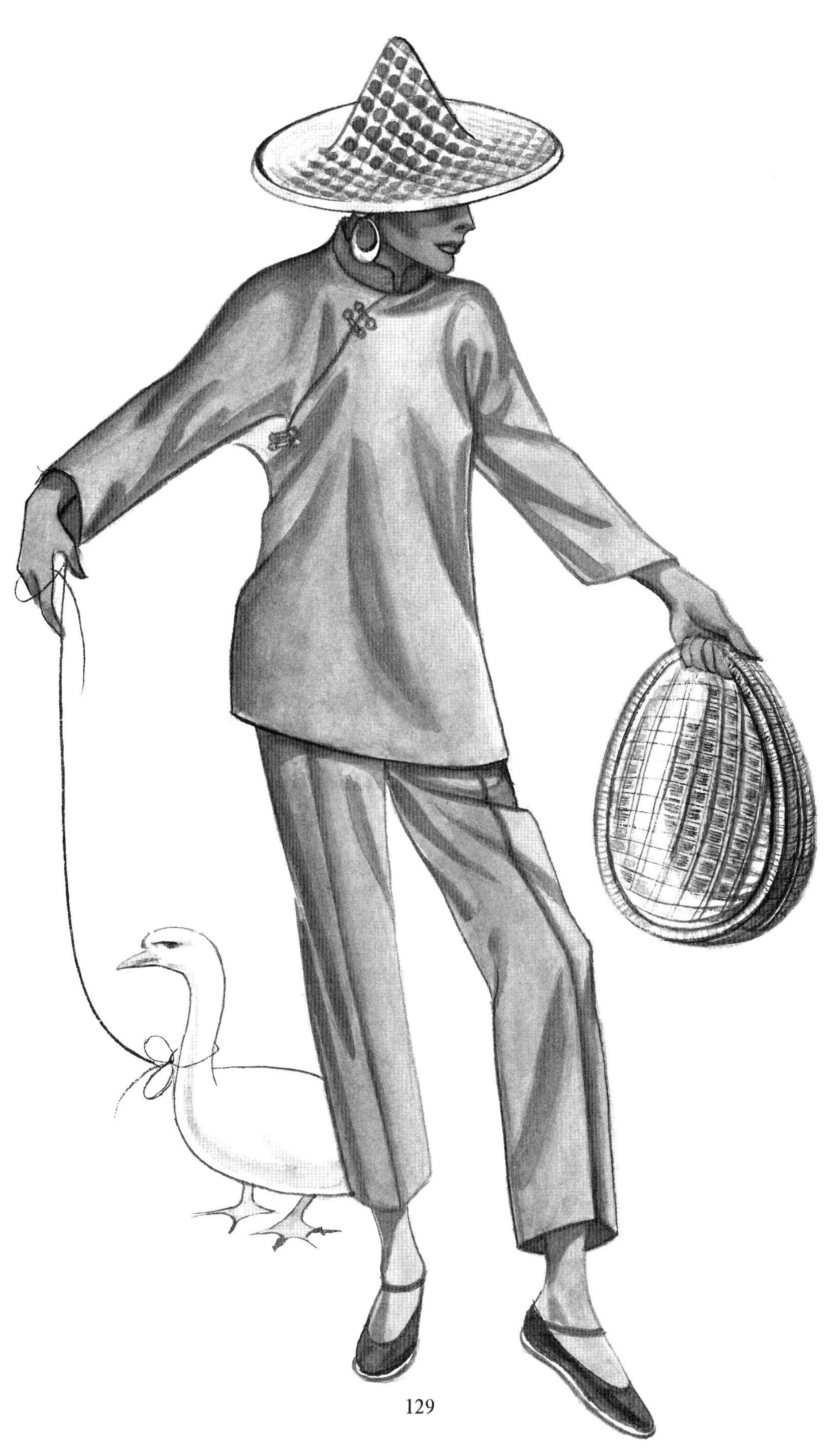

The Old Silk Road

The Silk Road was actually a caravan route, following the Great Wall, climbing the Pamir Mountains, crossing Afghanistan and continuing to the Levant. From there its precious cargo crossed the Mediterranean Sea. With the loss of Roman territory in Asia, this route became increasingly dangerous. It was revived under the Mongols and Marco Polo traveled the road to Cathay. Today the United Nations has plans to turn the Old Silk Road into a Trans-Asian Highway.

Xian, as the ancient city of Chang'an is now called, is in northeast China where the 4,000-mile Silk Road began. In 1974 a huge pit was uncovered in Xian, which was filled with over 6,000 terracotta soldier figures. They are life-size and in battle formation. It is estimated that they were made 2,000 years ago, in order to guard the emperor's tomb. Excavation continued, and in 1980 two sets of chariots and horses were unearthed. Each chariot has a driver, and gold and silver interlocking patterns are on saddles and bridles. Today, this city is a very popular tourist attraction.

Silkworms . . . 'Bombyx Mori'

Silk is the strongest of all natural fibers. One cocoon of good-quality, unbroken threads can be made into 600 to 1,000 yards of silk thread. In Chinese the words meaning mulberry, silkworm and silk have been inscribed on bones and tortoise shells, which are believed to date back to the biblical Great Flood. By the second century, silk was the mainstay of the Chinese economy. Sericulture, the fabrication of silk, had been a well-guarded secret for 3,000 years. A Chinese princess carried mulberry-tree seeds and silkworm eggs in the lining of her headpiece to her Indian bridegroom. At about the same time Emperor Justinian sent two monks to transport seeds and eggs in the heads of their canes to the Byzantine Empire. The secret was out!

Silkworms are treated as carefully as newborn humans and are raised under exacting temperature-controlled conditions. Even loud noises and strong odors can upset them.

In early summer the female lays from 300 to 500 eggs. She then dies within a few days. The eggs are placed on special strips of paper and put in cold storage, until the next spring when they are incubated to hatch. The hatched eggs are put on spotless trays with a fresh supply of mulberry leaves every two hours. They eat all day and all night until they are 70 times their hatched size and have shed their skin four times.

When these three-inch-long, one-inch-thick worms stop eating, they are placed in tiny wooden compartments, and attach themselves to a twig of straw and begin to form a cocoon. As they swing their heads in a figure-eight movement, a fluid which hardens into a fine silk thread is rendered. This filament is spun around the body of the worm until all the fluid is used, completing the cocoon in about three days. In the next stage the pupa becomes a moth, and would break through the cocoon if allowed to do so. Since the handlers do not want the silk thread broken, only enough moths to lay eggs for the next cycle are allowed to break through. The rest of the cocoons are kept intact by killing the moths inside. Wild silkworm caterpillars, which feed on oak and allied trees, are raised in a semi-domestic state. Shantung silk is made from this type of thread. There are saris in the collection made of the silk of both the cultivated and semi-cultivated caterpillars.

Scenic Treat and Terror . . . A Day in Guilin

The Li River flows in beauty for 437 kilometers, between Guilin and Hangzhou. Small boats take tourists to see the needle-like peaks, shimmering waters and garden-like fields. The rising sun gives a surrealistic feeling to the scenery, as though it were a part of a traditional Chinese misty landscape painting.

After lunch on the boat we had another treat ahead, a trip to some famous caves. We had just met our guide and driver, who were scheduled to take us to dinner and to the plane for Shanghai that evening. The cave was their idea, and we could not resist the opportunity to see something not many travelers get a chance to see.

We had all of our important papers with us, passports, credit cards and cash in our tightly clutched purses, as we joined hundreds of Chinese sightseers. We were the only foreigners. We entered the cave on a stone path, which skirted bottomless pools. In an awed voice the guide warned us that no one had ever found the bottom. The pools were covered with waterlilies and other growth, and the cave with its colored lights was truly magnificent.

The crowd was quiet and polite, yet persistent in pushing ahead. The path was uneven and frightening. We hoped we wouldn't have to test the depth of the `bottomless' pools. Jo was hanging onto the arm of the guide, and I on that of the driver; they were our only security.

We hadn't gone far when the lights suddenly went out. A cave with no lights must be the blackest thing there is. And such silence! No one moved. Our voices were a bit high . . . not hysterical, of course, but higher-pitched than usual. "Jo!" "Dorothy!" No one in the world knew where the two of us were, and there was not a single flashlight anywhere.

Our guide caught our panic, although he was perfectly calm. Perhaps this was not an unexpected occurrence, so what was he doing without a flashlight? He asked, "Do you want to wait until the lights come back on and see the rest of the caves?" What a silly idea! He said he knew a short way out and to "Hang on!" We had not considered letting go! We inched our way through the darkness and the crowd, somehow avoiding bumping someone into the wet abyss.   Suddenly we were in sunlight. What a wonderful relief!

Those caves created the most panic of almost any of our adventures. But what nice people were in that cave! In the midst of this throng, we didn't experience even a slight tug at one of our purses.

It was time for dinner but Jo and I had lost our appetites, so our guide and driver ate their dinners and ours, too. They ate for such a long time that we were afraid of missing our plane. It flew to Shanghai only twice a week. They insisted that the plane was always late. If we missed our connection in Shanghai, our group would continue to the States without us. To add to our worries, our guide in Shanghai had our return tickets. Passengers were boarding when we arrived at the airport, however, so all was well.

I wish I could remember the name of our Guilin guide, as a warning to anyone who might travel in that direction. However, we did give him an extra tip to buy a flashlight. It is most unlikely, though, that he would bother with anything so 'unnecessary,' when everyone in Guilin knows that those lights go out all the time, and always come back on . . . eventually.

The Chinese Opera Princess

Themes of Chinese operas are very romantic and rich in color, plot and style. The dances are not only lively, but often very athletic. In large cities hundreds of people patiently stand in line for hours to get tickets.

This costume is exquisite. It is made of pure silk, in a beautiful shade of red, heavily embroidered with flowers and the fabled phoenix bird. (This beautiful, lone bird is believed to live in 500-year cycles, at the end of which it consumes itself by fire, rising renewed from the ashes with youth and beauty, symbolizing immortality.) The phoenixes on this costume are embroidered in shades of blue, green, gold and aqua, and the flowers are in pink and blue with green leaves.

The jacket has a large phoenix on the back, one on the front and on each of the sleeves, as well as flowers all around. Bands around the bottom of the jacket and around the sleeves at the wrists are stripes of green, blue, aqua and gold. Over these bands are rows of flowers , topped by clouds, in shades of aquamarine. These striped bands are typically Chinese, and are found on many handicrafts. The hand covers may be worn over the hands or turned up as cuffs. At the opera in Shanghai, they were worn long, covering the hands.

A floor-length skirt has two panels, decorated with flowers of pink and blue with green leaves. The panels and hem are outlined in black and dark green in a geometric pattern with small flowers on the borders. The rest of the skirt is accordion pleated.

A yellow-fringed cape with a phoenix embroidered on each shoulder is worn over the jacket. Since this is the dress of a princess, the yellow color of the long, hand-tied fringe is in keeping with the rule regarding yellow to be worn only by royalty. The cape has the usual stiff Oriental collar, but it has a straight, center-front closing.

The blue hat is of papier-mâché and cardboard, decorated with silver paint and hundreds of pearls. A black, handwoven cap of horsehair is worn under this remarkable headdress to hold it in place on the head and to make it more comfortable for the wearer. The earrings each have seven long strands of pearls, with a total of 254 small and eight large pearls on each earring. The black velvet sandals (with inch-wide platform soles) are trimmed with white braid and pink satin.

It took the manager of an opera shop, two clerks and our Chinese tour guide, as well as a patient driver and tour group, to enable us to assemble this costume in Hangzhou, China, on beautiful and historic West Lake. Jo, Grace and I wandered away from the group and the area where the bus was parked in order to do some shopping. Seeing that our allotted time was expiring, we were about to start back to the bus when we saw Sue running toward us, waving her arms to come quickly. We didn't think we were *that* late!

She had found an opera shop and had persuaded our driver to let us have some more time to look over what appeared to be a treasure-trove of costumes. She had told him about the collection and, as was true in every country, he was enchanted by the idea of showing one of his country's examples of ethnic dress in a museum in the U.S. Even the other tourists on the bus were interested and did not complain about waiting. This generosity of spirit was one we encountered everywhere. We were expected to show our purchases to our tour group, and always did so. Later, seeing a replica of this costume on the princess in the opera in Shanghai, added to our delight.

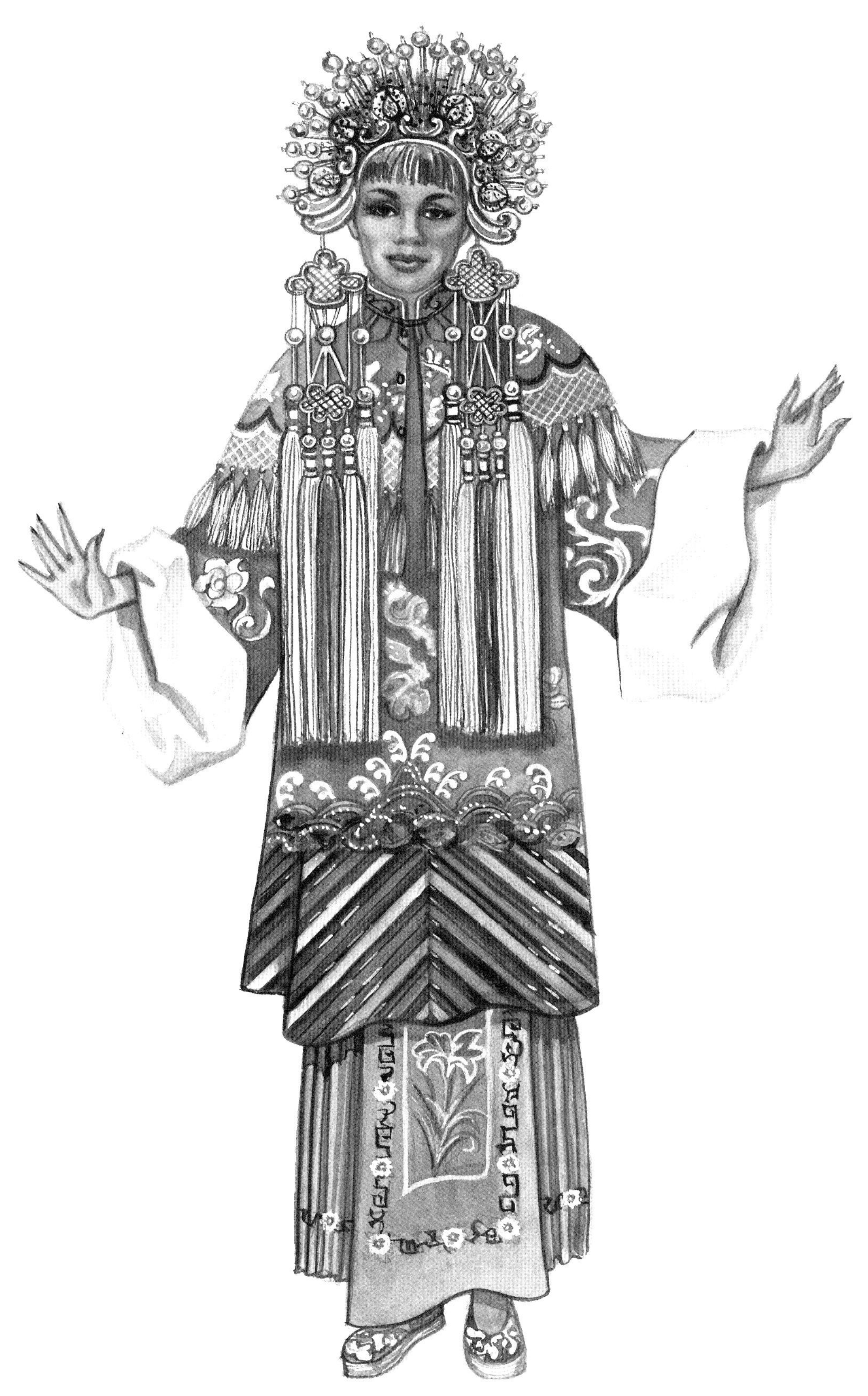

Be not afraid of going slowly, be afraid of standing still.
Chinese Proverb

Who is narrow of vision cannot be big of heart.
Chinese Proverb

If one word does not succeed, 10,000 are of no avail.
Chinese Proverb

A kind word is like a spring day.
Russian Proverb

There is more light than can be seen through a window.
Russian Proverb

Put things into their places, and they will put you in your place.
Arab Proverb

Northward from the Himalayas

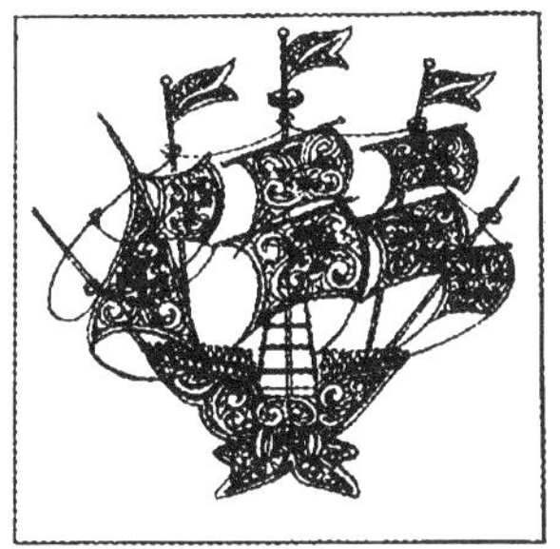

Bhutan
Tibet
Mongolia
Russia

"We live very close together.

So, our prime purpose in life is to help others,

and if you can't help them at least don't hurt them."

The Dalai Lama

Kingdom of Bhutan . . . Druk-Yul

In the fourth month of the Wood-Tiger Year, at the auspicious Hour of the Serpent, June 2, 1974, at 9:10 a.m., a handsome teenager rose from his golden throne and placed on his shoulders his great-great-grandfather's four-colored scarf. Jigme Singye Wangchuk had formally become the fourth hereditary king of Druk-Yul, the Dragon Land, or Bhutan. He was 19 years of age.

Bhutan is a country high in the eastern Himalayan Mountains. It is bordered by Sikkim (a state of India) on the west, by Assam (also an Indian state) on the east and south, and by China (Tibet) on the north. This is a land 200 miles long and 90 miles wide, and its Chinese border is the main ridge of the Himalayas. It is said that if you are going uphill you are in Bhutan, and if you are going downhill you are in China.

Vermont and New Hampshire combined, both in area and population, are roughly the same as Bhutan. The capital is Thimphu, 8,400 feet in altitude, with a population of 20,000 in 1987. There is one medical doctor for every 8,969 persons, and the literacy rate is 15 percent. The currency is the ngultrum.

Tibet ruled Bhutan in the 16th century. British influence grew in the 19th century, and it became a British protectorate by a 1910 treaty. In 1949 independence came, with India guiding foreign relations and supplying aid. At the present time it is a monarchy.

This is a rugged, mountainous, deeply-forested land, with so many waterfalls that one is rarely out of hearing range of running water. Before 1950 there was little contact with the rest of the world. It is a fact that before 1960 most of the people had never seen a wheel, but by the early 1980's there was a one-lane road running the length of the country, and an airport was under construction. By 1994 a road network had strengthened the linkage of the country to India, and the airport was completed.

The people are a branch of the Mongolian race. Three-quarters of them are Buddhist, with a Tibetan background, and one-quarter are Nepalese and Hindu. The Buddhists are constantly repeating the four-word prayer "Om mani padme hum," meaning 'the jewel of the lotus.' They believe that if they utter this prayer often enough they may escape the cycle of birth and death and be taken directly to paradise. Their religious beliefs are very strong.

On the road to Paro we saw farmhouses that looked surprisingly like Swiss chalets. However, upon closer inspection we discovered that the farm animals live on the ground floor and the family on the floor above. The views were magnificent, and we saw yaks in the mountains. We encountered a rock slide on our way to Thimphu. The workers clearing the rocks were all Nepalese. It seems that they do the heavy work in the country. In no time at all they had broken huge boulders into ones small enough to roll over the side of the road and down the mountain. The first vehicle through was an ambulance, and the second was a sleek Mercedes with the king, wearing a modern sport shirt, sitting beside the driver.

We were told to get postage stamps, as they were a great buy. To our surprise, they had a picture of our first man on the moon, Neil Armstrong. The transition from an age before the wheel to the world of the astronaut in 20 short years is a giant leap in history, and a rare privilege to share. This world of ours is indeed a strange and wonderful place.

Claudia Visits Bhutan

Bhutan, at the stage of development it had reached in the early 1980's when we visited, was heaven for the young and adventurous. Claudia Taylor was both. Her notes about our tour there should prove of interest to anyone looking for a really new experience.

September 13: In the early morning, the Indian train kept stopping for long periods of time. It was 11 a.m. when we finally reached Calcutta. Our plane to Bagdogra left at 1:10 p.m. Mom and I were looking forward to getting our mail and a bath in the room we had reserved for the day, but knew we didn't have time to go there and get to the airport. We had heard that traffic jams in Calcutta could tie up the roads for as long as eight hours, with all of the cattle, camels, donkey carts and trucks and cars that break down for one reason or another. We offered our taxi driver all of the rupees we had left if he could get us to the airport on time. We drove in the median and on the sidewalk, honking the horn the entire hour. Finally, racing into the airport, we saw Dorothy and Jo at the ticket counter and knew we had made it! We must have looked awful - dirty, disheveled and exhausted. But we all arrived in Bagdogra on time, where our guide, Mim, and driver, Peter, were waiting for us. Fellow travelers, Wayne, Mary, Wyche, Brooks, and Soshana were already on the bus.

September 14: It was a three-hour drive to Phuntsoling, at the Bhutanese border. When we had our passports checked we had to sign a paper promising we would not take antiques, ammunition or bear bile out of the country. Everyone laughed. The next morning after breakfast we started our ride up into the mountains. I sat with Wyche and Brooks, two American brothers on vacation from jobs in Saudi Arabia. They had Sony Walkmen with headsets and really good music. Listening to the Doobie Brothers and seeing all of that scenery at the same time was an unbelievable experience. It takes seven hours to get to Paro from Phuntsoling over winding, one-lane mountain roads. We passed huge waterfalls, some of them flowing over the road, and we would just drive through them. The wildflowers were gorgeous. When we reached a point where we could see Paro Valley below us, the view took our breath away.

September 15: Our hotel in Paro consisted of small bungalows, each with two rooms. Jo, Dorothy, Mom and I shared a bungalow and celebrated our arrival with a small cocktail party with the rest of our traveling companions. With our fare of fish-shaped crackers and nuts, as we sat at a long table, I felt like we were in an Agatha Christie novel.

September 16: We spent all day touring Paro. The farmhouses were quaint and attractive, with unusual architecture. They all had red peppers drying on their roofs. We stopped for a visit at our guide's home and met his mother and grandmother. The kitchen stove was wood-burning and made of iron. Pots, pans and other utensils hung from the walls. The living room had no furniture at all, but a whole room was devoted to an altar to Buddha. The upstairs was a storeroom for hay and supplies, and it looked as though about five people slept in one room.

September 17: The best day so far! Mary and I went with Wayne, Wyche and Brooks on a climb to Tak Tsong Monastery, or Tiger's Nest. I wore Dorothy's Indian moccasins and three pairs of socks, since I didn't have the right shoes. We bussed to the river and crossed the bridge to where the horses were waiting for us. We climbed for more than two hours up a steep trail that wound up the mountain. We were each taught a different call to make the horses move. Mine was 'Ah Cho!' The lower altitude was covered with forests and moss that hung all over the trees and rocks. It was creepy. I was glad when we could get off the horses and go the rest of the way on foot. We started climbing straight up a huge cliff. I could not have made it without the long, strong grasses to hold on to. It was exhausting! I thought, 'I really must quit smoking.' Reaching the monastery was the greatest! We were so high and there I was with a crown of wildflowers in my hair. How they ever built Tiger's Nest up there among the rocks with Paro so far below is a mystery.

I turned a huge prayer wheel until the bell rang. It was like being at the top of the world, and hearing that bell made me feel that I was on heaven's doorstep. I decided I would take up trekking when I got home. I felt so free, and felt I had learned much about myself. Coming down the mountain there was music and I was dancing from foothold to foothold. At the bottom we waded through shin-deep mud in some rice fields. The moccasins and socks stayed in the mud. Kids came out of somewhere and laughed at our dilemma.

We found our bus, got our lunch out and took it to a nice spot on the bank of the river. Brooks and Wyche dunked their heads in the river and the cold, cold water felt so good on my feet. Brooks bent over to get a drink and there, between some rocks in the river, was a dead baby. Later our guide told us that if a child under six dies it is thrown in the river, because it is so expensive to have a cremation. This custom we did not like one bit!

September 18: We took malaria pills and headed on to Thimphu, the capital. Everyone in this country is still wearing their traditional dress. The women's dresses are long, and the men's are knee-length wrap-around skirts. Many men wear plaid, knitted heavy socks and high-topped laced boots. Mary and I were stiff and sore at first as we visited some more Buddhist monasteries called Dzongs. At one of them we saw one of the younger monks get lashed with a leather whip on his bare bottom. Did he scream! We think a lot of that goes on here - no insubordination is tolerated. I, for one, had been Dzonged enough!

Prayer flags were flying everywhere. The people call the country Druk, rather than Bhutan. It is ruled by a very young king, age 26 and single. The guides seem to like him a lot. His father died of a heart attack in 1972 while hunting in South Africa. The people seem to be trying very hard to keep the country as it is, both physically and religiously. Back at our lodge we were glad to sit in the sun and watch the folk dancers in their lovely, colorful costumes. Dorothy was in heaven.

September 20: We left for Phuntsoling. Sharing Bhutan with our new friends made it all even more exciting. Brooks and Wyche would trek back to Paro Valley before returning to their jobs. We loaded them down with peanut butter and crackers, a flashlight and the rest of our cookies. I took their film to have it developed. They said Saudi Arabia is bad about losing film. We boarded the bus and waved goodbye to Mr. Green Jeans, as we had named the man dressed in green who followed us at some distance everywhere we went. We never did know who he was.

How I hated to leave Bhutan! Tourism will change this country. We were so lucky to be able to see it as it has been for centuries.

Bhutanese Kira - Woman's Ethnic Dress

Everyone in Bhutan, men, women and children, wear their country's native dress. This is one of the few countries left where this situation still exists. As Bhutan is drawn more and more into the outside world, this will undoubtedly change, but in the early 1980's, before construction of the airport, being in this country was like visiting another world in another century.

Women's dresses are made of pieces of hand-loomed textile, 18 inches in width and close to three yards in length. Each piece consists of three bands of weaving stitched together. The result is called a 'kira.'

The background color of this wonderful example of weaving is a natural or off-white color, which forms a four-inch fringe on each end. There are two-inch-wide stripes in colors of pink, red, blue and green. At the top and hem of this kira, when it is wrapped around the body, there is a five-inch finely woven border, striped in brown and navy and yellow, with red and green embroidered designs every six inches along the border. This is one of the most exquisitely woven pieces in the entire collection.

Wrapping or folding this piece of cloth is difficult, as its weight is necessary for warmth in the high altitudes of this mountainous country. It must be wrapped into a full-length, sleeveless dress, with an inverted pleat on the right side. All is held in place by two large pins at the shoulder. These pins, two inches in diameter, and roughly crafted of imitation gold and silver, are on a 16-inch chain of the same metal. They were difficult to find, since we were not prepared to pay the price of the beautifully worked gold and silver 'koma' or 'jabtha,' as they are called. It took Mim, our very nice, obliging guide, three days of searching to locate pins at a price that was practical. They are correctly made, which was most important.

The dress is held at the waist by a belt, or 'kera,' two and a-half inches wide and 68 inches in length, with nine-inch fringe on each end. There are stripes every two inches in red, blue, orange and white. Heavy embroidery in a triangular-shaped design decorates 28 inches of the belt.

A black coat is typical, and is made of heavy synthetic fabric with a satiny sheen. It has long sleeves and a three-inch band which forms a collar and extends down the front of the coat. It can be worn either inside the kira, as a blouse, or on the outside as a coat.

Young girls usually wear their hair in a 'Dutch bob' with bangs. This is very fetching with the small, triangular-shaped, pointed-top straw hat perched on their heads.

This kira was found in a handicraft shop run by the Bhutanese government in Thimphu.

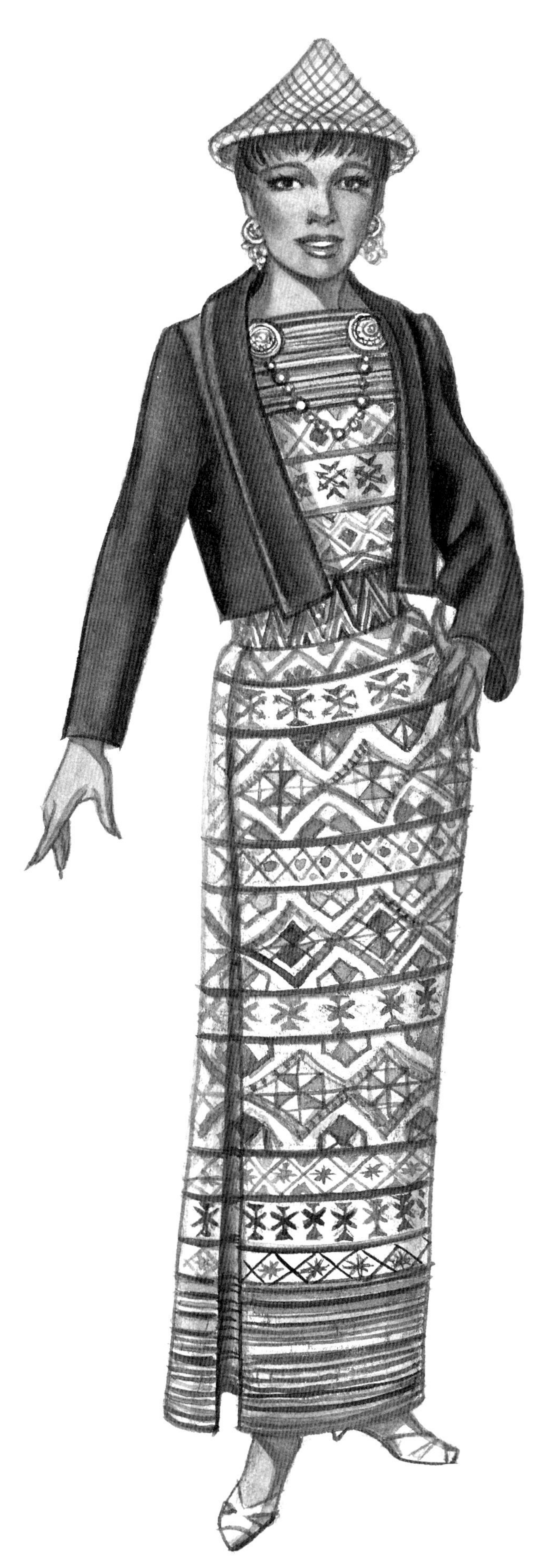

Tibet, or Bod

Padmasambhava, in the eighth century, wrote:
"When the iron bird flies and horses run on wheels, the Tibetan people will be scattered like ants across the world and Dharma will come to the land of the Red Man."
(Dharma means universal law or religion.)

Tibet is a remote land in south central Asia, often called the 'Roof of the World.' It is a region of China and its capital is Lhasa. The population in 1990 was 2.1 million, and another four million Tibetans form the majority of the population in adjacent areas that are now a part of China.

This is a land of superlatives. It occupies more than 470,000 square miles of mountains and plateaus and shares with Nepal claim to the world's highest peak, Everest, which is 29,028 feet in altitude. It is a fact that the valleys of Tibet are higher than the mountains of most of the rest of the world. The average altitude of this land is 15,000 feet. Jiachan, at 15,890 feet, is believed to be the highest inhabited town on earth.

Lhasa, the capital of Tibet, lies at 11,830 feet altitude and, because of the temperature variations, it is possible to freeze and roast in the same day. As a result of the cool, dry air, grain can be safely stored for 50 to 60 years, dried raw meat and butter can be preserved for more than a year and epidemics are rare.

Early in the seventh century, Slon-Brtsan-Sgam-Po established Tibet as a military power. Around 775 A.D., the Indian Tantric (a form of Buddhism) master, Padmasambhava, came to Tibet. Among other accomplishments, he established the first Buddhist monastery and the first Buddhist university in the country. The Buddhists and Shamanists wrestled for power, and in the ninth century the Kingdom of Tibet dissolved into factions. With the Muslim invasion of India, Tibet was cut off and developed its own kind of Buddhism. Kubla Khan, the grandson of Genghis Khan, became a Tibetan Buddhist.

The first Dalai Lama appeared in 1578. Dalai means 'oceans,' and Dalai Lama means 'oceans of wisdom.' The Great Fifth Dalai Lama instituted a blend of religion and politics, known as a theocracy. He also completed the building of the magnificent Potala, the winter palace of the Dalai Lamas on Red Mountain in Lhasa. With its position between India and China, Tibet was a pawn of both these countries and withdrew into itself as a cultural and religious whole, welcoming isolation.

Since the 18th century, China ruled Tibet until 1911, then gaining control again in 1951, and crushing a rebellion completely in 1959. All land was collectivised and the Dalai Lama and 100,000 followers fled to India, where a government in exile was formed in Dharmsala, not far south of the Kashmiri border. This government is an embarrassment to China, whose solution is to get rid of as many Tibetans as possible, substituting Chinese residents. In Lhasa, for example, which has grown recently to 400,000 inhabitants, most of the newcomers are Chinese civil servants and military personnel. The remaining Tibetans are restricted in movement from one zone to another, even in Lhasa itself. Until 1979 independent travelers were not allowed into the country.

When the Dalai Lama dies, his succession is maintained by the discovery of a child into whom the leader's spirit is believed to have entered. The present and 14th Dalai Lama is Tenzin Gyatso. He was born of Tibetan parents on the fifth day of the fifth month of the Wood-Hog Year of the Tibetan calendar, which is June 6, 1935, in Amdo, Qinghai province. Search parties scoured the land to find this child, doing so with the help of significant 'signs.' This will be his position for life.

The people of Tibet are of the Mongolian race, short and sturdy, and their main food is barley meal. The most important animal in the country is the yak, a sort of hairy buffalo. It supplies milk, butter, cheese, meat, cloth and transportation. One of the delicacies of the country is yak-butter tea. This rancid butter tea is not appreciated much more by the average visitor than is Mongolian kumiss.

Because of their strangeness to our culture, some of the major exports of Tibet are of interest. They are yak tail, camels, musk, bear bile, deer horn, mice, incense, medicinal herbs, mules, marmot fur and that well-known commodity, gold.

Buddhism has permeated every facet of life in Tibet. It wraps the people like a cloak and is three-quarters of their culture. Prayer flags wave from every possible high point, and prayer wheels are always turning, kept going by a flick of the wrist. Inscribed on the wheel is "Hail to the Buddha in our hearts." Every home and nomad tent has a yak-butter lamp that is never allowed to die out. 'Kjangchang,' or prostrating oneself, is commonly seen at shrines and temples and is a popular activity during the months of Buddha's birth, the fourth month of the year. Prostrators throw themselves face down upon the ground, spread-eagled, with hands and arms outstretched. They can then arise and prostrate themselves again from the place where their hands have last touched the ground. Supplicants often do this in a clockwise direction around a monastery or sacred place. They believe that they are revolving around Buddha in the way planets move around the sun.

A charming Tibetan greeting and show of respect is the gift of a white ceremonial scarf called a 'khata,' during visits to monasteries or shrines. It is also offered during marriage and death ceremonies.

The winter residence of the Dalai Lamas crowns Potala Hill, or Red Mountain, in Lhasa. It is without doubt one of the most impressive religious monuments of the world. As an architectural achievement the Potala has been said to equal the building of the Egyptian Pyramids. Built of wood, earth and stone, it is 13 stories high. There are more than 1,000 rooms, 10,000 shrines and 200,000 statues. No steel or nails were used in the construction of this monument to Buddha. The huge stones were carried on the backs of donkeys or people, since there were no wheels when the Potala was built. On the top floor are the apartments of the present Dalai Lama, left as they were 'when the clock stopped' and he fled the country in 1959.

This 'Land of Snows' is a land of legend. A favorite is the tale of a Christian monk who found himself in a country called Shangri-La. (Even a movie, *Lost Horizon,* was based on it.) The monk attempted to convert the people he found there but was himself converted to Buddhism. He is said to still be alive, 200 years later. Another legend says that somewhere north of Tibet there is a wondrous, misty land surrounded by impenetrable snow-covered mountains. Its name is Shambhala with a city called Kalapa. Poverty, sickness and crime are unknown in this land, and people live to be over 100 years old. About 300 years from now, according to the legend, Lhasa will be covered with water, and war and chaos will pollute the earth. When the last barbarian thinks he has conquered all men, the mists will rise and the King of Shambhala will ride forth, destroy the forces of evil and a new Golden Age will reign for 1,000 years.

Tibetans are a gentle people who abhor violence against any living creature. Perhaps someday they will again be able to live in 'Shangri-La' by regaining control of their beloved homeland.

Tibetan Ethnic Dress

Woman's Baku

This woman's long, sleeveless jumper dress is called a 'baku.' The apron is a 'punther.' It was a gift of Madam Tendu-Fla of the Windamere Hotel in Darjeeling, India. She loved the baku, her native dress, and we saw her wear it all the time we were in Darjeeling. The fabric is a dark gray synthetic, with an apron that has horizontal stripes in red, black and greenish blue. There are metallic triangles at the waist of the apron where the ties are attached. A fullness above the waistline of the jumper is used for carrying packages and is typical of Tibetan ethnic dress. Since all Tibetan women wear aprons, a sash is not needed to reinforce this carrying pouch. The blouse is of green silk with long sleeves and a soft collar.

A pure silver key ring with nail clipper, nail cleaner and a tiny spoon to clean the ears makes an interesting piece of jewelry. It is secured to the dress by a hook. Five turquoise and two coral stones decorate this unique piece.

A large ring worn on the first finger of the right hand is a Tibetan engagement ring. It was found in an antiques shop in Srinagar. It is not of great value, and the stones are glass, but the type is unusual and difficult to find today.

With this baku, ornamental boots can be worn indoors. They are of wool and reach halfway up the calf of the leg, with multi-colored braid trim down the back. There is floral embroidery in blue, pink and white on the toe. The sole is white and about an inch wide, with three layers of leather, all stitched on with heavy woolen thread.

'Sambo' is the name of the hat, which either a man or woman can wear. It has a six-inch crown, covered in a metallic cloth with rick-rack braid. There are four flaps covered with a soft, brown fur, one each in front and back and over each ear.

Young Girl's Dress

This small, pink satin, sleeveless garment is for a young girl. The textile is Chinese satin, with a pattern of circles in an Oriental design. The dress is worn without a belt or apron. Apparently young girls do not carry enough parcels to need a carrying pouch. The blouse is a sheer blue-green silk chiffon with a satiny narrow stripe. The sleeves are long and there is a soft, rolled collar.

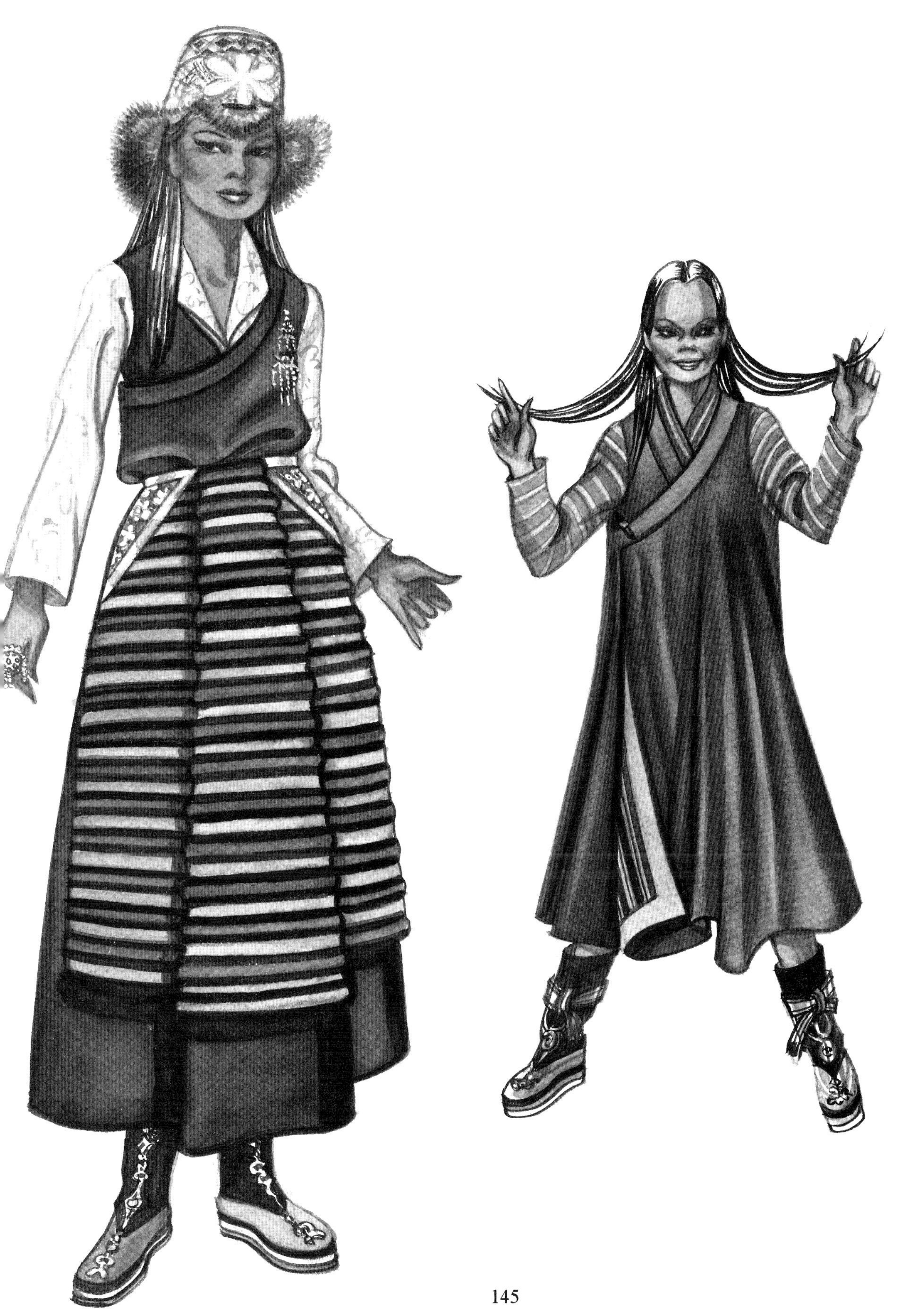

Man's Chuba

The man's ethnic dress, a 'chuba,' is of brown satin with embossed Chinese medallions. Bright-blue silk lines the collar, the neck opening, the cuffs of the long sleeves and the ties at the waist on the right side of the garment. Typically, a loose fold makes a pouch when the robe is tied. A red sash is 45 inches long and makes the pouch more secure when wound around the waist.

Boots with a decorated band at the top are worn with regular men's trousers. The red string hat is round, with a four-inch fringe falling from the brim. This hat can be worn by either a man or a woman. It is held on the head by metallic cloth bands.

The Tibetan articles of clothing were found in Lhasa, Tibet, when my husband toured that country.

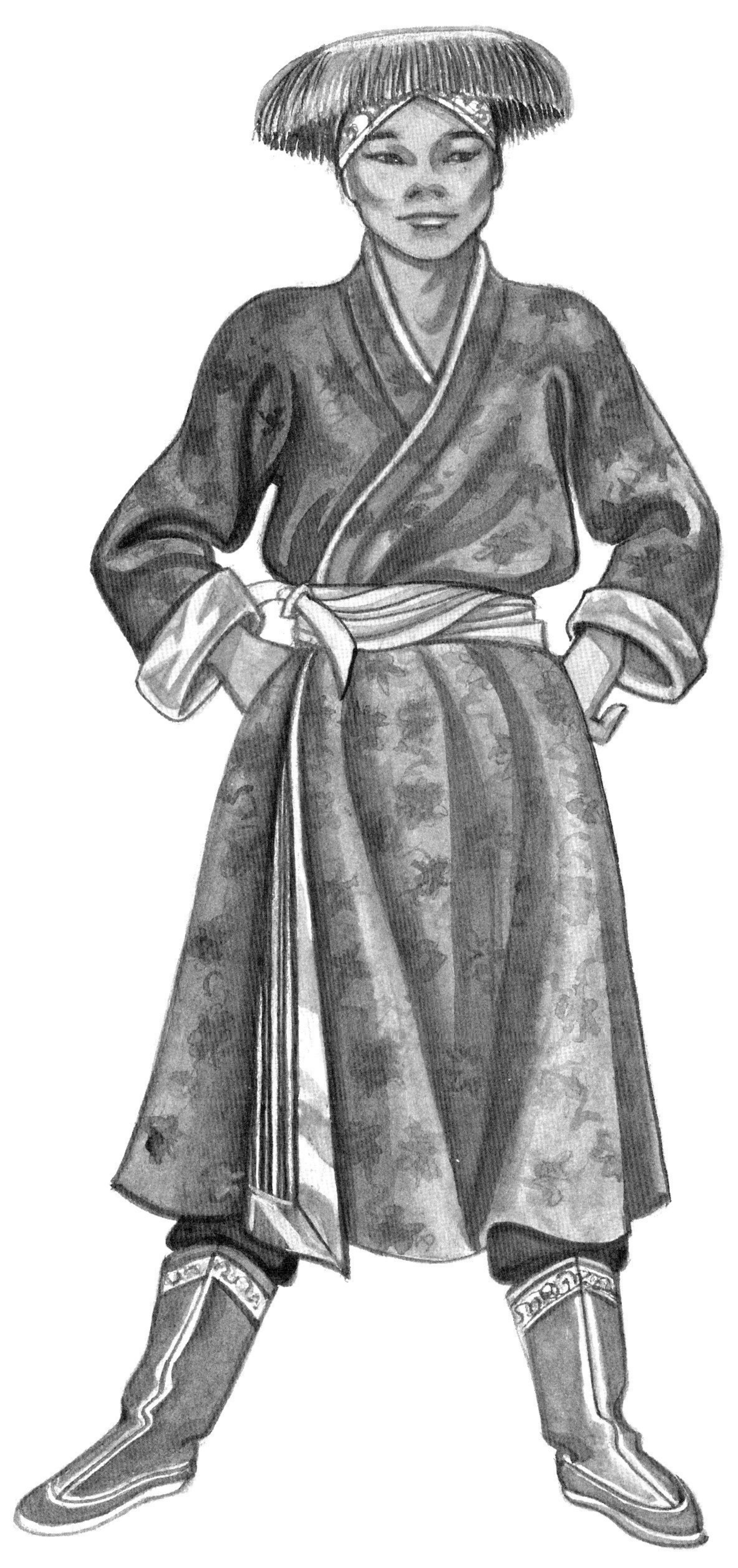

Tibetan Buddhist Monk's Robe

Our monk's robe is an important addition to the collection. It was acquired with the help of the Office of Tibet in New York, taking a full year of persistent effort before the robe was in our hands.

We went to a program given by Tibetan monks who were touring the United States. They were very friendly and helpful when they understood that the religious robe of their beloved, lost country would be exhibited in a case in a museum in America. They allowed us to take pictures so that we would know how to wrap the costume properly.

This outstanding acquisition consists of a top, skirt, shawl and a wonderful hat. The top, skirt and shawl are made of a dark red synthetic material and the hat is the color of gold. The top is shaped like a T-shirt with short, cap sleeves with blue binding. The skirt is a tube, one and one-half yards wide and two yards long. It is folded into three pleats, two in front and one in back. The shawl is over three yards long, intricately wrapped around the body and draped over the left shoulder. The body of the hat is made of a deep-pile fabric, with an ornate crown and fringe of heavy gold-colored thread. Ordinary men's sandals are worn.

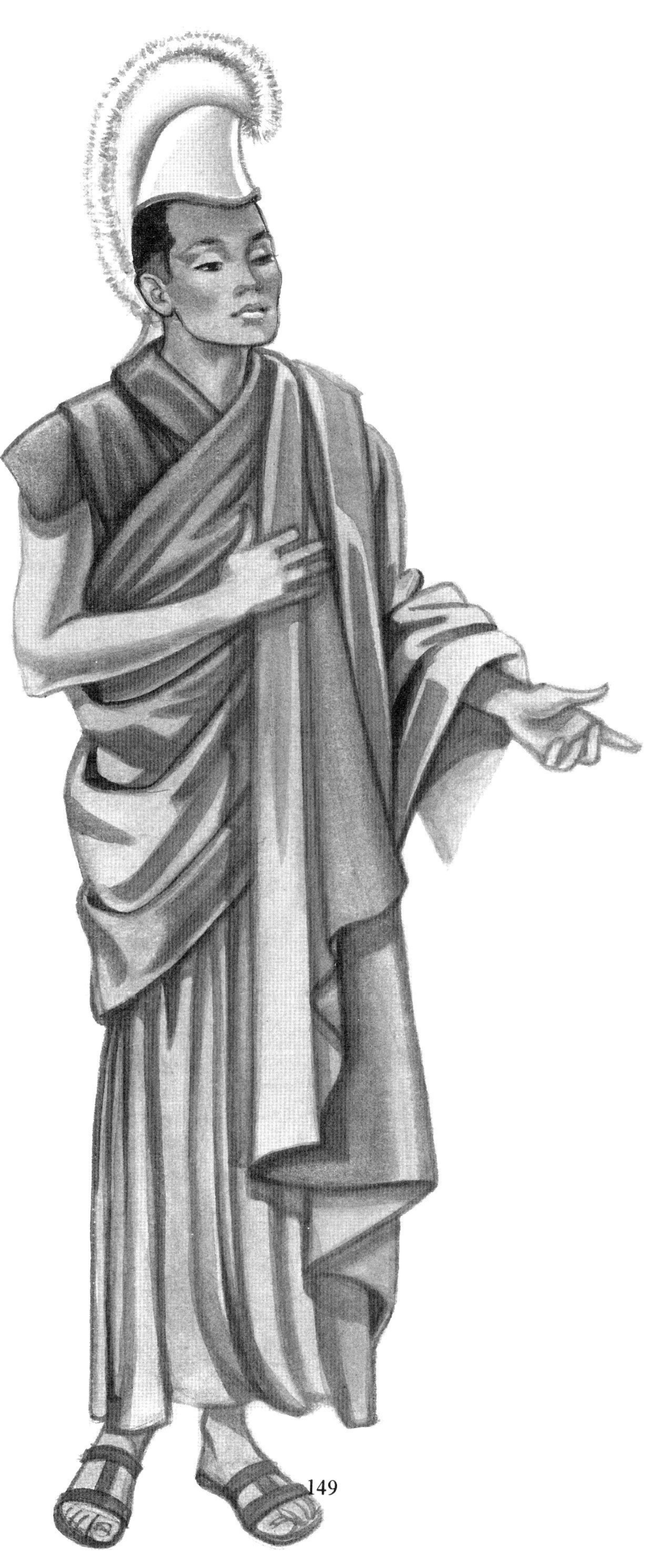

Mongolia

Mongolia, also known as Outer Mongolia, is in east central Asia.   It is bordered on the north by Russia and to the south by China. The Gobi Desert cuts a wide path across this southern border. The country is twice the size of Texas, with a population one and one-half times that of Houston. Ulan Bator is the capital. Nearly one-quarter of the nation's population now lives in this city. The tughrik is the monetary unit and literacy is 89 percent.

This is one of the oldest countries in the world. It reached the height of its power in the 13th century when Genghis Khan conquered China. In later centuries Mongolia bccamc a province of China, until declaring independence in 1911. In 1921 it became communist. When free elections were held in 1990, the communists were re-elected. Today, the government is described as `in transition.' Although 50 countries have diplomatic relations with Mongolia, the United States is not one of them.

Seventy-five percent of the people are Khalkha Mongolians. While the religion is traditionally Buddhist, only one of the 600 Buddhist lamaseries that were once in the country remain. Of the former 100,000 lamas, just a few hundred are left, and most of them are elderly. The problem of the 'living Buddha' was solved when no successor was found.

The indigenous religion of the Khalkhas is Shamanism. A shaman is a person believed to be able to heal the sick by appeasing the spirits in behalf of the ill person as he communicates with the world beyond. He is currently a prominent figure in both the religion and the medicine of Mongolia. It is estimated that there is one conventional medical doctor for 340 people.

Mongols have always been nomadic, moving their livestock and camps as much as 100 miles at a time, in search of better pastures. Sometimes they make as many as 10 moves a year, folding up their felt 'yurts,' or tents, and transporting them with cattle, horses, camels, sheep or goats. However, with economic change, over half of the employment is non-pastoral.

Beijing to Ulan Bator

Jo and I traveled north from China into Mongolia by train. At the Chinese border there was a delay of several hours. Not only was the paperwork copious, but the guards were slow in processing it. Also, each car was lifted while the wheel assembly was changed from the standard gauge of Chinese trains to the five-foot gauge of Russian trains used for rail travel through Mongolia. All of the car windows had been recently washed, so there was nothing to obstruct the views of the Great Wall, which we followed from Beijing on our way to Ulan Bator. We agreed that this monumental architectural achievement of nearly 2,000 years ago is equally awesome from both sides.

The Gobi is one of the great deserts of the globe. It is about 1,000 miles long and three to six hundred miles in width, mostly in Inner and Outer Mongolia. The word Gobi means 'waterless place,' and much of it is bare rock, not sand. Wild camels, horses and asses roam free, but vegetation is scarce. There were occasional clusters of felt yurts when we reached Outer Mongolia, and our train was raced once by what appeared to be youngsters molded to their small ponies. Had it been a short race, they might have won.

It was here that we met Eva and Mike (Mihaly). The train was crowded, and they were in line for a seat in the dining car. They looked very nice, and Eva looked tired. We invited them into our compartment to rest. This young couple was combining an architectural convention in

Beijing with a holiday in Mike's native Russia. They had bread, cheese and sausage with them, as did all properly seasoned travelers in this part of the world. Since our tour guide had given us a bottle of wine, we all decided it would be more fun to dine in our quarters and avoid the overworked dining car waiters. We shared pictures of children and grandchildren. Eva and Mike had two beautiful ash-blond little girls back home in Budapest, where their grandparents were sharing care-taking. We even talked politics, or rather, I did, while Jo kicked me under our small window table. However, they seemed as eager to hear about our culture as we were to learn of theirs. I suspected they enjoyed hearing a different point of view, so I ignored Jo, and we all became friends anyway.

Mike was the son of a Russian diplomat and had been raised in Africa and India. He was a communist and told us, frankly, that he saw trouble ahead for his country. Eva had a brother living in New York. She had visited him recently and had enjoyed the United States very much. We saw this couple again in Budapest, but as I often say, that is another story.

As we traveled north the skies clouded and began spitting snow. We were told that our planned trip by bus out of Ulan Bator into the Gobi Desert might be canceled. We would hate to miss what was most kindly described as the 'greasy' taste of kumiss, which is brewed from fermented mare's milk, and must be tried by all visitors. And who ever heard of visiting Mongolia without being in one of those felt yurts the Mongols live in while in camp?

The warning turned into reality, and the next morning the ground was covered with snow, so driving would have been hazardous. However, our local guide in Ulan Bator turned out to be exceptionally knowledgeable about the history and culture of the area. She was a Deel and loved the idea of her native costume being shown in an American museum. She promised to take us to the very best places in her city to find ethnic dress. We would go where the natives shopped. She herself wore a becoming version of the deel, with a magnificent fur coat and hat. We noticed that the wearing of animal furs did not have the stigma in cold Asian countries that it has in the West.

Is There a Shaman in the House?

The Mongolian guide and I went shopping. Jo did not feel well and decided to remain in bed. We found excellent examples of the dress of a Deel woman and man, as well as Buryat costumes for both sexes and perfect accessories of all kinds. I was enchanted by the beautiful, pointed satin hats of the Deel men and the tasseled ones of the women. A Mongolian wrestler's suit and a bonanza of other treasures exceeded my expectations.

Upon returning to our room, I found Jo coughing constantly, and she felt alarmingly warm. Having felt the foreheads of many children and grandchildren, I considered myself an expert and pronounced her very ill. This was the first time that either of us had been seriously ill on a trip, and it could not possibly have been at a worse time. Without an American embassy we had no way of locating a good doctor. Our guide assured us that she knew of a top-notch shaman, but Jo made her own decision. She said that as a good Lutheran she did not need a shaman to appease any bad spirits in her behalf, and that she had no intention of being left behind the next morning. She suggested that I go through my medicine case and find some of those antibiotics I was always reminding people to take along. Luckily, I had some extras. Jo assured me that she wasn't allergic to them, and the next morning she was comfortably ensconced in our train compartment, sipping hot tea. By the time we reached our next stop she pronounced herself well, and she was!

The Khalkha Mongols of Mongolia

Man's Deel

This man's ethnic dress, or 'deel,' is made of fine quality wool. It is a coat-type garment, calf-length, worn with regular men's trousers and tied with a long, orange sash. There is the Asian stiff collar and the usual left-over-right closing. Three buttons fasten the garment at the top and two at the waistline. The neck binding, buttons and buttonholes are of a red, gold and metallic fabric.

Deel and Buryat men and women all wear the same type of sash. The sashes in the collection are orange and green, and all are three yards long and over a foot wide. They are tied by holding one end and winding the rest of the sash tightly around the body. The loose end is tucked into the sash, or 'bus,' at the left side of the waist.

Mongolian riding boots called `Mongol gutal' have turned-up toes as their distinguishing feature. They are highly decorated around the top of the instep and there is a green leather strip up the front and back of the boot.

Brown quilted heavy flannel socks are trimmed with a decorated leather band at the top. These socks serve two purposes, that of protecting and cushioning the foot while the boot is being worn, and as indoor footwear in the home or yurt. They are called 'dimesiin turii.'

A spectacular orange satin hat has a wide, scalloped, black velvet brim. The satin crown comes to a point in the center and is covered with blue and gold metallic cloth.

Woman's Deel

This woman's deel is of green satin with an Oriental design of large, lighter-colored circles. It is floor length, with a high, stiff collar and a right underarm closing. There are seven button-and-braid fasteners down the right side of the garment. An inch-wide band of metallic fabric decorates the long sleeves at the wrists.

The hat is a green satin skullcap trimmed with an orange metallic cloth band around the hairline. Four narrow strips from the brim to the crown end at a button-like ornament on the top. A long tassel of orange yarn flows from this button.

The ethnic dress of the Khalkha Mongols and the Buryats of Mongolia and Siberia are very much alike. They are another excellent example of the regional, rather than national, character of the folk order. Both tribes have survived governments unfriendly to individualism and have kept their identities as a people. However, the Buryats of Mongolia are more traditional than those of Russia.

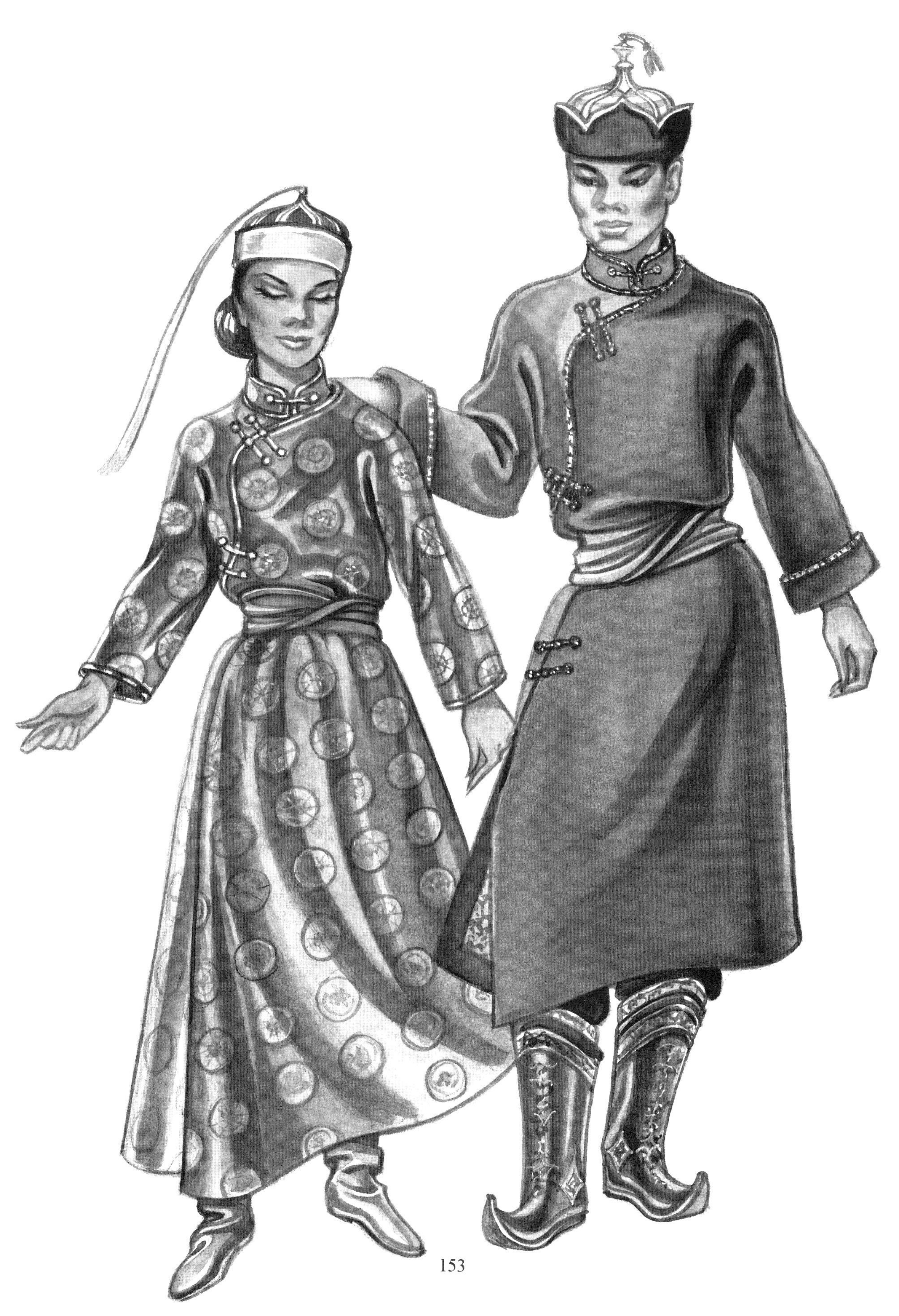

Mongolian Wrestler

The most famous celebration of traditional ways in Mongolia is the annual Naadam festival of the Three Manly Sports (wrestling, archery and horse racing), beginning July 11 of each year on National Day. This festival has recorded roots going back 2,300 years, with wrestling being prominent since ancient times at religious festivals. All the horse-racing contestants are children from seven to twelve years of age who race cross-country for 20 miles.

At these festivals there is an impressive entry of several hundred participants, clad in their 'dzodog' and 'shudog,' or brief top and shorts. They are made of a satin fabric. The dzodog is blue with long sleeves. The stomach and chest are bare. The shudog is red. Embroidery in gray yarn outlines both garments around all edges, with a large diamond-shaped embroidered figure in the center. Ties made of heavy, braided yarn with tassels on the ends hold the garments on the body.

Finding this unusual example of athletic wear was an unexpected stroke of luck, due to our clever Mongolian guide. Unique to the world of sports, this wrestler's outfit is well known among professional athletes.

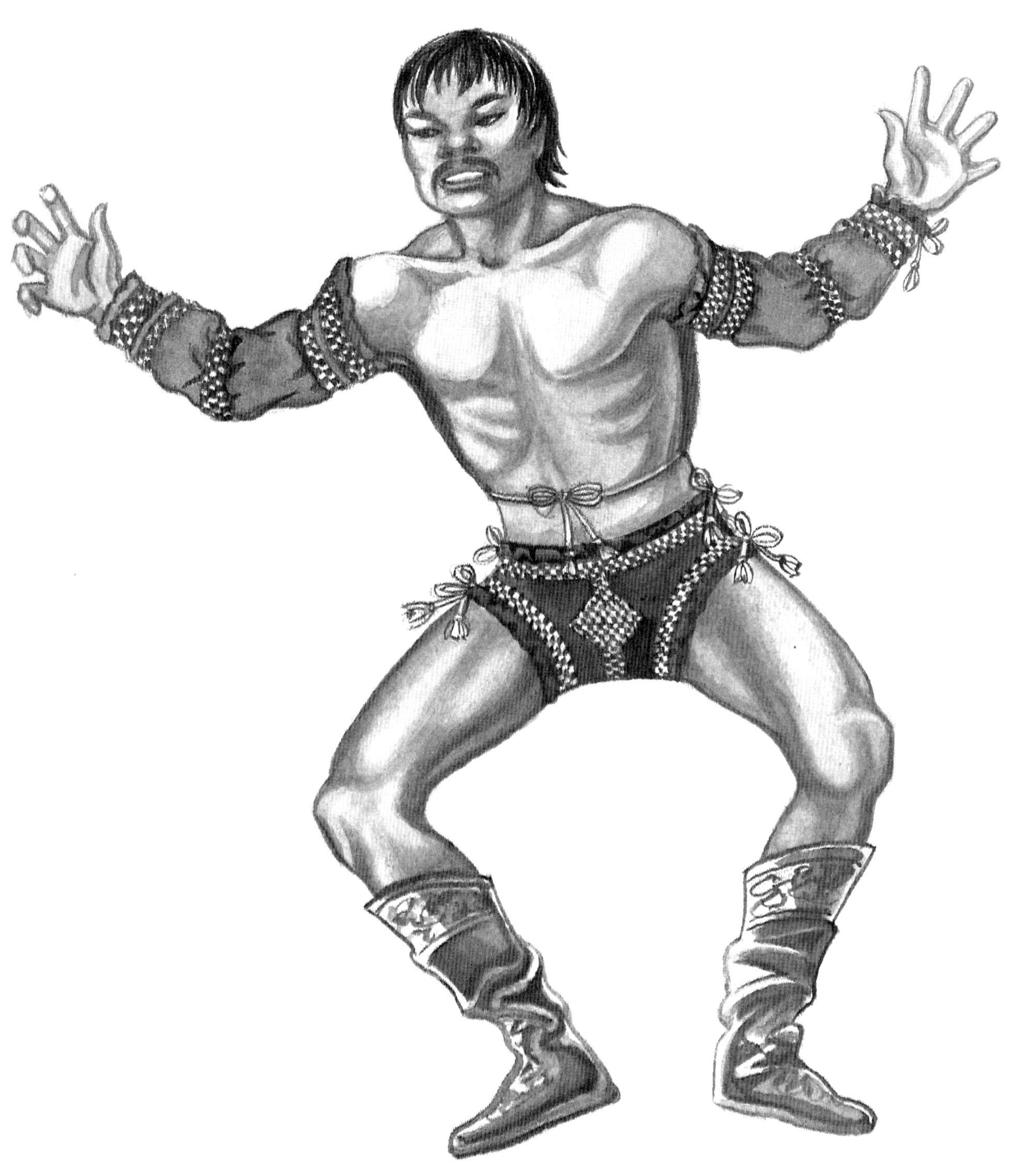

Russia is a riddle

wrapped in an enigma.

Winston Churchill

The Russian Federation

The Russian Federation, although it comprises 76 percent of the area of the former Soviet Union, is still the largest country in the world. The population is almost 150 million, and it stretches from Eastern Europe across Northern Asia to the Pacific Ocean, covering more than six and one-half million square miles. It is almost double the area of the United States, which has 100 million more people. Moscow is the capital, and the currency is the ruble. Literacy is 99 percent. After 1917, all religion was discouraged, and it is estimated that 25 percent of the people are Russian Orthodox and 60 percent are nonreligious at the present time.

In the ninth century the first Russian state was established by Scandinavian chieftains. In the 13th century the Mongols overran the country, and in 1480 Russia freed itself. Ivan the Terrible was the first czar and Peter the Great founded the Russian Empire in 1721. Vladimir Ilyich Lenin led a coup in November of 1917, and the country came under communist control. The hammer and sickle flag flying over the Kremlin was lowered and replaced by the Russian flag on December 26, 1991, ending the domination of the Communist Party over every aspect of Russian life since 1917. This federation now consists of 20 autonomous republics, 49 oblasts and six krays.

We made three trips to Russia in four years, and had many interesting experiences in our search for ethnic dress in this huge, militarily powerful, overwhelming and sometimes disturbing country that was the Soviet Union.

Russia, September 1983 . . . A Surprise Ending

We knew before we went to Russia that there might be problems ahead. A South Korean 747 had wandered off course and Russia retaliated by shooting it down, killing all aboard.

We had around-the-world tickets and multiple visas, all paid for. Jo, Grace Taylor and I planned to hit the really `way out' places this time. Jo and I were grandmothers, and Grace was planning to retire, turning her travel agency over to her daughter. To see it all we had to keep moving; after all, it is a big world out there.

Russia was our goal, and we were leaving in just a week. My Marine son said, "Don't go, Mom." After years in Vietnam he had a dim view of communist governments. My husband asked, "Can you get your money back?" We checked and found that if we decided to drop out now we would lose everything, because it was too late to cancel. However, if the State Department were to say it was not safe, we'd get every penny back. What a dilemma! We knew better than to ask the opinion of our friend, a professor of Russian Studies. Four years before, when we'd planned a trip to Afghanistan, and the American ambassador was assassinated, the professor had advised us not to risk traveling there. Tourist safety turned out not to be an issue, and our only chance thus far had been thwarted.

Our plan was to spend several days in Copenhagen, Denmark, before going on to Leningrad. We would check with the State Department while there. At least we'd get that much of a trip, and Jo wanted to purchase some silver bracelets at Georg Jensen's like the ones she'd lost. (These were very special bracelets her husband had given her on their last trip together, before he became terminally ill.) Also, we wanted so much to stroll the beautiful Tivoli Gardens once again. Grace would meet us in Moscow. She had already been to Leningrad and wanted to visit friends in London. She would also bring the additional tickets and visas that had been slow in arriving.

Nina was our guide in Leningrad. She was a nice girl, and we had lots of fun with her. We did all the tourist things . . . museums, churches, Petrodvorets, (built for Peter I in 1721, with its galaxy of fountains). Since we didn't want to miss a thing, we went to the Peter and Paul prison, which was a czarist prison. Communists didn't show off their own prisons, of course.

We were enjoying ourselves immensely, until we ran into a Colorado friend who had flown to Russia in a private plane for a banker's convention. He hailed us and asked, "Have you heard? No commercial planes will be flying into Russia starting tomorrow. I hope you have your own plane."

We weren't bankers and there were no private planes in our lives, but we were leaving the next day for Tashkent, which was within Russia, so we didn't have a problem. It did seem strange, however, that we hadn't heard a word about this, either in the papers or on television. We could see by the look on Nina's face that she was shocked. Our banker friend assured us that he would tell my husband that we were safe - so far. We decided not to worry. There was a wonderful adventure ahead, the celebrated night train from Leningrad to Moscow, with a first-class compartment. Grace was to arrive the next day on Aeroflot. Surely Russia wouldn't stop flying its *own* planes.

That train ride was a memorable experience, the ultimate of luxury for Russia. It lived up to its reputation, except for one small detail . . . the latch on our door was not working properly, and we got locked in. No one could hear us pounding; the train was noisy, and the soundproofing in our compartment was complete. A note shoved under the door finally brought the 'car lady' who fixed everything and brought us hot tea. We made it in style into Moscow (properly pronounced Mosco, with a long o, our guide told us).

The Intourist Hotel was across the street from KGB headquarters, and we could see the ornate towers of the Church of St. Basil the Blessed in Red Square. We settled in and worked on reservations, deciding to take a short tour to a lesser museum that day, saving the big sightseeing trip around Moscow so Grace could go with us the next day.

When we arrived back at the hotel the phone was ringing. It was the American Embassy, with a cable from Grace, informing us that she could not get out of London. Aeroflot would not honor her ticket. The British were the first to stop flying into Russia because of the bombing of the 747, and she could not even get to Paris or anywhere from which to fly into Moscow. She was trapped. And so were we! The cable concluded, "Tell the ladies to leave!" She didn't say how.

We had found a note on our door telling us that the Russian government was warning all guests to leave their rooms when their reservations expired. No extensions would be given. Any luggage found in the room would be removed to storage (wherever that was). Our reservations were to end the following afternoon, when we were to leave for Tashkent.

No money would be refunded from the expensive tour we had booked for the next day. We knew enough to not even bother thinking about that. It was going to be necessary to watch our expenses. We had no plane tickets to anywhere, since Grace was to bring them. But that evening was not wasted; it turned out to be very interesting and exciting. The American girl who had called us from the embassy lived near our hotel, and our Moscow guide lived in the same hotel, so we all got together and talked far into the night. We learned that our embassy people were very nervous because there were 10,000 American tourists in town, and when their reservations expired they would expect their embassy to take care of them.

Our new friend told us to be at the Aeroflot office by eight the next morning. It was close enough to walk. Still there was not a word on television. Americans are not prepared for dead silence in the news media about important issues. Jo said not to worry, that God would take care of us. She dropped off to sleep immediately. I envied her her faith, but I had a less restful night. At 5 a.m. I was up packing and woke her. She informed me that having a nervous breakdown was not going to solve anything.

By 8 a.m. we were at the airline office door, ready to battle the mob. The sign said it opened at 9 a.m.. Just a few Russians (no panicked tourists) were waiting. It was cold, even with our indispensable long underwear on. We saw people drinking coffee in the small hotel next door, but they wouldn't let us in because we didn't have the necessary hotel card. A few more people arrived by 9 o'clock, but no one spoke English. Once we finally got inside the Aeroflot office a pretty blond girl wanted to know why we were changing our plans, adding that it wouldn't do any good, because everything was 'booked.' That did it! I decided to continue with my nervous breakdown . . . what did we have to lose? In a very loud voice I said, "Don't tell me that even you don't know that international flights aren't coming into Russia."

Her answer was "Shhhhh," and in a low voice she asked if we would like to go to Frankfurt that afternoon on Lufthansa. We were weak with relief, but it wasn't over yet. They didn't take American Express. Luckily, Jo had a Visa card, so we got our tickets, rescued our luggage and sat in the lobby of our hotel waiting for our ride to the airport.

No one seemed to know about the flying ban . . . not even the girl at the Intourist desk. She didn't say a word when we told her, but when we left her, she picked up the telephone and talked excitedly for a long time.

There was Red Square and the Armoury, that magnificent museum in the Kremlin, just a few blocks away, but we felt it was unwise to leave the hotel and our luggage. After a five-hour wait, our taxi finally arrived.

The Sheremetyevo Airport was bedlam. Everyone there knew what was happening and lines of people fighting for tickets stretched for what seemed like miles. We thankfully got on the last Lufthansa plane to land in Moscow for the duration of the strike, leaving hundreds of frantic people behind us.

"Thank God! Where are you?" my husband yelled over the phone.   We were relaxing calmly in what seemed to us the most beautiful hotel in the world, the Intercontinental on the Main River in Frankfurt. The TV was blasting the news about the problems tourists were having in Moscow. We were later to learn that our plight made the papers at home several times.

We didn't want to go home yet. We knew we'd get a full refund, and both our Visa and American Express cards were good here, so we chose Italy by train. We didn't even need an Italian visa. Lufthansa was sympathetic to our plight and obtained small, inexpensive, delightful hotel rooms, with train tickets from Venice to Florence and on to Rome.

In Rome we re-lived history in the Colosseum, a huge amphitheater, built in the first century, where hand-to-hand combat was engaged in between gladiators and between men and animals. We visited the subterranean cities that were the Christian catacombs and the Pantheon, dedicated to 'all the gods.' How thrilled we were to see Michelangelo's ceiling fresco in the Vatican's Sistine Chapel. The artist began this painting in 1508, and when my husband and I first saw it in 1967, it was faded by more than 450 years of aging. Now, 16 years later, Jo and I saw it as it was being restored to its former brilliance.

After tossing some coins in Trevi Fountain, we did what any discriminating women would have done: We bought Italian shoes from a shop near the Spanish Steps.

When we were ready to leave Rome, a three-block ride from the hotel to the train station was a surprise, since on our arrival that same trip in reverse had taken over an hour and lots of liras. When we had not reacted to the taxi driver's casual remark that our hotel was a long distance from the station, he'd made the most of it!

After Rome, we went to Morocco, but that's another story.

Second Trip: Eastern Russia and Siberia by Ship and Train

There were many young people on the ship from Yokohama, Japan, to Nadhodka, Russia. All of them were graceful, slim, agile and long-legged in their tight jeans and heavy sweaters. How could every one of them be so beautiful? This group was the Kirov Ballet. They had been on tour and were returning to Leningrad.

We boarded in Yokohama in a rainstorm and the weather did not change until we had nearly reached our destination. The ship was a German World War II survivor and not very stable. Just a few of us showed up for meals, and Jo was not one of them. I fell off my chair one night. Fortunately, no bones were broken, because we never did see evidence of a doctor on board.

The icy-eyed bar girl told us she had no bottled water to sell us, and yet we could see it on the shelf. She just didn't like Americans. Jo bribed the room stewardess with a silver bracelet, so she brought us a huge container of boiling water which was perfect for tea and for drinking when it cooled.

She helped us with a little Russian:

    Spasiba - Thank you

    Nyet (Neeyet) - No

    Da - Yes

This wasn't for credit, so we dropped the course right there.

Because of the weather the ballet group could not practice, but when it cleared the last afternoon aboard, they played ping-pong on deck. That was pure poetry in motion. Not everyone has a chance to see members of one of the world's finest ballet companies leap for ping-pong balls.

The creaky old ship made it, luckily for us. Some time later an article in the *Wall Street Journal* reported that 300 Japanese children were rescued from that very ship when a serious problem developed in the Sea of Japan.

To Khabarovsk by Train

Jo and I had a four-bed compartment on the train and felt very lucky. Jim, our guide for the whole trip, found himself rooming with an unfamiliar woman, the wife of a concert pianist whom she was joining in Khabarovsk. She had tons of luggage, which had to be moved around to find space to sit or to go to bed. At least we had a place for Jim to sit, so he joined us for tea. The train was packed.

Apparently, when space is allotted on Russian trains, there is no consideration of gender. The next morning, Jo whispered that in the middle of the night there was a knock on our door and a young woman asked if she could sleep with us. I hadn't heard a thing, nor did we see much of her in the overhead berth. She was exhausted and slept most of the way to Khabarovsk. Her name was Betsy, and she had just left her husband and Japan after deciding to divorce. She was going home to Tennessee - the long way. She was looking for adventure, but not the kind she almost had. She had found herself in a room with a burly 'Romeo' who she said was odorous as well as boorish. His leers had so frightened her, that she was afraid to sleep. She had asked the car lady to find her a room with women. We all learned what Russian women already know . . . that traveling alone overnight on trains in that country is not without risk.

Khabarovsk

This is a major industrial center on the Amur River, in Eastern Russia. Many plush Russian jobs were located here and in Irkutsk, Siberia. Communist-party faithfuls were sent to these cities as rewards, and Americans were not particularly welcome there. We were thankful to be with a tour group. One of the men asked to disembark from our bus at an area about 10 miles from our hotel and had to walk home as no taxi driver would pick him up.

A young man named Pavel, who was in training to become a tour guide, sat behind us on the bus. He had a college degree and spoke beautiful English. It was fun sitting near him because he was always contradicting our city guide, under his breath. For example, when the 'medical school,' was pointed out, Pavel would inform us that it was a military training school. And when a very long line was pointed out as being people who wanted some special kind of scarce product, he told us that it was a vodka line. He was refreshingly frank.

To Irkutsk on the Trans-Siberian Railroad

On this train we were not allowed to linger in the aisle outside our compartments. I was on my way to get water for tea, enjoying the view of the dense forest outside the aisle window, when a wooden log structure came into view. It looked like the pictures I had seen of stockades built by settlers of the American West, as protection against the Indians. Those walled compounds had to be the Siberian prisons we had heard so much about. There were gun turrets at the corner of each of the four walls. Now I knew what we were not supposed to see. A harsh voice reminded me of where I was, and I dashed to my room and shut the door. Jo got the hot water.

An American-flag pin always adorns my lapel while traveling, and the only unpleasantness that has ever resulted from wearing it in over 100 countries occurred in Irkutsk, Siberia. Our hotel had a lovely park with a path along the Angara River. It was great to be able to get a morning walk again after all those days on ship and trains. However, young couples pushing baby carriages along the river path covered tiny faces with a blanket so that I could not see them. It must have been that pin! I got the message.

Irkutsk is a surprisingly modern city. Many of the apartment buildings looked quite new and each was loaded with television antennas. This was a city of well-dressed people. The women wore beautiful fur coats and hats and custom-made high-heeled boots. Jim said, "If I didn't know better, there are times when I'd think I was in Paris."

We went to a circus-in-the-round and sat in the top row. The women were dressed in cashmeres, Scottish plaids and, of course, many kinds of furs. Men wore tailored leather jackets, and little girls looked like they were dressed for a party in black velvet frocks and big white bows in their hair. The teenagers looked much like teenagers everywhere.

In every country we have visited with the possible exceptions of Myanmar, Bhutan and some Muslim countries, teenagers were dressed similarly. A party was in progress in our hotel in Irkutsk, Siberia, and the teens looked exactly like groups of young people I have seen at the homes of my grandchildren. Their hairstyles were the same, and the music as ear-splitting. Western influence, with the help of Hollywood and television, is causing Westernization of dress all over the world. Conformity is a 'must' for teenagers and even younger children.

Lake Baikal

This lake in western Siberia is the world's deepest. Its depth is 5,315 feet, and it covers 12,162 square miles. It is said to contain about one-fifth of the fresh water on the earth's surface.

In 1970 there were approximately 315,000 Buryats living in Siberia, about half of them in Buryatiya, which borders the eastern side of the lake. By tradition the Buryats are a nomadic, pastoral people who herd horses, sheep, goats and camels. Their religion is a combination of Buddhism and Shamanism. Their origins are not clear, but they belong to the Mongoloid group of peoples. They have ceased being nomadic and have become farmers, with most of them living in the typical run-down wooden houses of Siberian peasants.

We drove to a lovely restaurant on the shores of Lake Baikal in late fall of the year, and saw elderly women breaking the ice in ponds to do their laundry. We enjoyed immensely the delicately-flavored fish of the lake . . . a special treat of the area. We did not enjoy the ladies' restroom in the restaurant, however. It was spotlessly clean, but consisted of a very fancy marble cube over two feet high, which had to be climbed to reach the hole in the middle of the top.

Man's Ethnic Dress of Buryatiya

The dress of the Buryats is similar to that of the Khalkha Mongols. This man's costume is of dark gray wool, with the same right shoulder-closing as the man's deel, but the binding is of black satin. There is a stripe each of red and green satin across the chest of the garment, and black satin edges the calf-length hem.

Sleeves are very long, with cuffs that turn up to show a lining of bright blue plush-like fabric. These sleeves, when turned down, keep the hands warm in the bitterly cold winters. A sash, called a 'bus,' is wrapped in the same fashion as those of the deels. Regular men's trousers are tucked into the riding boots, which may or may not have turned-up toes.

Grandson Andy is pictured in this costume.

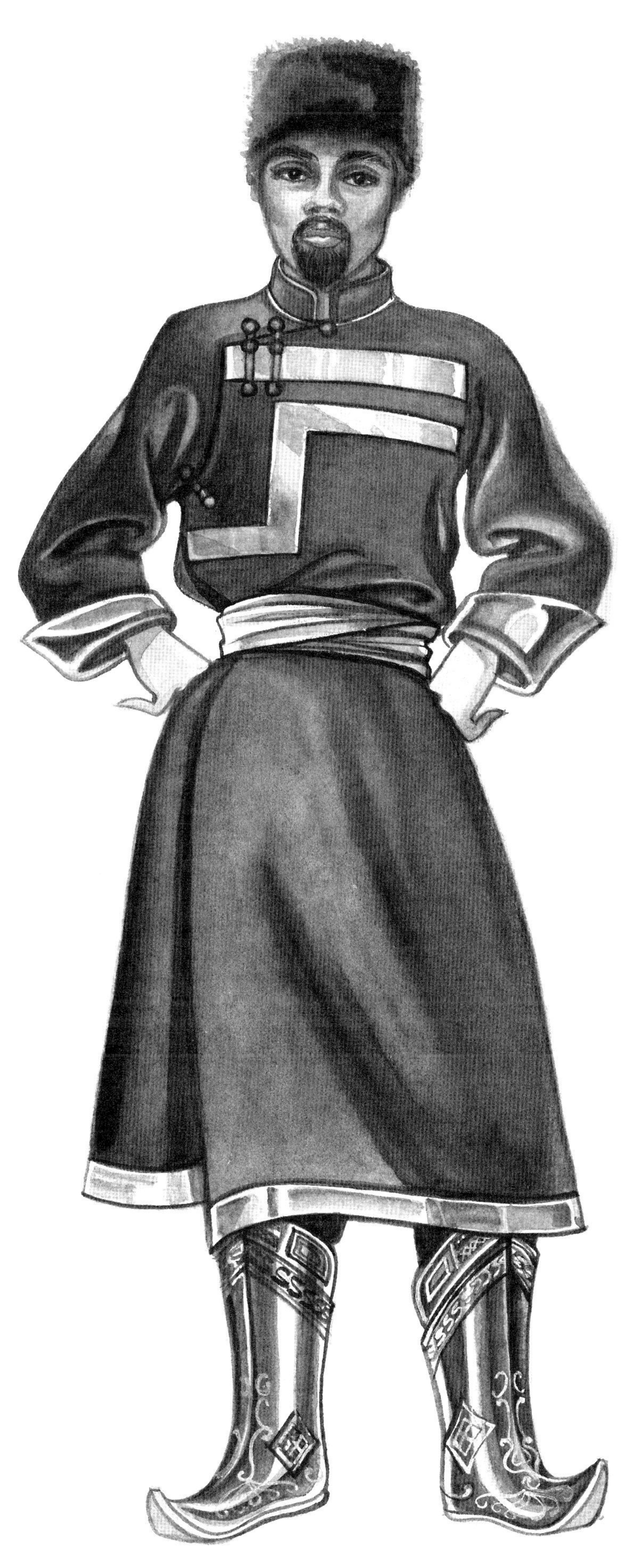

Buryat Woman's Ethnic Dress

This floor-length dress is dark red, and the synthetic fabric has a random leaf design in a darker red. The neckline has a high, stiff collar made of bands of red and silver. The same silver band trims the long sleeves as well as all dress openings. A properly wrapped sash completes this costume.

Both the man's and the woman's outfits were found with the help of our Mongolian guide, in Ulan Bator, in a shop where the Buryats of that area buy their clothing. Although we saw some natives in Siberia wearing this type of dress, we found no shops to purchase it except in Mongolia. This was another amazing example of the good luck we have had in collecting.

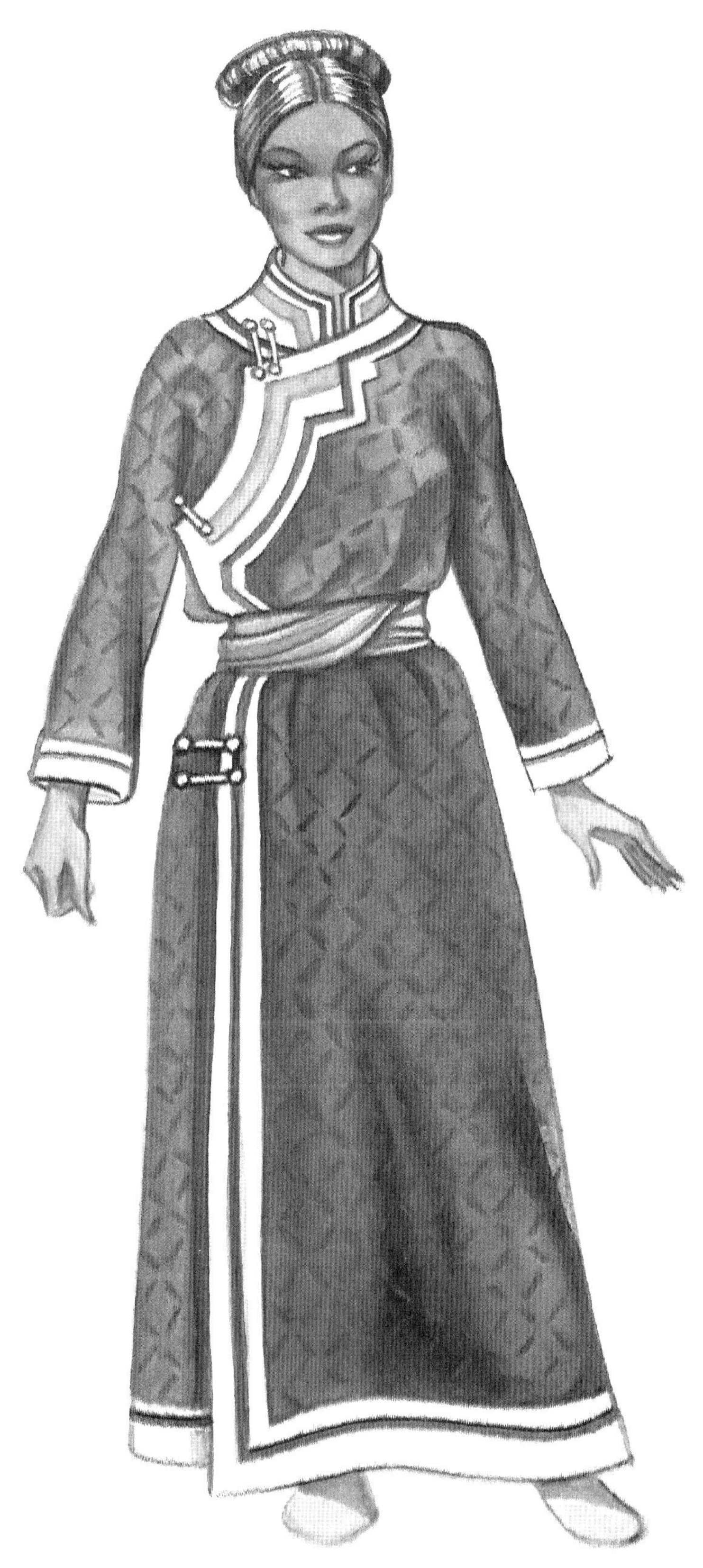

To me it seems a dreadful indignity

to have a soul controlled

by geography.

George Santayana

Moscow to Moscow - Third Trip

We took a comprehensive art treasures tour of Transcaucasia and Central Asia. Our tour guide and lecturer was a professor from the University of St. Andrews in Scotland.

The morning after our arrival in Moscow we left for Georgia, Azerbaijan and Armenia, the three collectively known as Transcaucasia. Our Russian guide, Raisa, a Georgian who lived in Tbilisi, wanted us to know that she was a good communist. She took us to an excellent restaurant for a typical Georgian dinner, which included beef wrapped in grape leaves and Georgia's fine red wine.

We saw the Roman baths and went by cable car to the top of a nearby mountain to see the view. A row of well-kept homes over a century old looked very much like historic homes we can still see in some cities in the United States.

On our drive through Azerbaijan we were told that before the revolution this country provided 51 percent of the world's oil. At the beginning of the 20th century the Baku oil field was the largest in the world. Azerbaijan is about the size of Maine. Its population is predominantly Muslim.

Armenia is a treasure house of old Christian churches and monasteries. At one partially restored Christian church a wedding was in progress. With the antiquity of the church and the panoramic background of Lake Sevan, it was a picturesque ceremony. The bride, groom and guests were in modern Western clothing. We drove to Arinberd, a town that was built in 782 B.C.

In driving around Armenia, we were often within sight of the peaks of Mt. Ararat, just across the Turkish border, where Noah's Ark is believed to have come to rest at the end of the biblical great flood. There are two peaks, about seven miles apart, the highest being 17,000 feet in altitude. This mountain is sacred to Armenians, who consider themselves the first race of people to be found after the flood. A Persian legend calls Ararat the cradle of the human race. Some explorers claim to have viewed the remains of the ark, but there is no conclusive proof of this.

Before flying to Uzbekistan we visited a ruined fortified castle, built in the first century B.C., and the cathedral at Fchmieadzin, which has been the seat of the Catholic Church of all Armenia since the 14th century. Armenia was a stronghold of Christianity, even during the anti-religion Soviet communist years.

Uzbekistan, October, 1987

Uzbekistan is the largest of the republics in the Russian Federation. It is slightly larger than California.   Alexander the Great captured Samarkand, an important city in Uzbekistan, in the fourth century B.C. Genghis Khan destroyed it in 1220 A.D., and Tamerlane, a Turkic conqueror remembered for his cultural contributions as well as his barbarity, rebuilt it in the 14th century. His goal was to make Samarkand the most beautiful city in the world, and he may have come close to that achievement. He was also responsible for constructing in Isfahan, Persia, 18 pyramids of skulls, 1,500 skulls to each pyramid. He was instrumental in bringing the Islamic faith to Uzbekistan. The people of the area are mostly Sunni Muslims.

According to our guide Raisa, there was complete freedom of religion in Russia and in Uzbekistan. Jo asked, "Then why do we never hear the call of the muezzin?" We missed the hauntingly beautiful calls to prayer heard five times a day from mosque towers in Muslim countries. Raisa answered at once, "Because they can all tell time now. No one needs it anymore."

Every time we passed a flower stall I would be handed a flower and the seller would point to my American pin with a smile. (Quite different from Irkutsk, Siberia.) We suspected that it was because the U.S. was helping Afghanistan resist the Soviets. The Uzbeks are blood brothers of the Afghans.

A dinner party was given by Raisa for our tour group at the hotel in Samarkand. It happened to be on October 19, my birthday. Another important event that day was a 500-point drop in the New York stock market. (We only learned about that later.) The dinner was memorable. It consisted of caviar, fried chicken, mashed potatoes, borscht, brown bread with butter, red cabbage and cucumbers, fresh apples with heavenly cheese, an assortment of Russia's wonderful yogurts, Danish beer, tea, cognac, chocolate candy and champagne for toasting. An Epicurean feast!

Since I maintained the party was in honor of my birthday, a speech was demanded. I managed a few non-political words, held in check by Jo's warning look. I knew better than to bring up controversial subjects while in a communist country. At the summer institutes I had attended for many years at our state university, I heard lectures by important political figures from all over the world, including Soviet defectors.

While we were in Tbilisi, Georgia, I had asked Raisa where Joseph Stalin's daughter lived when she came back to that city with her daughter after her father's death. Raisa had lived in Tbilisi, but she didn't even bother to answer my question. A bit annoyed, I casually mentioned that I'd been in Svetlana's home in Arizona. That did it! I had her attention, more of it than I wanted. Raisa kept wanting to know what was said about Stalin. "Nothing," was not an answer she could accept. My only contact with Svetlana amounted to a Coca Cola in her home on a hot day and time spent playing with Olga, her baby daughter. We did not discuss her father, although that would certainly have been an interesting subject. She had rented a home in my neighborhood for a short while after her divorce from her American husband, the ex-son-in-law of Frank Lloyd Wright. That was it!

The morning after our dinner party, our Uzbeki guide arrived with the car and driver we had requested to go shopping for Uzbek ethnic dress. Raisa had other ideas. She dismissed the girl and said she would go with us. Upon my protest the frightened girl whispered, "Don't get me in trouble."

Raisa knew where we should go and escorted us to a department store in Bokhara where there was a large selection of traditional clothing for both men and women. She stayed a few feet away, examining everything and trying to help with the choice of 'kurtas,' 'lozims' and 'chupans,' about which she obviously knew nothing. Jo and I finally wandered away to a jewelry store in the shopping center and bought some earrings for ourselves. Raisa arrived and asked to see, in fact, demanded to see what we had bought. She then spoke quietly to the manager. There is no doubt that 'good communists' take their protestors seriously, and Svetlana was an important one. Her break with her father and leaving Russia created a great furor in the country. I was happy to put an end to my involvement on that subject.

We were not able to fly to Moscow on time because of a heavy fog that enveloped most of Europe. It was wonderful to have time to see more of the incomparably beautiful mosques of Samarkand and Bokhara. Our visas expired, but Raisa said that was no problem.

When the fog lifted enough for us to fly into Moscow we had one night at the Intourist Hotel, the same one we had left so precipitously four years before. All tours were ended for the day, and we had to catch our plane the next morning. It was still daylight, and Jo and I were determined that we would not be the only tourists ever to visit Moscow three times and not see Red Square or the Armoury. They were only a block away and our luggage was secured this time.

The Armoury lived up to its reputation, with the spectacular costumes of the czars and czarinas, their horses and carriages, and fabulous jewelry. There were the Fabergé eggs, studded with diamonds and precious gems, as well as icons and paintings of former days. A feast of history and beauty.

It was getting dark and, enroute to our hotel, we turned in the wrong direction. When a policeman approached, Jo whispered, "We must have a death wish." (Remember, our visas had expired!) Clicking his heels, the dashing officer said politely in excellent English, "Ladies, please stay within the yellow line." We recovered in time to ask him for directions back to our hotel, and he walked part of the way with us.

We missed dinner, but were not too late to join the group for a performance of the Bolshoi Ballet. As we came out of the dreamlike atmosphere of the performance, the streets were filled with tanks and soldiers. Russia was not at war . . . the soldiers were rehearsing for a huge military parade. We sat on the window seats in our room and watched them far into the night. It was exciting - and troubling.

Kurta and Lozim of Uzbekistan

This beautiful example of Uzbek ethnic dress is of pure silk in a jagged, lightning pattern called 'all the colors of the rainbow.' The tunic, called a 'kurta,' has long sleeves and a turned-back collar with a yoke. It is knee length, worn straight, without a belt, over wide-waisted trousers called 'lozim,' that taper down to the ankles. A narrow, handmade braid is sewn around the bottom of each leg. The fringe at the end of the braid always ends up on the inside of the leg, where it is tied and stitched.

To Uzbeks color coordination is not an issue. What is important is the brightness of the colors. The kurta and lozim do not have to match and rarely do, except for dress wear and theater costumes. This outfit matches.

A waist-length, sleeveless vest is made of dark red velvet. The heart-shaped embroidery design around the neck and over the garment is of real gold and silver thread. The Gold and Silver Shop, where the vest was found, is well known for the beauty of its work.

The shoes and hats were found in a Beriozca Shop in the Intourist Hotel in Samarkand. They are both of purple velvet, with embroidered designs in gold and silver, with red and green velvet inserts. The shoes have open toes, and the hat is a four-sided skull cap, which perches on the head in a very attractive fashion.

Young girls in Uzbekistan were wearing their hair in many long, tight, waist-length braids. Our Uzbeki guide must have had nearly 100 braids.

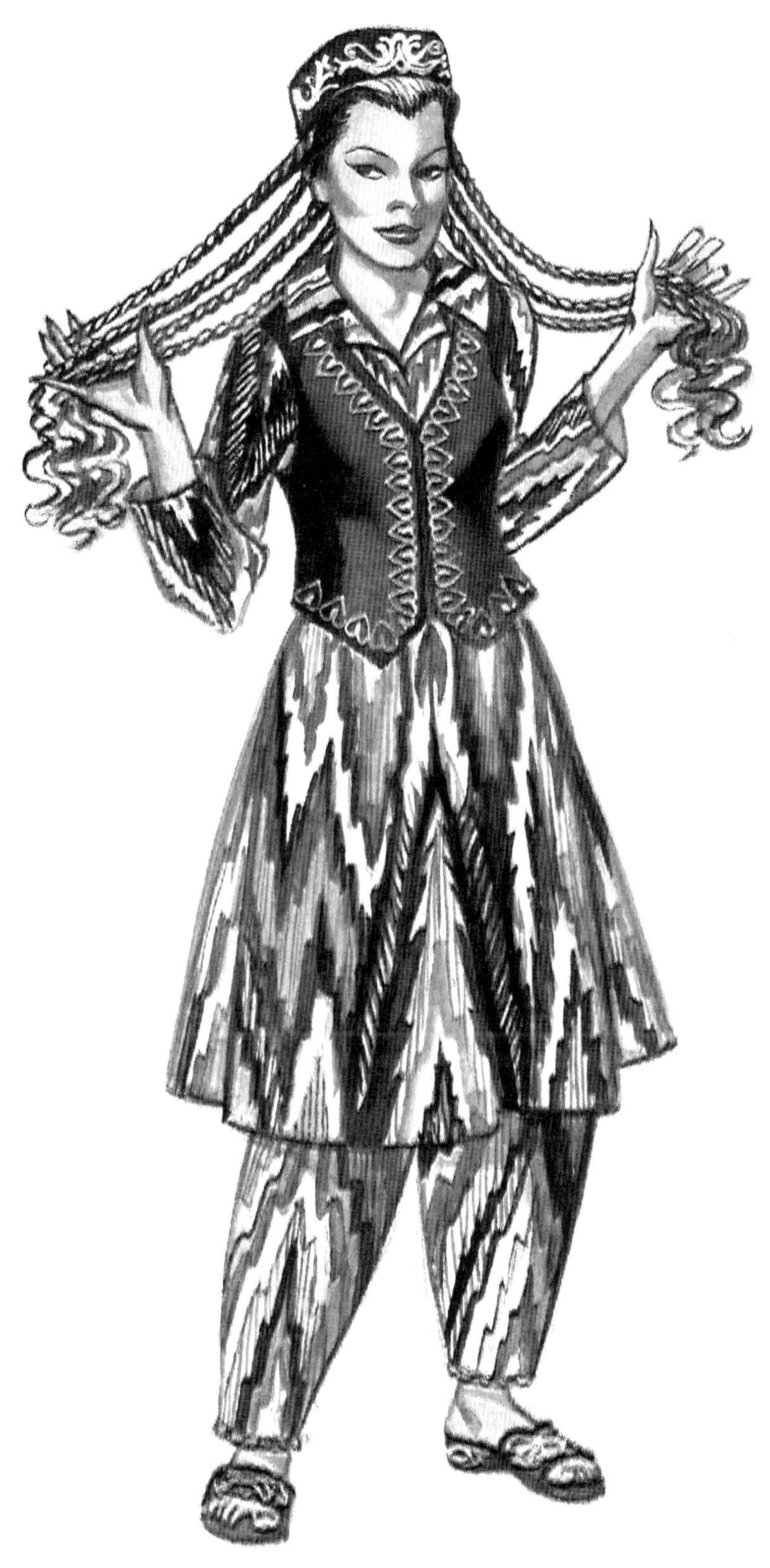

The Chupan
Man's Costume of Uzbekistan, Russia

This man's coat is made of a horizontally striped heavy silk. It is long and is worn over regular men's trousers, sometimes with boots. A two-inch band of self-trim outlines the neck, extending 18 inches down each side of the front opening. This band is outlined in purple, white and black embroidery thread, as is the entire garment. There are no fasteners on this coat. It is held together by crossing it in front and securing it with a large scarf that is used as a belt.

The scarf is a red cotton square folded diagonally and tied in front at the waist with a double knot, but not a square knot. The ends are always of uneven length. The scarf has a blue embroidered design in the center and a two-inch embroidered band around the edges that is outlined with gold thread.

A black, square skullcap is embroidered with white designs, and is several inches in height. It is worn by all Uzbeki men when out-of-doors. It is called a 'tyubetevka.' This hat was a gift from a Russian tour leader we met in Calcutta. He insisted that the wearing of this hat means that one is a member of the Uzbek tribe.

My grandson Alan is wearing this chupan.

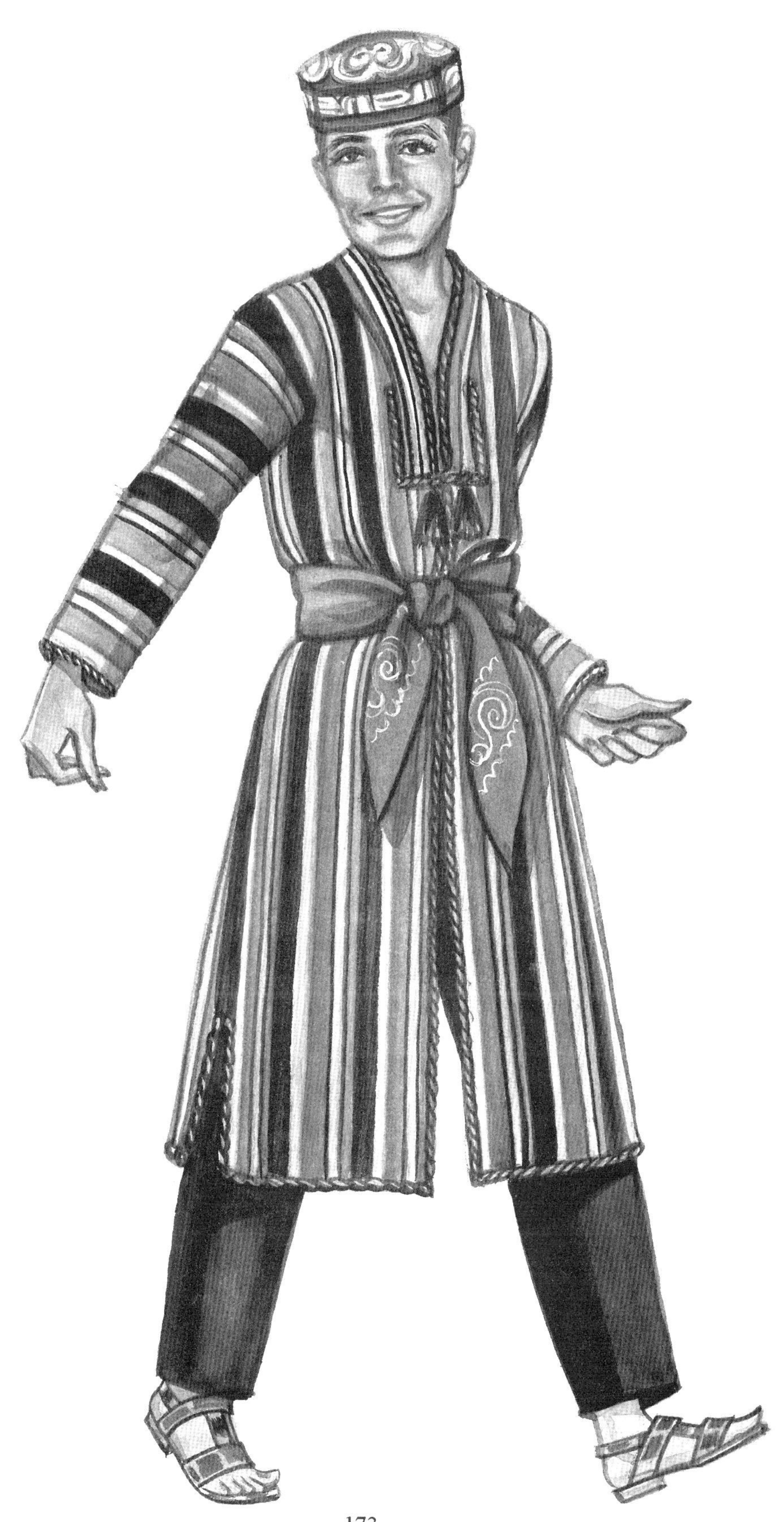

Nearly all the traditional costumes

of Eastern and Western Europe

are worn primarily for festivals

and important events.

Europe has largely replaced its ethnic dress

with modern Western wear.

Chapter Eight

Festivals of Europe

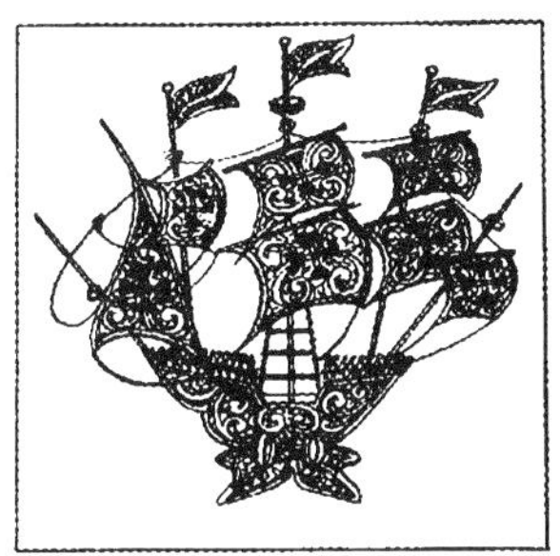

Scandinavia
Great Britain
The Netherlands
Germany
Eastern Europe

Scandinavia

The Kingdom of Sweden is on the Scandinavian Peninsula in northern Europe. It is a constitutional monarchy with a head of state and a head of government. It is larger than California, but California has more than three and one-half times the population of Sweden. The capital is Stockholm, the currency is the krona, and literacy is 99 percent. The vast majority of the population are Evangelical Lutheran, with 94 percent of the people of that religion.

The Swedes have lived in this land for at least 5,000 years, longer than nearly any other European people. They had the earliest parliament on the European continent, with all classes of society represented. By the 17th century Sweden was a major European military power. During the Napoleonic Wars, it acquired Norway, which became independent in 1905. Sweden has participated in no armed conflict since that time, maintaining neutrality in both world wars.

The Kingdom of Norway, on the west part of the Scandinavian Peninsula, extends the farthest north of any European country. It is a little larger than New Mexico, with a population almost three times that state's. The capital is Oslo, currency the krone, and literacy is 99 percent. The religion is 88 percent Evangelical Lutheran.

The first ruler of Norway was Harald the Fairhaired, or 'Finehair,' who came to power in the ninth century at the age of 10. The Vikings of Norway raided and occupied parts of Europe for two centuries. Although Norway remained neutral during World War I, it was attacked by Germany during World War II and held until 1945. After that, Norway abandoned neutrality and joined N.A.T.O. Norway's merchant marine is one of the world's largest. Norway has abundant hydro-electric resources and its standard of living is generally conceded to be one of the highest in the world.

The Republic of Finland is bounded on the north by Norway, on the west by Sweden, and on the east by Russia. It is slightly smaller than Montana, with a population six times that of Montana. The capital is Helsinki, the currency is the markka and literacy is 99 percent. The religion is 89 percent Evangelical Lutheran.

Early Finns probably migrated from the Ural area at the beginning of the Christian era. Finland became a republic in 1919, but in 1939 the Soviet Union invaded its neighbor, forcing the Finns to cede 16,000 square miles of land to Russia. In 1992 a pact was signed between the two countries. Finland is an integral member of the Nordic group of five countries, which, along with Norway and Sweden, includes Denmark and Iceland.

Scandinavian Scrapbook

A very special occasion deserves a very special celebration. Our 50th wedding anniversary was approaching and we decided to celebrate it in a different way, by taking a trip. We had never been to Scandinavia. Reportedly there was an ethnic group there that had a unique costume that had developed through the centuries and was still worn. Luck, which had not failed us yet, would help us find it. This turned out to be a good choice . . . a super-deluxe trip with super-nice people. The occasion warranted it!

Our guide Vibeke was a dream. My husband confessed to being hypnotized by her sparkling blue eyes. She was Norwegian and a "Miss Norway" 10 years earlier. She hadn't aged a minute nor had she put on one pound. She was also bright, and had planned everything meticulously.

We drove through Finland to the music of Sibelius' "Finlandia" and through Norway to "Song of Norway," reminiscent of Edvard Grieg. Vibeke had the right tape for every occasion. She introduced us to whale stew and cloudberry pie and roast reindeer. We always knew where the men were...consulting with Vibeke about the itinerary.

We went by ship from Copenhagen to Stockholm and to Helsinki, and then set out by bus for the very northern tip of the European continent, Norway's North Cape. From there we traveled south through Norway to the fjords and then to Bergen, Vibeke's home town and our last stop. This coincided with the date of our anniversary and provided a wonderful excuse for all of us, now good friends, to celebrate.

The setting was perfect! We had a tour of Vibeke's lovely home and met her charming parents. At our table in the beautiful hotel we found a magnum of champagne awaiting us. It had been sent by Grace and Claudia Taylor, from Colorado Springs...a nice touch from home. Those travel agents know how to do everything just right. After an announcement from Vibeke, the orchestra played "Anniversary Waltz" for us. I'm grateful we could still waltz! A handsome young man tapped me on the shoulder. I was flattered, until I had a few minutes to think and reality set in. When I questioned why he had asked me to dance, he replied with a smile, "You looked like a nice lady."

As a grandmother of eight and having had a bit of experience with flattery with a purpose, I asked him to tell me the real reason. "Well," he answered rather shyly, "did that beautiful girl at your table used to be 'Miss Norway'?"

Aha! "Would you like to meet her?"

"Oh, yes, ma'am, please!" Of course he would...and did. They danced the rest of the evening, and just watching them was fun for us all.

It should be mentioned that being in 'The Land of the Midnight Sun' isn't really that exciting when it's as light at 2 a.m. as it is at 2 p.m., and people are singing just below your hotel window. We oldsters needed our sleep, and North Cape, Norway, is not the place to get it in June.

The Gissi Goftee, Gapper and Nuftaga of Lapland

Lapland is a land of reindeer and cloudberries, a region above the Arctic Circle that stretches across Sweden, Norway and Finland and into Russia. The Lapps, an ethnic group numbering around 35,000, are believed to be a remnant of some archaic Caucasoid-like people who have been in this area for over 2,000 years. It is interesting to note that the Lapps are among the world's shortest people, with a mean height of five feet, while the natives of the rest of Scandinavia are among the world's tallest. There are three types of Lapp culture, mountain, coast and forest. The mountain Lapps are nomadic reindeer herders for whom the animals provide food, clothing, implements and transportation. Every year there is a reindeer roundup at which the herds are separated and marked. A high point of this event is the selection of the Miss Reindeer Roundup Queen for that year.

This costume was found in Rovaniemi, the capital of Finnish Lapland, an all-new city with beautiful, modern buildings. It sits exactly on the Arctic Circle. It was burned to the ground by the Germans during World War II and entirely rebuilt with the help of Alvar Aalto, the renowned Finnish architect.

Our Lapp dress, or 'gissi goftee,' is made of navy blue wool. The sleeves and hem are trimmed with a red stripe sewn to a red and white strip of fabric with embroidered edges. The red and white belt, or 'aveh,' was hand woven on a narrow loom. The weavers of Finland are very skilled.

Of interest to the world of costume is the fetching 'gapper,' a red woolen hat, trimmed with lace and tied under the chin. A two-foot square shawl is of silky synthetic with a red-orange background and blue flowers. The fringe is long and has five hand-tied rows. A gold-dipped silver pin, which is large, round and intricately made in a typical Lapp design, fastens the scarf. The reindeer-skin fur boots called 'nuftaga' have ties of braided yarn with tassels. They are worn over slacks or ski pants.

The Lapps are proud of their native dress, which is still worn in the countryside and in some large cities on important occasions. My husband saw this costume in the window of a folkloric shop near our hotel. By the time he had located me it was time to leave Rovaniemi, but everyone in our tour group said they did not mind waiting while the purchase was completed. As usual, they showed interest in the project. They seemed to feel that they were lucky to be able to travel and wanted others to have an opportunity to enjoy some of the cultural beauties of countries they may never get to see, except in a museum.

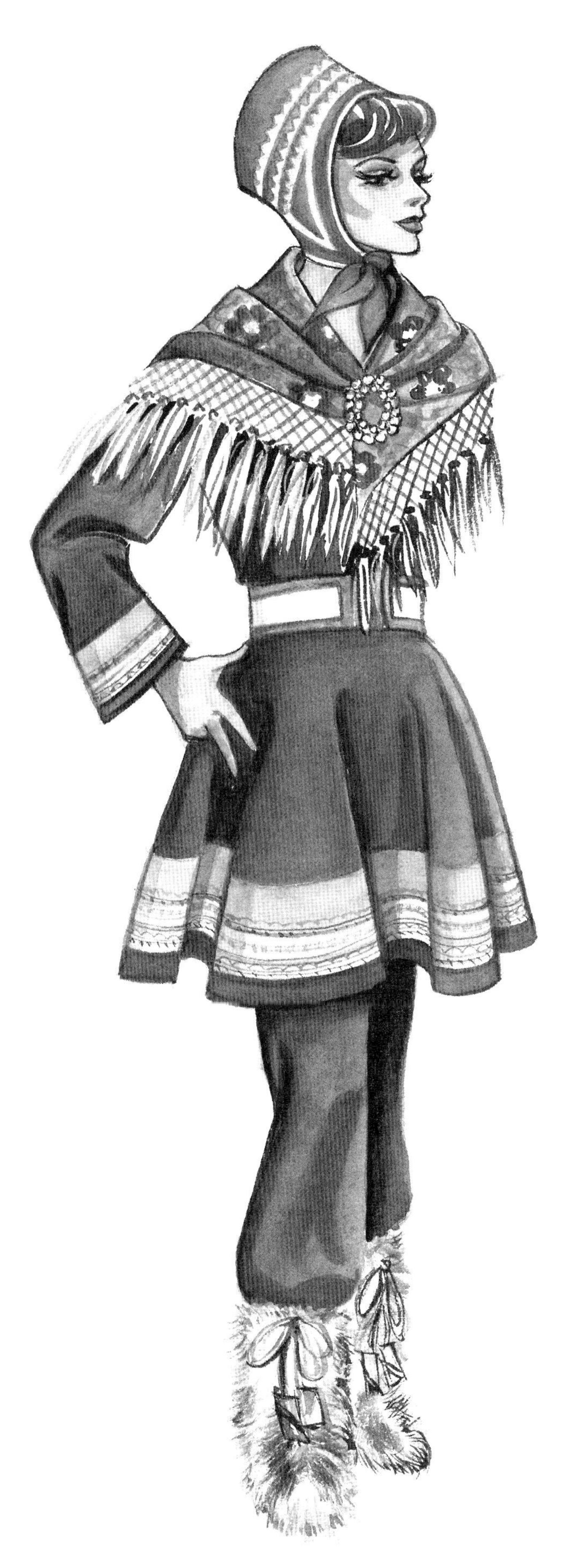

I traveled among unknown men,

In lands beyond the sea;

Nor, England! did I know till then

What love I bore to thee.

William Wordsworth

United Kingdom of Great Britain and Northern Ireland

The United Kingdom of England, Wales, Scotland and Northern Ireland cover an area about the size of Oregon, with 20 times the population of that state. The capital of the United Kingdom is London, the monetary unit is the pound, and literacy is 99 percent. The religion of the Church of England is Protestant Episcopal.

The government is a constitutional monarchy. Queen Elizabeth II is the head of state, and head of government is the prime minister. Parliament is the legislative governing body, consisting of the House of Lords and the House of Commons.

Until 6000 B.C., Britain was part of Europe. The Celts arrived 3,000 years ago and their language survives in Welsh and Gaelic enclaves. In 43 A.D., England was added to the Roman Empire. From 410 A.D., through the 11th century, Danish raiders fought for control. In 1215 the Magna Carta was signed, guaranteeing rights and the rule of law.

Under Queen Elizabeth I, England became a major naval power, which led to the founding of the colonies in the New World. In the 18th century the North American colonies were lost, but were replaced by growing empires in Canada and India. With the defeat of Napoleon in 1815, Britain became the world's leading power. Under Queen Victoria large parts of Africa and Asia were added to the Empire. In 1921 Ireland became a British dominion, an Irish Free State. Northern Ireland remained part of the United Kingdom.

Wales is a principality in western Britain, which is administered as a unit with England. It is 8,000 square miles in area, with a population of nearly three million. Cardiff is its capital. Edward of Caernarvon (1307 to 1327) was made the first Prince of Wales.

Scotland is a kingdom now united with England and Wales in Great Britain. It comprises 30,000 square miles and has a population of five million. Edinburgh is the capital. In 1603 the son of Mary, Queen of Scots, became James I of England and the crowns were united.

Castle Welsh Crafts and Cardiff Castle

The most desirable costume from the British Isles for the collection was that of Wales. A native of Scotland had promised his kilts to the museum in his will, and Britain's dress is completely Western, except for new citizens or visitors from foreign countries.

The Welsh Embassy in New York recommended a folkloric shop, Castle Welsh Crafts, in Cardiff, Wales. Not only would we be in Cardiff just one night, but to get there we were leaving Waterford, Ireland, that morning, driving to Rosslare, crossing the St. George's Channel by ferry to Fishguard in Wales, and then driving to Cardiff. This was a bus ride of nearly 200 miles. Also, it was a Sunday and we were leaving for Exeter, England, early the next morning. And that was not all!

That evening a private tour of Cardiff Castle had been arranged, with dinner at the ancient manor house, called Kemeys Manor. One could travel all of one's life without being invited to dine in the home of the owner of a real castle. Oh, well, I had at least an hour to get to Castle Welsh Crafts, buy the costume, if it was satisfactory, get dressed and get to the castle. That is, barring delay or incidents on the road or on the water. All of my costume shopping had been lucky so far, so why would Wales be different? And it was not!

We pulled into our hotel in Cardiff early. This was a 'first' for the entire trip. There is reason to suspect that our guide, who found the costume search interesting, had something to do with this.

My call to Mair (Mary in English) was recorded on an answering machine, but with my luck, I could not fail. She was waiting at the door when our taxi arrived. The costume was perfect! Mair had it made from real Welsh flannel, and it was colorful and beautiful as well as authentic. She had also made one for her small daughter, for photo post cards to be sold in the shop. That shop was a folkloric dream; the embassy in New York knew what it was recommending!

Cardiff Castle dominates the town. It seems that Henry VIII encouraged royalty to build manor houses when they found their castles very uncomfortable places in which to live. Cardiff Castle has been redecorated rather recently. Many artists have voiced disapproval of the results, feeling it should have been actually *restored*. The present owner of Kemeys Manor was among those who disapproved - quite vocally.

Since I was the only person in the group who had Welsh blood (on my father's side), our host asked my name. When I said my maiden name was Owen, he shouted, "We're related!" His name and that of his wife are Eifion and Beti Owen. Owen is like 'Smith' in the United States. Our bus driver's name was Owen also.

Have you ever taken a bus tour? If not, you have missed the opportunity to see EVERYTHING. Here is the itinerary we followed for a 21-day bus tour of the British Isles.

At the heart of a bus tour is the daily notice on the hotel bulletin board. Daily, for 21 days, it read:

"Wake-up call - 6:30 a.m.

Bags out and breakfast - 7:15 a.m.

On the bus by 8:00 a.m."

It should always be remembered that being late is penalizing at least 28 people, who by obeying the rules, were on time. One's slothfulness is not easily forgotten.

Day 1: Fly to London on an all-night flight.

Day 2: See Royal Albert Hall, Kensington's Museum, Chelsea, Knightsbridge with Harrods, Houses of Parliament and Big Ben, Westminster Abbey, Changing of the Guard, Tower of London and a cruise of the River Thames. Time in the afternoon for independent activities. (It actually said that.)

Day 3: London Stratford: Henry VIII's Hampton Court Palace, Runnymede (where the Magna Carta was sealed), visit Royal Windsor, take a stroll in the university town of Oxford, go to Sir Winston Churchill's burial place, drive to Cotswold Hills, visit Stow-on-the-Wold.

Day 4: See Ann Hathaway's cottage and Shakespeare's birthplace. On to Coventry, Sherwood Forest and York, England's most complete medieval city.

Day 5: See Hadrian's Wall, drive through Northumberland to the Scottish border, to Jedburgh to see the abbey ruins and Mary, Queen of Scots' house, the Floors Castle, and then arrive in Edinburgh in time to trace your Scottish ancestors on the archive computer at the Clan Tartan Centre (about 20 minutes).

Day 6: Princess Street and the Royal Mile, Edinburgh Castle and Holyrood Palace. Afternoon at leisure. Scottish evening ahead (optional).

Day 7: Through Fife to St. Andrews Gold Club, Braemar, Royal Highland Games and Balmoral Castle. Scenic route through the Grampian Mountains, visiting whisky distillery and a lecture on producing this drink...with samples.

Day 8: Battlefield of Culloden to Inverness, Loch Ness with its monster, Loch Oich to Fort William, then to sinister Glen Coe, where Macdonalds massacred Campbells, to the bonnie banks of Loch Lomond and on to Glasgow.

Day 9: South through Moffat's Tartan Tweed Center via Gretna Green, Lake District, Wordsworth's Grasmere. Spend time at the Merseyside Maritime Museum.

Day 10: Peak District of Liverpool, Haddon Hall, Chester on the River Dee, another optional dinner tonight.

Day 11: Follow coast of North Wales to Conway, panoramic route through Snowdonia, via Betws-y-Coed and Llanberis Pass. Caernarvan Castle, across Britannia Bridge to Isle of Anglesey to visit Llanfairpwllgwyngyllgogerychwyrndrobwllllantysilliogogogoch. At Holyhead board ferry to cross Irish Sea.

Day 12: Dublin orientation drive, Trinity College, Old Library. Afternoon at leisure. Typical Irish outing tonight.

Day 13: Across the Currah to the Irish National Stud at Kildare. Rock of Cashel, where St. Patrick preached, Tipperary, Limerick, St. Mary's Cathedral, King John's Castle and the Stone where the Treaty of Limerick was signed in 1691.

Day 14: Cross Shannon estuary by ferry, a 100-mile panoramic drive around the Ring of Kerry, after seeing audiovisual show and museum. On to Killarney.

Day 15: Clare coast from 668 Cliffs of Moher, then across the Burren to Galway. See Lynch Stone, Royal Tara China Factory, Connemara Marble Factory. Irish celebration tonight.

Day 16: Visit to Blarney to kiss Stone of Eloquence, then via Cork to Waterford, Viking stronghold. See Reginald's Tower and remains of original battlements.

Day 17: By ferry from Rosslare across St. George's Channel to Fishguard in South Wales, Cardiff Arms Park and Cardiff Castle, evening traditional Welsh fare at manor house of owner of the castle.

Day 18: Orientation tour in Bristol. Then elegant Georgian city of Bath and Roman baths, then Cheddar Gorge and King Arthur's Glastonbury.

Day 19: From Exeter to Plymouth, see Mayflower steps and lecture on Sir Francis Drake, cruise on Plymouth Sound. Cross River Tamar by ferry to smuggler's port of Looe. Return to Exeter by way of Dartmoor. Stop in quaint Weidecombe-in-the-Moor.

Day 20: Exeter to London, to Stonehenge and Salisbury.

Day 21: Home, after a night and a day on the plane.

The purpose of including this itinerary is to show just how hardy we travelers really are. At the end of the tour the guide took a poll to see who could correctly guess the miles we had traveled. One of the four teenagers on the trip guessed 120,000, while another said 250,000. (It was actually 3,500 miles.)

This trip was a real challenge, and we were fortunate no one became ill. One reason the older members of this group survived is that the bus was comfortable and not crowded. The unfortunate part was that our very well-educated guide lectured to a sleeping audience for most of those 3,500 miles.

The British Isles have much evidence of their importance in history as well as scenic interest. I've left out many memorable features, like the roads where treetops form a canopy for miles, the millions upon millions of black-faced sheep, the Scottish tattoo, the Irish papal deer, the broom, the gorse, the heather, the bracken (fern) covering the forest floor, the Roman and Norman history, World War I and World War II and how the British Isles survived . . . these are the things one remembers when rested up after a strenuous holiday.

Ethnic Dress of Wales

There is no solid evidence that this dress is a traditional costume of Wales, since it seems to have been based on the 18th and 19th century peasant dress of Britain and Europe. However, early in the 20th century, it was worn in Wales for festivals and folk dancing, and is now considered Welsh ethnic dress. It is included as such in costume collections. Because of the beautiful voices of the Welsh people, there are wonderful choral groups, many of them dressed in their 'betgwn' and 'aberpergwm.'

The breeding of sheep is one of Wales' most important industries, and wool is used in clothing. The wool flannel from which this dress is made comes from the Cwumllwchwr Mills at Ammanford. This hand-loomed wool is made in many combinations of small checks and stripes, as well as in solid colors.

The skirt of this costume is floor length and made of red flannel. The betgwn, which means bedgown, is a kind of outer garment or coat. The language of this country has spelling strange to Western eyes, and is difficult to pronounce, but very musical when spoken or sung. This bedgown has a round, lace-trimmed neck, long sleeves and four cloth-covered buttons from the neck to the waist, where there is an opening for the skirt to show through. The back is gathered and slightly longer than the front, and the hems are bound with narrow black wool. The flannel in this bedgown is of small black and red checks. There is a 'fissu,' made of white, lace-trimmed crepe, that can be worn around the neck if desired.

A shawl, or aberpergwm, is made of a yard-and-a-half square of red, black and white small-checked flannel, with self-fringe on all sides. A lace-trimmed apron made of fine white cotton with satin ties is worn over the red skirt. A black felt hat, with a seven-inch crown and a wide brim, is trimmed demurely with white lace which frames the face. Shoes with large silver buckles are worn to complete this colorful outfit.

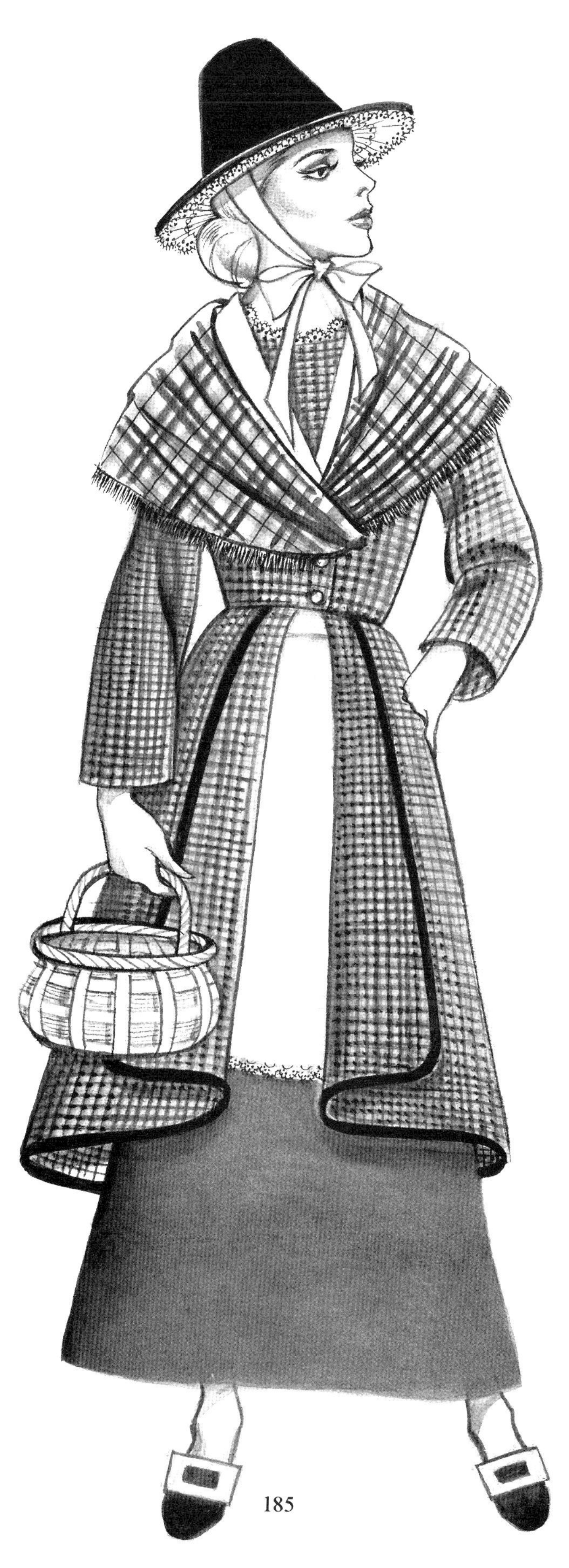

185

To men of other minds my fancy flies,

Enbosomed in the days where Holland lies.

Methinks her patient sons before me stand

Where the broad ocean leans against the land.

Oliver Goldsmith

Kingdom of the Netherlands

The Netherlands is a country on the North Sea in Northwest Europe. It is the size of Massachusetts, Connecticut and Rhode Island combined, and the population is one and one-half times that of the three states. The capital is Amsterdam, the currency is the guilder, and the religions are 36 percent Roman Catholic and 27 percent Protestant. Literacy is 99 percent.

The topography of the Netherlands is flat, with an average altitude of 37 feet above sea level, although the western part of the country is sometimes as much as 22 feet *below* sea level. Flood control and the building of dikes and sea walls, to protect the coastline against the ravaging powers of the North Sea, started as early as the end of the Dark Ages. It is now protected by 1,500 miles of dikes. Since the 12th century approximately 3,000 square miles of land have been reclaimed from the sea.

The government is a parliamentary democracy, under a consitutional monarch. The head of state is Queen Beatrix, and a prime minister is the head of government. The seat of government is The Hague.

Julius Caesar conquered this region in 55 B.C., when it was inhabited by Celtic and Germanic tribes. After the empire of Charlemagne fell apart, the Netherlands (Holland, Belgium and Flanders) split among counts, dukes and bishops. It passed to Burgundy and then to Charles V of Spain. Holland fought an 80-year war with Spain (1568-1648) for independence and freedom of religion. The rise of the Dutch Republic to naval, economic and artistic eminence came in the 17th century. This 'Golden Age' produced great artists such as Rembrandt and Vermeer, philosophers Erasmus and Spinoza, and scientist Leeuwenhoek. The country was affluent, ranking high among sea-faring nations, and becoming a world power. The East India Company was established and the Dutch East Indies and West Indies were colonized. Trade was at an all-time high. During World War II the Netherlands maintained neutrality, but they were invaded and brutally occupied by Germany from 1940 to 1945.

Horticulture, which began at the end of the 1500's with the planting of tulips, is still an important part of the economy today. Many flowers, plants and vegetables are grown in highly sophisticated greenhouses. The Flower Auction in Aalsmeer is a popular tourist attraction, along with the countless windmills that can be seen from the 3,200 miles of canals.

Woman's Ethnic Dress
from Volendam, Holland

The national character of the Dutch people is reflected in their costumes, which show considerable differences between regions and even villages. Some are still frequently worn, while others only appear at festivals or other special occasions. A costume can reveal the religion and marital status of the wearer and his or her social position. It can show whether the wearer's background is agricultural or fishing, and it can also indicate a state of mourning.

This example is probably the best known of the women's costumes in Holland today. The black wool top, worn tucked into the skirt, has a square, low neckline, outlined by inch-wide braid with woven windmills and tiny tulips. A cotton neckpiece has rose and blue flowers with green leaves.

The ankle-length skirt is of heavy flannel, with wide, orange vertical stripes, alternating with narrow red, white and blue stripes.

Six to fourteen skirts may be worn, one on top of the other, depending on the wearer's financial status. There are two aprons. The 'work' apron is of heavy cotton, with colorful stripes, while the 'dress-up' apron is of the same black wool as the top of the dress, with a wide band matching the flowered material of the neckpiece.

A narrow, hand-knitted, fringed scarf is blue with red and white design. A small hat is of starched lace, with distinctive points that are indigenous to the costume hats of the Volendam region. This costume is not complete without a two- or three-strand red coral necklace, as coral is regarded as being lucky in Holland.

Wooden clogs called 'klompen' are an important feature of the dress of the Netherlands. At one time it was the custom for young men to present clogs they had carved and decorated to their fiancées. Dutch women are fastidious about the cleanliness of their homes, and clogs are worn only outside the house.

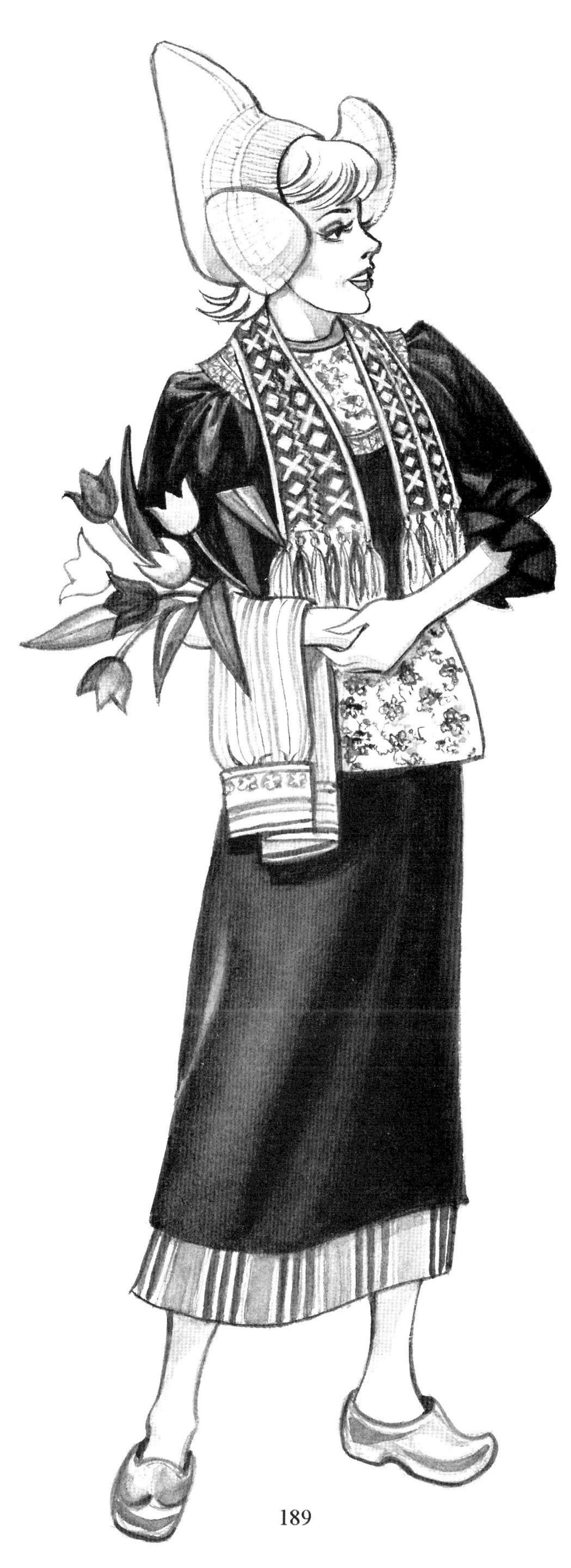

The world is moving so fast these days

that the man who says it can't be done

is generally interrupted by someone doing it.

Elbert Hubbard

The Federal Republic of Germany

Germany, prior to World War II, was comprised of numerous states with a common language and traditions, united into one country in 1871. After World War II it was split into two parts. Together, West and East Germany are the size of Wyoming and Virginia, with a population almost 12 times that of those two states. The ethnic makeup is German. The religions are Roman Catholic, 37 percent, and Protestant, 45 percent. The capital is now Berlin, the currency is the mark, and literacy is 99 percent.

Germanic tribes were defeated by Julius Caesar in 53 B.C., but Roman expansion north of the Rhine was stopped in 900 A.D. Charlemagne consolidated lands that became the Roman Empire. The Thirty Years' War, 1618 to 1648, split Germany into small principalities and kingdoms. Otto von Bismarck formed the German Empire, which reached its peak in 1914, before World War I. After losing that war, the Republic of Germany elected Presidents Ebert and General von Hindenburg. The latter named Adolf Hitler chancellor. Hitler became Fuehrer (leader) the day after von Hindenburg's death. Hitler abolished freedom of speech and assembly and began the persecution of Jews and opponents. In World War II, with total defeat near, Hitler committed suicide.

After the war greater Berlin was created in, but not part of, the Soviet zone of East Germany. A wall dividing Berlin was built in 1961. The border was reopened on November 9, 1989. A year later the formal unification of East and West Germany took place.

In 1967, on our trip around the world, my husband and I took a detour to Berlin. We had to fly through a narrow corridor of apartment buildings that flanked our landing pattern. There wasn't much sound from the passengers as we descended.

The next day, on a bus trip into East Berlin, I noticed a young girl whom I had seen at breakfast in our hotel. She was traveling with her mother and said she was in Berlin to marry a young U.S. Army lieutenant. When I told her our son was the same rank and was married to a girl from Dayton, it turned out that this girl had gone all through school with our son's wife, Sue. We had lots to talk about, and put this coincidence high on our list of 'small world' happenings.

On our way out of East Berlin everyone had to leave the bus, while mirrors were used to scan its chassis. It seems that defectors would often tie themselves in unlikely places in order to leave the country.

In September of 1989, on my second crossing into West Berlin, we sailed through with no problems . . . a sign that significant change was on the horizon.

German Dirndl

The first Oktoberfest was held in 1810 in Munich, in the German state of Bavaria. It was in celebration of the engagement of Crown Prince Louis to Princess Theresa. Every year, from that time on, a huge fair is held in a place called Theresa's Meadow. It lasts for 16 days and takes place in large tents, decorated in Bavaria's colors of blue and white. Bands play, and people enjoy German specialties such as bratwurst, pig's knuckles, strudel, pretzels and dumplings, washing it all down with beer from any of 1,200 breweries. The atmosphere is roaring and sometimes rowdy, but everyone seems to be having fun. Each year 30,000 students turn out.

In a recent poll three out of four Germans would prefer living in Munich over any other city in Germany. Although it is completely modernized it still retains a touch of the old royal Bavaria. It is just 30 miles from the edge of the Alps. Louis I, the crown prince who became king, planned and created a style of romantic classicism, which is a unique aspect of today's Munich.

This dress was purchased to wear to an Oktoberfest. It was found by a Pan American flight attendant, who bought it just for that purpose. The airline's employees helped support a children's hospital, and I was invited to do a costume show fund raiser.

The dress is blue, with a small white print. Its style is that of a typical German dirndl. The neck is square, with a white lace ruffle and an inset with several ruffles of the same lace. The apron is pink, with a white vertical stripe.

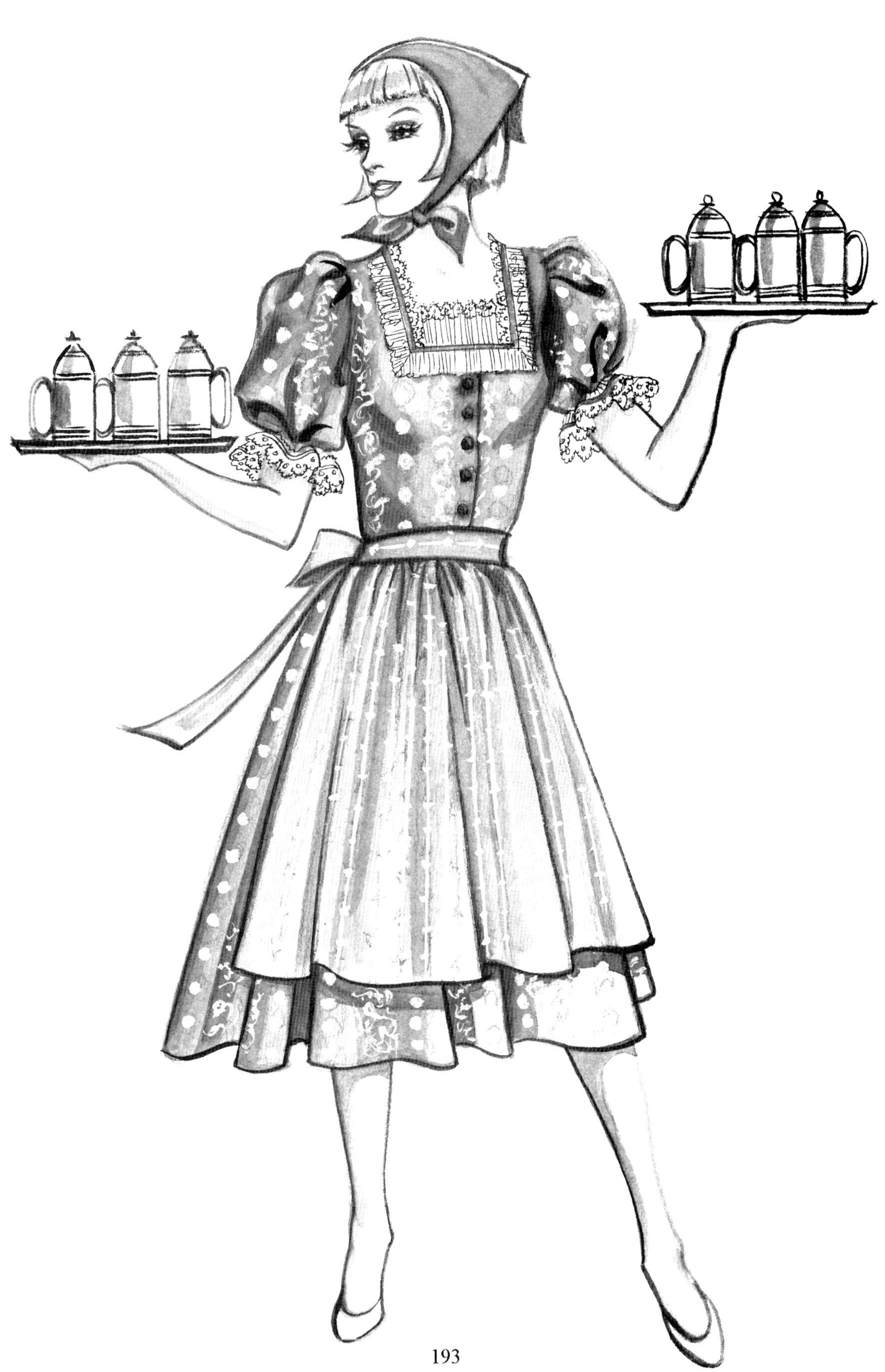

Kaleidoscopic View of Eastern Europe
The German Democratic Republic (GDR)

The GDR became part of the Soviet sector of Berlin in 1949. The East German government decreed a prohibited zone three miles wide along West Germany's 600-mile border and a fortified wall was built in 1961. Berlin's telephone system was cut in two.

We all knew that something big was happening when we went through 'Checkpoint Charlie' at the border between East and West Germany. The border guards were polite, which was a definite switch. Alex, our tour guide for the entire bus trip through Eastern Europe, said that he had never seen anything like it, and he had been taking travelers on these tours for 20 years. Into East Germany we drove, without a hassle, past the Brandenberg Gate, over wide boulevards of that famous thoroughfare, Unter den Linden, with a memorable stop at the Pergamum Museum.

Pergamum was an ancient Greek city in northeast Anatolia, created in 180 B.C. It was known as the most beautiful of all Hellenistic cities. In 1878 the Berlin Museum reconstructed Pergamum's Altar of Zeus, with its great 400-foot-long by 8-foot-tall frieze. The huge figures in the frieze represent the battle between the gods and giants, and it is carved in such a fashion that they seem to leap out of their background. It is impossible to observe this work without feeling the physical and emotional violence of the struggle.

Before crossing the border into Poland we visited Dresden, which was devastated by Allied bombing in 1945, and has since been rebuilt. We were able to see the pride of its art collections, Raphael's "Sistine Madonna" and priceless Meissen porcelains.

The Republic of Poland

Poland, located in east central Europe, is a little larger than the state of Arizona, with a population nearly 10 times that of that state. The capital is Warsaw, the monetary unit is the zloty and literacy 98 percent. The population is 95 percent Roman Catholic.

From the 14th to the 17th centuries Poland was a great power, stretching from the Baltic to Black Seas. In the late 18th century it was divided among Prussia, Russia and Austria. In 1919 independence was regained under the Treaty of Versailles.

After the Hitler-Stalin pact of 1939, Poland was invaded by both Germany and the USSR. It was the first country in Europe to stand up to Hitler. During the course of World War II, Poland fought against both the Nazis and the Soviets, losing six million citizens. Despite written and verbal assurances at Yalta in 1945 that Poland would be free after the war, Russia occupied the country from 1945 to 1989. From 1989 to 1993 a weak, semi-democratic government existed, but in 1993 the communists came back to power. Economic reforms in Poland are ahead of political reforms. Nonetheless, it will take some time before heavy industry is privatized and a market economy is established.

Warsaw, a 1,000-year-old city, was nearly destroyed by bombing in World War II. The reconstruction of this city is of great importance to Poles throughout the world. There is a statue of a lovely girl, in the form of a mermaid, carrying a sword and shield. While this mermaid is not as well known as the one in Copenhagen, Denmark, it is equally beautiful, and is symbolic of the Polish spirit. The model for this statue was killed the first day of the ill-fated 1944 resistance uprising. The motto of Warsaw is "Contemnit Procellas," which means 'Defies the Storm.'

Krakow is an interesting and delightful city, which suffered little bomb damage during World War II. This city goes back to the Stone Age, when its inhabitants lived in limestone caves around the present site. For five centuries the seat of the Polish kings was Krakow. It is the city of the 15th century astronomer Copernicus and home of Poland's oldest university. John Paul II was Cardinal of Krakow before he was elected pope in 1978.

Musical geniuses Frédéric Chopin and Ignace Paderewski were Poles. Among others worthy of note are Nee Sklodowska, the discoverer of radioactive elements, and the winners of Nobel Prizes, Marie Curie (who won two), and Lech Walesa.

The Magnificent Mazowsze

The Magnificent Mazowsze is a dance company, named for the great plains area of central Poland that surrounds Warsaw. Mira Ziminska, one of Poland's leading actresses, married Tadeusz Sygietynski, a composer and student of folkloric songs and music. They formed a colony for the purpose of finding and preserving the costumes, stories and dances of regional areas of Poland and using them with authenticity on the stage. Of 5,000 who were auditioned, 180, their ages averaging 16, were chosen to begin the program. By 1950 the young people were ready to perform inside Poland, and then travel to Paris a year later for their first program abroad. Since that time the dance troupe has toured the world, returning to the United States a number of times.

Mira continued this work after the death of her husband, and today has approximately 100 trained dancers, singers and orchestra members. More than 1,000 authentic costumes are worn, representing most of Poland's regions, with every detail carefully chosen. During a tour 98 trunks are required just for costumes and props. The countryside is scoured for original representative clothing. Some of the older folk-dresses weigh as much as 20 pounds. Mira has become a folk heroine for her work in the preservation of the cultural heritage of her land.

While in Poland a few weeks before the Berlin Wall came down, we saw the younger dancing group at a restaurant where they were performing. Even the beginners in the Magnificent Mazowsze Dance Company are superb.

Bluzka and Spudnica from Lowicz, Poland

On holy days, holidays, baptisms and other celebrations, this charming dress is still worn in Lowicz in central Poland. The blouse, or bluzka, is a black velvet sleeveless jumper. The front and back of the bodice are hand embroidered with red flowers and green leaves that have touches of blue and yellow. The attached skirt, or spudnica, is made of a heavy, hand-loomed wool textile in horizontal stripes of blue, orange, green, red, pink and off-white. The stripes vary from six inches to very narrow. The bottom of the skirt is edged by a wide black velvet band, with floral embroidery every 12 inches. The apron is made of the same fabric as the skirt, with an embroidered black band around the bottom. The effect is that of layers, since the apron is shorter than the skirt.

The pure linen, off-white blouse has cut-out embroidery on the edges of the sleeves and collar. A band of embroidery in red and green is on each shoulder. A scarf of fine red wool, with long, hand-tied fringe, has a red and green flower-and-leaf print. It is 30 inches square and is worn folded diagonally as a headscarf unless a headdress of flowers is worn in its place. A five-strand, red-bead, costume-jewelry necklace is traditional.

This dress is very popular and has been in every one of the Mazowsze performances I have seen. It is typical of the authenticity and distinctiveness of each costume chosen from the regions of the country. Dr. Edward Rozek, a professor of political science at the University of Colorado, is responsible for our being able to acquire this excellent example of ethnic dress. Dr. Rozek fought for Poland in the tank corps for the Free Polish-Government-in-Exile in England during the war. While on a recent trip to Poland he was a guest in the home of President Lech Walesa.

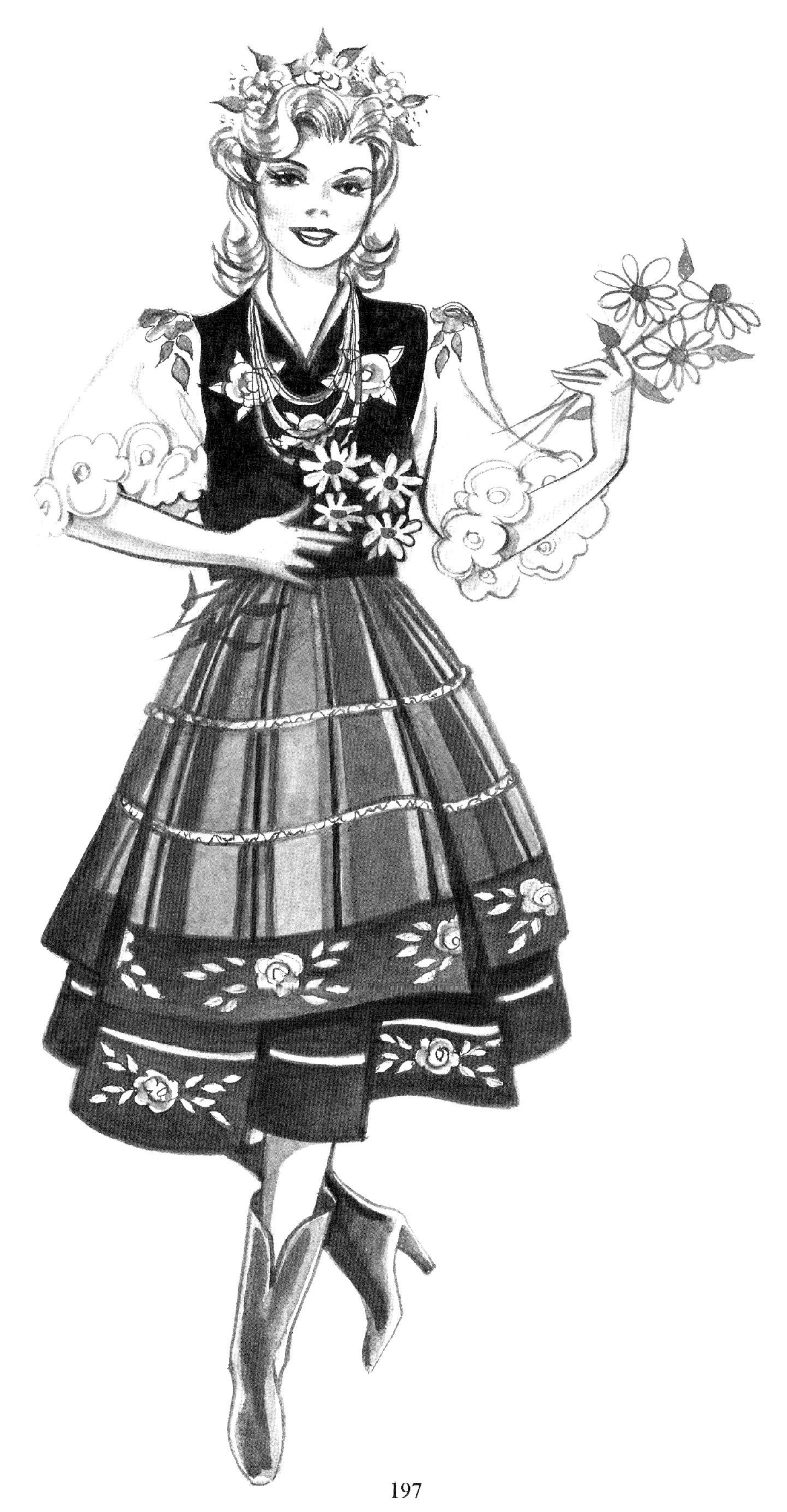

The Czech Republic

Czechoslovakia is in east central Europe, south of Germany and Poland. It is almost as large as the state of South Carolina, with about three times its population. The capital is Prague, the monetary unit the koruny, and literacy is 99 percent. Religion is about evenly divided between Catholicism and the atheism of communism.

In the ninth century Moravia and Bohemia became part of the Great Moravian Empire and then part of the Holy Roman Empire. In 1939 Hitler dissolved Czechoslovakia, making protectorates of Bohemia and Moravia. In 1948 the communists seized power before the elections and declared themselves victors. When 700 leading intellectuals signed a human rights manifesto, it was ignored, and a governmental crackdown followed.

In 1989 Vaclav Havel, a playwright and human rights activist, became president. He was reelected in 1993 when the country split into the Czech Republic and Slovakia.

Prague was known as the 'Golden City' because of its gold-plated rooftops. It is also called the 'City of 100 Towers.' Like Rome, it is spread on seven hills and has long been considered one of the world's most beautiful cities. Wenceslaus Square is in the heart of Prague. Good King Wenceslaus, who is extolled in the Christmas carol of that name, is the patron saint of the Czechs. He was a prince-duke of Bohemia, who took over the government in 924 and was murdered by his own brother. His remains were placed in the St. Vitus Cathedral, which became a pilgrimage site during the Middle Ages.

History is proving that Czechoslovakia was the only country in eastern Europe that was prepared to handle democracy after the fall of communism.

The day we drove to Budapest was confusing, to say the least. We had passed hundreds of cars and trucks lined up at gasoline stations, but our guide Alex had handled the situation so well that we didn't even realize that there might be a serious problem. This day we were deposited at a ski resort in the Carpathian Mountains, and Alex and our driver disappeared. Luncheon and lots of coffee later, Alex dashed into the lodge with his hands full of passports. He and the driver had been begging travelers for gasoline and finally had enough to get us into Hungary, where right across the border there was a Shell gas station.

Everyone was given their passport to present to the Hungarian border guards, that is, everyone except Jo. Hers had disappeared. Every square inch of the area was searched by all of us . . .futiley. We filed onto the bus, Jo anticipating all kinds of dire consequences. It didn't take long to realize that Jo, in the excitement over the lost passport, had left her good, warm, London Fog raincoat on the back of the chair at the ski lodge. It was starting to snow. While searching through the baggage piled up in the back of the bus, the passport was discovered under a seat. All was well! What was losing a coat, compared to losing a passport in Eastern Europe?

The border guards seemed to have no idea that they might be out of a job soon. As soon as our nearly-empty tank received its allotment of fuel, the driver turned up the heat, and we were happily on our way to Budapest.

The Republic of Hungary

Hungary is a country almost the size of Indiana, with nearly twice as many people as that state. It lies to the south of Slovakia. The capital is Budapest, the monetary unit is the forint, and literacy is 98 percent. This is a predominantly Christian country. It is a parliamentary democracy.

The earliest settlers, mostly Slavic and Germanic, were overrun by Magyars from the east. They are of the Finnish-Ugrian race. After many Turkish invasions, Hungary was dominated by Austria and in 1867 became a dual monarchy under the emperor of Austria. Russian troops took over the country in 1944. In 1956 opposition to communist rule turned into open revolt, which the communists met with a massive attack. Imre Nagy, the premier of the 1956 revolutionary government, was tried and put to death, and thousands were arrested. The last Soviet troops left the country in 1991, after the fall of communism.

Budapest is built on two sides of the Danube River, with Pest on the left bank and Buda on the right. The city is an artful melding of the exotic and cosmopolitan. Hero Square is one of the main attractions with its magnificent statues representing historical events. There is an old Turkish bath that is still functioning, with natural hot springs that reach 108 degrees Fahrenheit. The second subway to have been completed in Europe is in Budapest. Elizabeth Bridge connects Buda and Pest, crossing the Danube in a single span. It was reconstructed as a suspension bridge after being demolished by retreating German forces at the end of World War II.

Waiting for us in the lobby of our Budapest hotel were our Hungarian friends Eva and Mike, whom we met on the train ride through Mongolia. They presented us with a bouquet of flowers. We resolved to remember, for our own future guests, how welcome the flowers made us feel. They took us to lunch the next day and Eva knew exactly where to find the kind of raincoat Jo was looking for. After shopping, Eva and Mike joined our group for a Hungarian dinner, complete with gypsy music, and then took us to their home for after-dinner coffee.

This was a first for us, as we had never been in a communist home in a communist country. Their meager furnishings surprised us, because this was a privileged home in a 'politically correct' area of Budapest. We were reminded that 85 percent of all the buildings in the city had been demolished in World War II. We Americans need to visit less fortunate areas of the globe to fully appreciate our good fortune. While admiring their two young sleeping daughters, we all admitted to wondering what is wrong with a world that cannot get along when there is much more that binds us than separates us. As Mike drove us back to our hotel he said that he saw chaos ahead for Hungary and civil war for Russia. He also said that he envied our good life in America and wished that he could raise his little girls in such a safe haven.

Romania

Romania is a country almost as large as Oregon, with eight times Oregon's population. It is in southeast Europe on the Black Sea. The capital is Bucharest, the currency is the lei and literacy is 96 percent. The religion is 70 percent Romanian Orthodox and six percent Roman Catholic. The government is a republic.

Wallachia and Moldavia, under Turkish domination, became Romania in 1861. Independence was claimed from Turkey in 1877, and four years later a kingdom was formed under King Carol I. Five years later a constitutional monarchy was established. In 1947 the communists occupied the country. Internal policies became oppressive and the protests that followed caused great loss of life. President Nicolae Ceaucescu ruled until the end of 1989, when he and his wife were executed.

After crossing the Hungarian border into Romania we traced the caravan route of migratory gypsy clans through the Transylvanian Alps and deep, silent forests into Cluj. We felt that we had lost 100 years in time. Cars were replaced by horse-drawn vehicles and Brasov, a well-preserved medieval city, was a fitting background for Dracula's infamous Bran Castle. After climbing dozens of steps to the castle we saw no sign of Dracula . . . just massive, ancient-looking furnishings. The author of the legend of Dracula was Bram Stoker, who wrote in the form of diaries kept by principal characters about a Transylvanian vampire, who made his way to England and stayed alive by drinking human blood. The persons so victimized became vampires as well. The legend of Transylvania is still a popular source of horror fiction.

Our memories of Romania include the delicate, intricate lace curtains at the windows, the many storks that winter in Kenya and summer here, the multitude of geese, the water buffalo used to plow the fields, and the native version of Dracula. It differs from that of the British. The Romanians insist that in the 15th century a prince from Walachia, south of Transylvania, committed hundreds of savage murders. The family that owned Bran Castle imprisoned Vlad Tepes in the castle. Either version was acceptable to us. Romanians also claim that Bucharest once was the Paris of Eastern Europe.

The Republic of Bulgaria

The Danube River carves a natural border between Romania and Bulgaria. We crossed at the ancient Roman port of Rousse over the 'Bridge of Friendship.' Bulgaria is on the Black Sea. It is almost as large as Ohio, with about three-quarters of the population of that state. The capital is Sofia, the monetary unit the lev and literacy 98 percent. The religions are 85 percent Bulgarian Orthodox and 13 percent Muslim. It was settled by Slavs in the sixth century. Turkic Bulgars arrived in the seventh century, merged with the Slavs, adopted the Christian faith and, by the 12th century, had established powerful empires. The Ottomans, a Muslim power, ruled from the end of the 14th century for 500 years.

In 1944 Bulgaria was taken over by the communists, but in 1990 parliament revoked the role of the Communist Party. Todor Zhivkov, the party leader for 35 years, was convicted and imprisoned in 1992. Soviet troops were never stationed in this country, as they were considered unnecessary. According to our guide, Alex, 'profit' was considered a dirty word, and until 1992, the state determined everyone's living quarters as well as their salary.

Every Balkan city had balconies draped with drying clothes. Evidently, clothes dryers were unknown even in the late 1980's in these countries.

Federal Republic of Yugoslavia

Yugoslavia is on the Adriatic Sea, sharing borders with Hungary, Romania and Bulgaria. It is roughly the size of Kentucky, with about three times the population of that state. Present-day Yugoslavia consists of the former republics of Serbia and Montenegro, formed in 1992 into the New Federal Republic of Yugoslavia. The capital is Belgrade, the monetary unit the dinar and literacy is 90 percent. The religion is 65 percent Orthodox and the remainder are Roman Catholic and Muslim.

When the Austro-Hungarian Empire collapsed after World War I, the Kingdom of Serbs, Croats and Slovenes was created from the former provinces of Croatia, Dalmatia, Bosnia, Herzegovina, Slovenia, Voyvodina and Montenegro. The name was changed to Yugoslavia.

Nazi Germany invaded Yugoslavia in 1941 and Josip Bros, known as Marshal Tito, had gained control by the time they were driven out. In 1946 it became a federated republic with Tito, a communist, in control. He accepted military and economic aid from the U.S., France and Great Britain. President Tito died in 1980. In 1991 Croatia and Slovenia declared independence, and fighting began between the Croats and Serbs in Croatia. Serbia supplied weapons to the ethnic Serbs in Bosnia and Herzegovina, prompting the United Nations to impose sanctions. Two years later Yugoslavia said it was cutting off support for the Bosnian Serbs and the U.N. voted for a conditional easing of sanctions in 1994.

The Bosnian Mountains around Sarajevo were the site of the 1984 Winter Olympics, and there were many apartment buildings in the area erected for that event. The city has a strong Muslim character, with many mosques and an ancient Turkish marketplace. Sarajevo is the seat of the head of all the Muslims in Yugoslavia, also that of Serbian Orthodoxy and a Roman Catholic Arch-Bishopry.

Jo and I became trapped in an elevator on the sixth floor of the Holiday Inn in Sarajevo. We might have had a very long stay if a native of the area had not been in the same predicament. There were many buttons to push in case of trouble, but we couldn't read the directions. The 'Made in U.S.A.' sign didn't help a bit.

Everyone had to have their picture taken while standing in the cement supposed-footprints of Archduke Franz Ferdinand on the exact spot where he was slain by a Bosnian Serb student on June 28, 1914. According to our history books this was the shot that started World War I.

A mountainous, scenic drive took us to Mostar, an ancient city known for its Oriental traditions, colorful markets and single-arch bridge. From Mostar we followed the Neretva River Valley to the spectacular Adriatic coast, and then south to Dubrovnik. Central Yugoslavia is known to have the most beautiful coastline on the Mediterranean Sea, and in Dubrovnik was the best example of all European Medieval walled cities. This historic monument had been carefully preserved since the seventh century until, in a few hours, it was destroyed by shelling in the Serbian-Bosnian war. Recollecting walking tours in this ancient fortified town in its storybook setting, and realizing that it is no more, causes grief to anyone who has been there. The senselessness of such wanton, unnecessary destruction is difficult to fathom.

Our guide Alex was Yugoslav. He spoke with sadness about the situation in his country. "Several years ago I moved my family to Italy," he said. "I could see that the political situation here was hopeless. There are no limitations on private business, but there are over a million people unemployed just in Belgrade, and people are afraid to invest in this country. The land of my birth has become a feudal society."

Chapter Nine

African Adventure

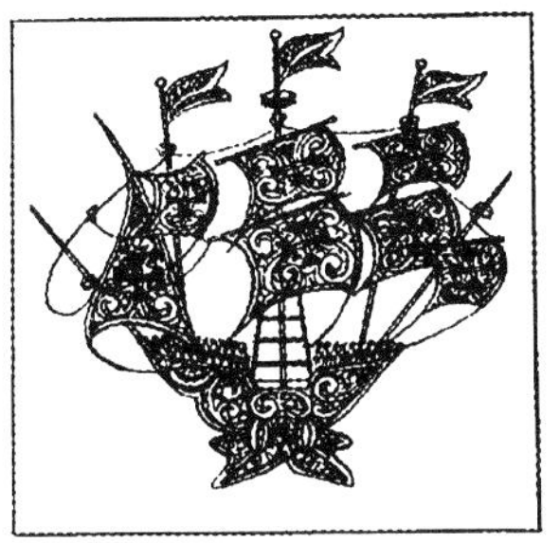

Morocco
West Africa:
Senegal
Côte d'Ivoire
Ghana
Togo
Benin

Kingdom of Morocco

Morocco, on the northwest coast of Africa, is bordered by West Sahara and Algeria. Although larger than California, its population numbers almost three million less than that state. The currency is the dirham and there is a 50 percent literacy rate. The religion is 99 percent Sunni Muslim, and the people are 99 percent Arab-Berber. The capital is Rabat. The government is a constitutional monarchy, with the king as head of state.

The Berbers were indigenous to the area, followed by the Carthaginians and Romans. In the 11th and 12th centuries a Berber empire ruled all of northwest Africa and most of Spain from Morocco. Part of Morocco was ruled by Spain in the 19th century, and by the early 20th century France controlled the rest. It was the Berber tribes that kept the French Foreign Legion busy until the warring factions were brought under control in 1933. In 1956 France withdrew from Morocco. Tangier, an international seaport, was integrated into the country, and Morocco became independent.

In 1976, 70,000 square miles of phosphate-rich land in the former Spanish Sahara was annexed by Morocco after Spain withdrew. A guerrilla group, Polisario, proclaimed the region independent and attacked with Algerian help. The U.S. acted militarily and economically, and in 1980 Morocco again occupied the disputed area. A cease-fire was signed in 1990. The United Nations will conduct a referendum in Western Sahara to decide whether it should become independent or remain a part of Morocco.

Moroccan Memories

Because it is closer to Europe than any other African nation, there is a fascinating blend of old and new here. Morocco is close to being a one-ethnic-group country. Since it was an ally in World War II, many former military and government personnel return to vacation there, remembering its ethnicity and color. Casablanca is especially popular with tourists. Beautiful, elegant, elaborately embroidered caftans are irresistible to women shoppers.

Sightseeing in Casablanca proved a disappointment. We knew that it was wise to get guides and cars from reliable sources, but we had arrived on a late flight from Rome with no time to make arrangements for the next morning. The hotel doorman was so insistent about his uncle's good English and his knowledge of the city, that we agreed. We were even told that the uncle was a registered guide. Upon being greeted the next morning with "Good morning, sirs," we knew we'd been had! He knew one other phrase in English, "That's the sea." We already knew that. So we saw the sea and never learned what else we saw, since everything was explained in Arabic. However, he took us to the Medina where we were able to find the man's and woman's djellabah, so the day wasn't a complete waste. Upon our return to the hotel we looked for the doorman, but he had disappeared. It was just as well for him that he had.

Jo was our driver in Agadir, and we got him the smart way, through an agency in the hotel. With two Jo's in one car, getting acquainted wasn't difficult. Jo the driver was enchanted with the idea of a female named Jo. He had never heard of such a thing.

There was a large fish processing plant in Agadir, so if you like the smell of fish it was a nice city. We left soon for Taroudant and Marrakech. Taroudant, an entirely-walled Berber village, was fascinating. There were many ethnic shops to roam through. When we couldn't find the right belts for the Berber dancing dress, the son of a storekeeper was sent to search for them while we ate couscous and drank refreshing mint tea. Couscous is the national dish, made with spiced semolina cooked with meat sauce. Our young shopper found the right belts for that complicated costume.

On our way to Marrakech we saw farmers tilling the soil with their camels, much as they have done for centuries, not disturbed by overhead jets. Berber nomads were herding their flocks, dressed in their djellabahs and carrying long canes.

Marrakech is a very sophisticated resort city, a favorite of Hollywood stars, Parisian designers and jet setters. With its red-ocher buildings, it is an oasis and gateway to the Sahara. In the 11th century it was one of Islam's great cities.

An exotic sight was Place Jema al Fna Square with its acrobats, jugglers, snake charmers and gaudily costumed water boys wandering noisily through the crowd with huge animal bladders full of water strapped on their backs. We didn't see any non-Moroccans buying water. At a Berber donkey fair outside of town an old man was seated on the ground with his wares spread out before him on a blanket. This is where the amber and silver necklaces were found. The black veils from our hotel shop completed the purchases.

This was the end of the trip that had begun in Moscow after the shooting down of the South Korean 747, that led to an international pilot strike. Instead of continuing through Uzbekistan and China and around the world, we were lucky to have been able to head south to Frankfurt, Germany, and from there through Italy and then Morocco - all on our own! It had been a long journey, and we were ready to go home.

Moroccan Man's and Woman's Ethnic Dress

In a shop in the Old Medina, the original Arab residential and commercial quarter of Casablanca, we found the woman's 'caftan' and the woman's and man's 'djellabahs.'

The man's djellabah is a long, white, cotton tunic. It is worn over a Western-style man's shirt and trousers. There is white, shiny crocheted braid around the neck and down the front, with 35 crocheted buttons and buttonholes. The sides of the garment are left open at the hem for ease in walking. A 'takiya,' or white crocheted skullcap, is very popular all over north Africa and the Middle East, as well as Asia. The yellow leather shoes with pointed toes are exactly like those worn in Egypt. The backs of the shoes are pushed down into the sole and are worn as scuffs.

A woman's caftan and djellabah are both full length and are beautifully made. The salmon-colored dress, worn under the djellabah, is fashioned from a silky, synthetic fabric. The neckline, long sleeves and hem are edged with a wide green and silver braid. A green djellabah is worn over the caftan, and a cowl-like headpiece snaps onto the djellabah. It is usually worn as a collar, but is a protection during sandstorms. A small, black, velvet shoulder bag has a quilted front.

Bangles, beads and colored yarns decorate the black, three-cornered 'tarboosh,' or headscarf. Each tiny appendage hanging from the tarboosh is wrapped with gold thread. The smaller sheer, black veil, a 'mandeel,' is also triangular and decorated, like the tarboosh. These veils were found in a hotel shop in Marrakech. The clerk was very kind and patient in her demonstration of exactly how they are worn.

The most attractive results are obtained when a native of the country is present to handle the finishing touches of any ethnic dress. Putting these veils on just right is a complicated process, as is also true of the saris of India, the sarongs of Indonesia, the woman's dress of Bhutan, the man's dancing dress of Thailand, and the West African woman's turban.

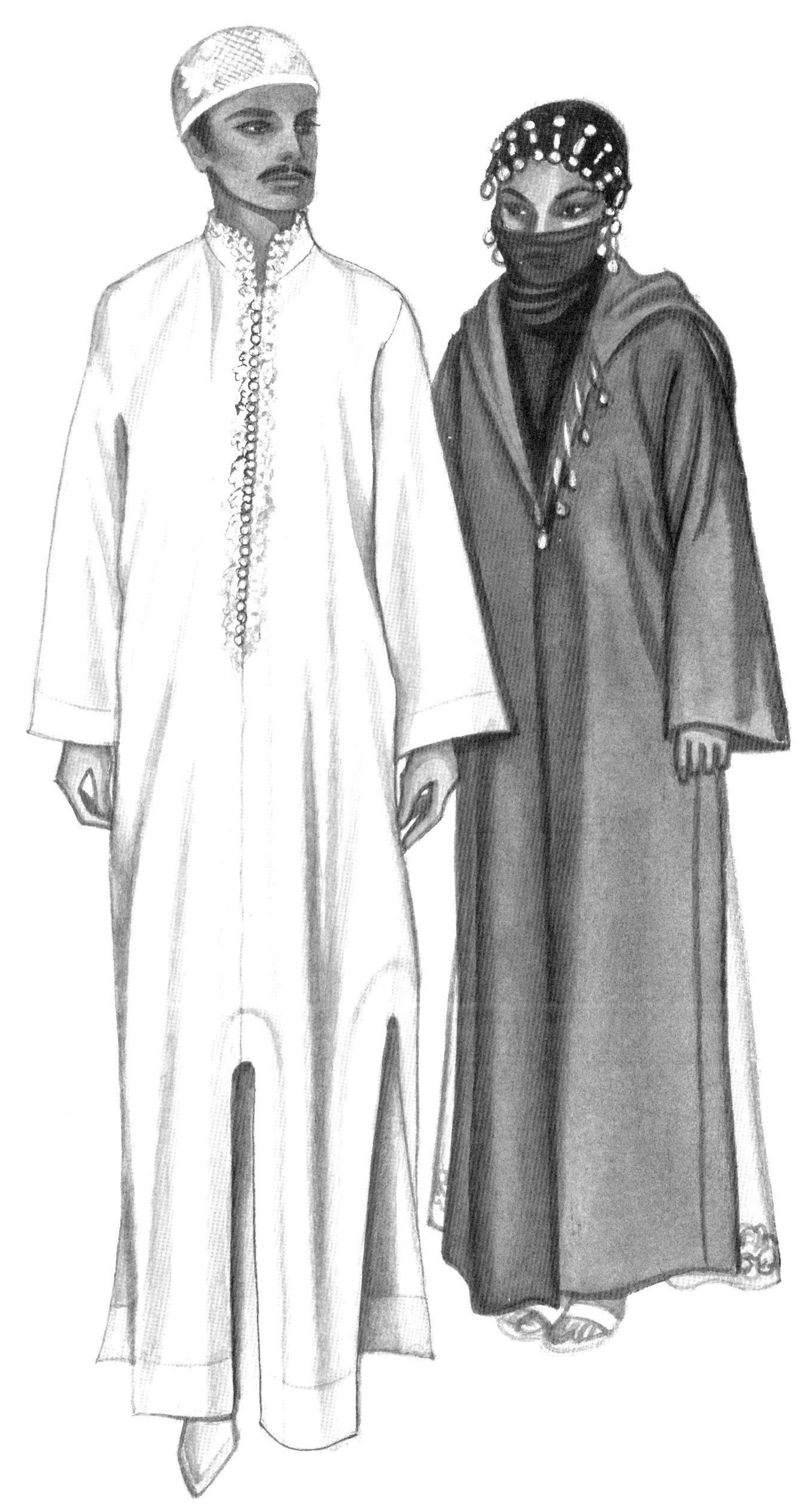

Man's Djellabah

This man's djellabah is made of brown and white vertically striped cotton. The long, loose, tunic-like robe is usually buttoned from the neck partway down the front of the garment. The sleeves are long, and there is an attached hood which is most likely worn during sandstorms, since we did not actually see it worn as headgear.

A jaunty, red felt 'fes' or 'fez' is cone-shaped, brimless and has a red tassel. This hat is popular in Morocco and in many other parts of the world. Until the 19th century the only place it was made was in the city of Fes, which is a center for traditional crafts and trade in north central Morocco.

The shoes are yellow leather 'scuffs,' still popular in this part of the world.

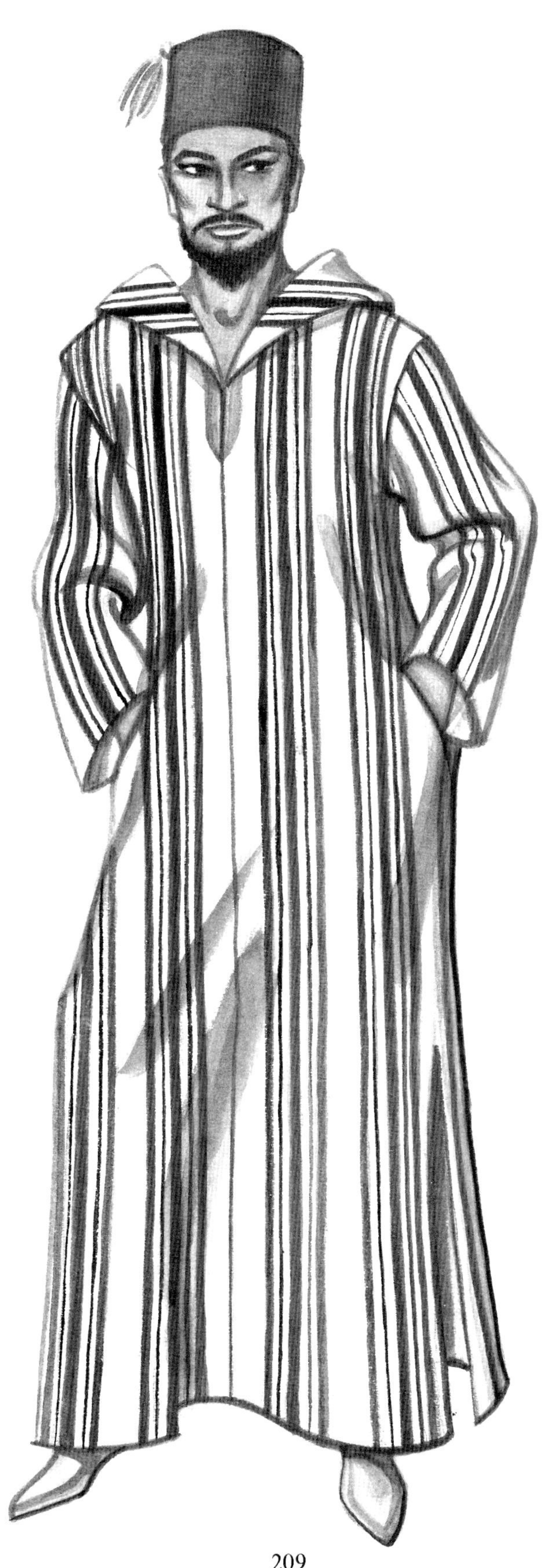

Berber Dancer of Morocco

This excellent example of a Berber dancing dress was found in a 'souk,' an Arabian shopping center, in Taroudant, a walled Berber village about 80 kilometers east of Agadir. There are two dresses, one worn over the other, often draped with three yards of black and white cotton cloth. Only the black was available at the factory in the village where the dancers bought their supplies.

Both dresses are long tunics, with long sleeves and slits at the hem. The overdress is open from the waist down. The dresses are made of the same sheer, silky, synthetic fabric, brightly printed with flowers in shades of pink on a creamy background, with three narrow gold stripes at two-inch intervals. Pink, gold and white braid trims the neck, wrists, skirt openings, shoulders of the overdress and the front opening.

Yard-long belts of braided green wool yarn are finished with two elaborately wrapped multicolored tassels. The shoes, of red and green Moroccan leather, have high backs and no heels. Designs are embroidered in purple and blue in a lattice-work design on the red toe area. A green and yellow tassel is at the instep of the shoe.

Complicated jewelry includes a five-inch headdress, with 36 beads inlaid in silver and 12 dangles, each with a coral bead, forming a fringe over the forehead. A long stickpin holds up the cotton lengths at the shoulder. The two necklaces of amber and silver, which were found at a Berber souk in Marrakech, turned out to be wonderful finds since the beads, when tested by a gemologist, proved to be genuine amber. Some of the honey-colored beads are an inch and one-half in diameter, and they are beautifully matched. This Moroccan amber is found in the waters off the country's Atlantic coast.

The black markings on the face of the dancer resemble the tattoos which are symbols of a lost language, still written, but no longer spoken.

Despite the extravagance of the costume and accessories, Berber dances are quite primitive.

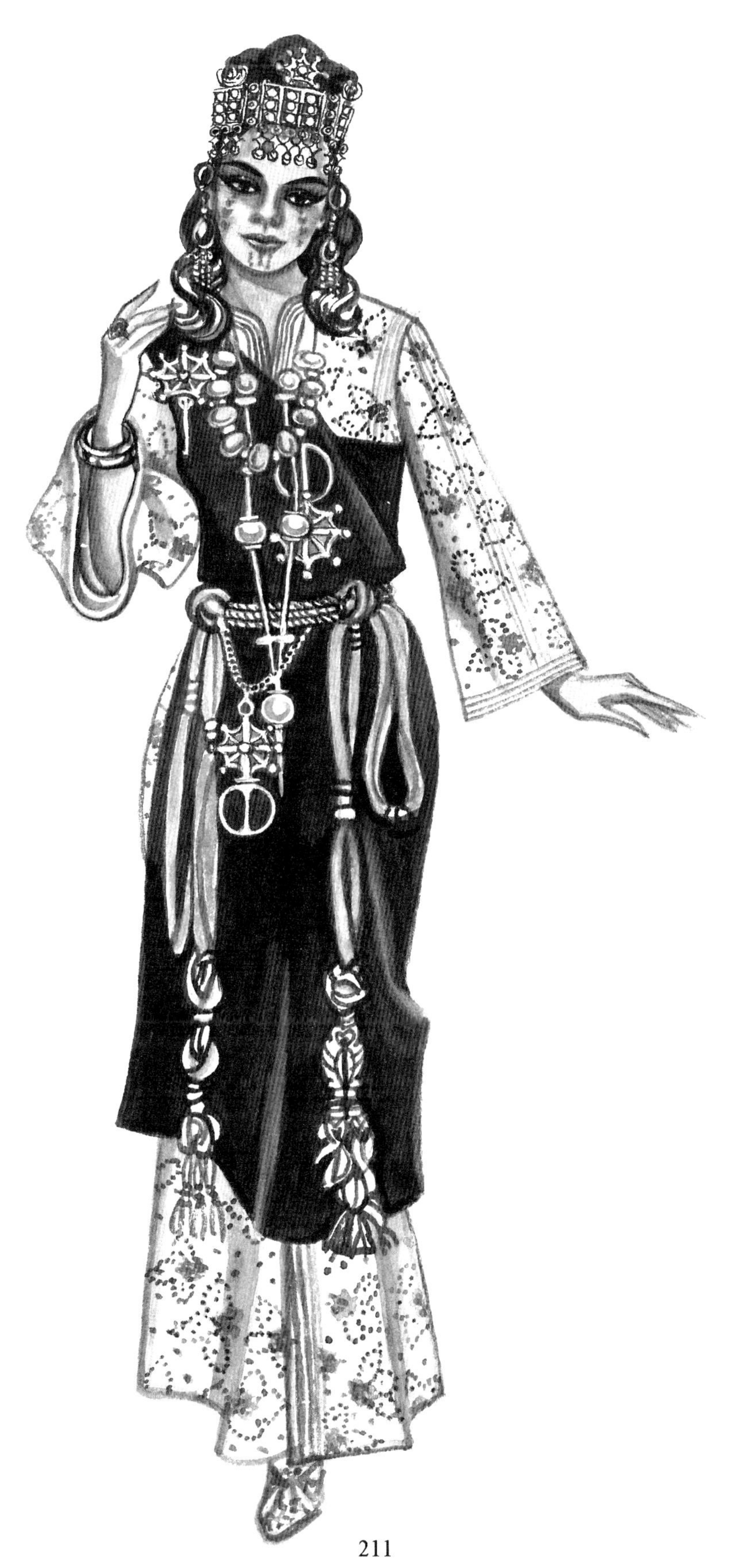

If you reject the food,

ignore the customs,

fear the religion

and avoid the people,

you might better stay home.

You are like a pebble thrown into the water,

you become wet on the surface,

but you are never a part of the water.

James A. Michener

West Africa

Call it mystique, adventure, or whatever you will, West Africa has a power of attraction which, despite its sometimes primitive conditions, continues to entice Westerners. The predominant European power in the area was France, so French is spoken throughout West Africa, along with native dialects.

We were there during the rainy season, but it only rained at night. Although near the equator, the heat was not oppressive. Malaria was supposed to be a problem, and a great fuss is made about taking medication for it, even for weeks after arriving home. However, we did not see so much as one mosquito.

Most religions in West Africa are based on animism, added to a belief in reincarnation and the existence of a supreme being. The people communicate through lesser deities. The Ewe of Togo have over 600 deities. Africans pray to these gods in order to gain health, good harvests and many children. This last request seems to be granted to all. Magic is important. Good magic keeps evil spirits away. The medicine man, or 'juju' priest, dispenses charms, tells fortunes and advises on religious matters.

Some cultural habits related to greetings are of interest. Africans place great emphasis on these. To get down to business immediately on meeting someone is considered very rude. Rituals must be observed. Some common salutations are: "Do you have peace?" "Thanks be to God." "Where are the people of your compound?" Not to take hands on entering and leaving a home is the ultimate act of rudeness. Cheeks are kissed three times, always first on the left cheek. Eye contact is usually avoided between men and women.

Eating traditions include forming the food into balls, always using the right hand. Using the left hand for eating is considered grossly offensive.

We had hoped to also go to Timbuktu in Mali to get a costume from the 'Blue Men,' who are descendants of the Berbers. It would complement nicely our Berber dancing dress from Morocco, but the flight to Timbuktu was canceled for some reason, and we would have had to rent a plane. That was definitely not in our budget.

Republique du Senegal

Grace, Jo and I went to West Africa via Air Afrique. Our first stop was Senegal, on the Atlantic Ocean. It is the size of South Dakota, with a population 12 times greater than that state's. The capital is Dakar, the monetary unit is the CFA franc, and literacy is 10 percent. French is the official language. The religion is 92 percent Muslim, blended with magic.

Senegal was one of the earliest inhabited regions of the world, dating back to 13,000 B.C. The Portuguese landed on Gorée Island in the 1400's and set up shop in the slave trade. The present-day dungeons on this island attest to the brutal treatment these slaves received. In the 1600's the French moved in and slave trading became a coastal operation. Powerful kingdoms in the interior conducted raids on each other to procure slaves. In 1815 the Council of Vienna forbade slave trading, and the main product of this country became peanuts, called groundnuts. In 1893 Dakar was named the capital of French West Africa. In 1960 Senegal achieved independence.

There are three Clubs Med in West Africa, and two are in Senegal. It is possible to travel in the southern Casamance region and live like a native - Club Med style. In a pirogue, or native motorized dugout canoe, we traveled through sand islands, lagoons, mangrove swamps, dunes, forests, huge ant hills and baobob forests for many scenic miles.

The Moors, once nomads roaming desert areas, are now very persistent merchants. They seem ready to arm-wrestle a prospective buyer to the ground to complete a sale. The tourist must learn to show no interest in an item, unless a decision to buy it has already been made, or it might have to be bought just to escape the seller.

There are a large number of Moroccans in Senegal, so the djellabah and occasional veils are seen, but many of the women wear the 'boubou,' as in the rest of West Africa. We attended a tea dance on the terrace of our hotel in Dakar, and the dancers wore short skirts, flowers around their necks and nothing else.

Republique de la Côte d'Ivoire

The Ivory Coast is on the south coast of West Africa. It is slightly larger than New Mexico, with a population nine times more than that state. The official capital is Yamoussoukra, and the de facto capital is Abidjan. The currency is the CFA franc, and there is 45 percent literacy. The religion is 63 percent indigenous and 25 percent Muslim.

This country was a French protectorate from 1842, becoming independent in 1960. In 1990 student and worker unrest led to the first multiparty presidential elections. Another election is slated for 1995. President Houphouet ruled with a firm hand. So many millions of dollars were poured into his native village, Yamoussoukra, that it became the butt of jokes. The four-star hotel has an occupancy rate of five percent, and the beautiful country club and golf course were nearly empty when we were there. The eight-lane highway leading into town stops dead-end at the jungle's edge. The cathedral is magnificent, and Pope John Paul II attended its dedication. There is also a presidential palace, which is protected by an alligator-infested moat. Live chickens, whose feet were tied, were thrown to these alligators by our guide. We did not find this at all entertaining, but when the alligator caught his dinner, the natives who were watching clapped.

Abidjan is the most vibrant city in West Africa. The best hotel in the country is the Hotel Ivoire Intercontinental, with an ice-skating rink, bowling alley, cinema, casino, grocery store and major art shop. This hotel is where I decided I would no longer be without cable T.V. If we could watch CNN in the Côte d'Ivoire, we could watch it in the United States.

We were disturbed to see the results of the students' trashing of their own university during a riot. We were never told the reason for the riot, but the school had to be shut down for months to be made habitable. All of the furniture had been chopped to pieces.

One evening we drove to a pagan dance in the forest, stopping for dinner at a popular restaurant, where we allowed our guide to order. The dish had a delicious aroma, and when Grace asked what it was, the young man replied, "It's a kind of rat, very special to this region." Without protest he happily finished off our entire meal. The ritual dance was held at a clearing in the jungle. Before the program began a man in a grass skirt and mask asked for the oldest person in the party. (This is considered to be a compliment.) Both Grace and Jo quickly pointed to me. So, surrounded by natives and pagan dancers, I had to sign a "Peace Treaty" with the natives. We decided later that television had brought Hollywood to the Côte d'Ivoire.

Ivory Coast Tribal Ceremonial Dress

The Korhogo region of the Côte d'Ivoire, an all-day drive north from Abidjan, is the home of the Senufo tribe. This area is famous for its cloth, a coarse, raw cotton, much like burlap, in an off-white or cream color. This cloth is painted in designs with a natural vegetable dye mixed with black mud, using a knife with a thick, curved blade.

An interesting example of the ethnic dress of this area was found in Abidjan, at a shop in our hotel known for its African arts and artifacts. The manager of this shop was well educated and knowledgeable about the history, art and native dress of his country.

This example of West African ethnic dress consists of a tunic, loose trousers and a tri-cornered headdress with a tassel on each corner. The cream-colored textile is coarse, but finer than a burlap. The painted design is in vertical rows about three inches wide. We were told that this was a ceremonial costume, used for pagan rituals.

The Senufo are the musicians of West Africa. Marimbas, tuned iron gongs, drums, horns and flutes are used. Drum and marimba bands are popular. The tribal rhythm is beat into the earth to call upon ancestors to join in the ceremony and purify the earth.

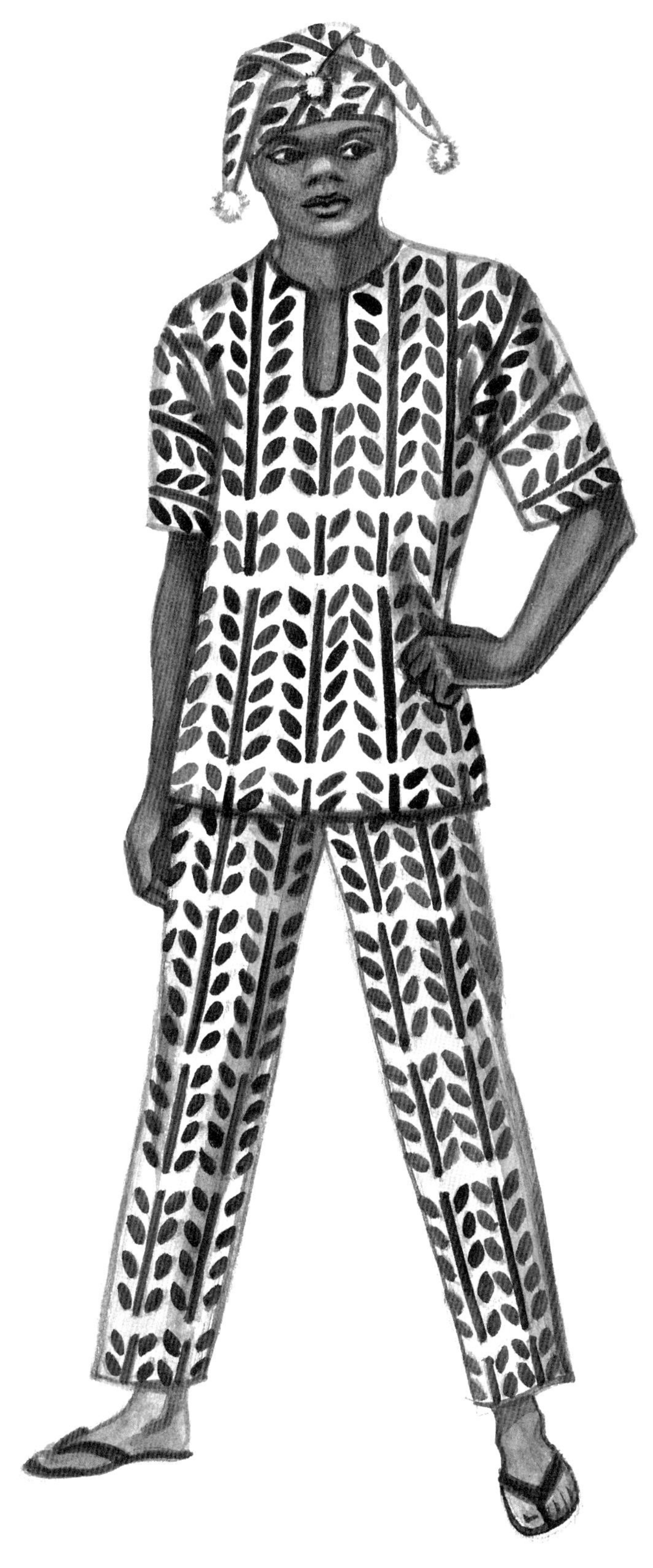

Republic of Ghana

Ghana is a tropical country on the southern coast of West Africa. It is not quite as large as Oregon and has a population nearly six times that state's. The capital is Accra, the currency is the cedi and literacy is 60 percent. Many tribal languages are spoken here, and religion is divided between Christianity, Muslim and tribal beliefs.

For centuries Ghana was West Africa's richest country because of its traffic in gold and slaves. The Ashanti tribes became the richest in the area. When the British outlawed slavery in the early 19th century timber and cacao became the main exports. For 113 years Ghana, then known as the Gold Coast, was ruled by Britain. It became independent in 1957 and gained status as a republic in the Commonwealth in 1960. Many coups have occurred within the military government. In 1992 a new constitution allowed for a multiparty political structure.

When we were in Togo we crossed the border into Ghana, just so we could have its stamp on our passports. The tour agency planned this without our knowledge. They are well aware of travelers' obsession to fill their passports with proof of countries visited.

Anago-Gbada from Ghana

Tunics and trousers like the 'anago-gbada' are presently popular with males all over West Africa. They are of heavy cotton with a design of green and brown elephants and impalas, with a sprinkling of baobab trees.

This costume was brought to the University of Colorado by Ghanian student Jonah Quist. He brought costumes along to show the International Club examples of his country's native dress.

The sandals, with soles made of rubber tires, were found in Ghana, when it was still the Gold Coast. They were donated to the collection by a former Pan American Airlines flight attendant.

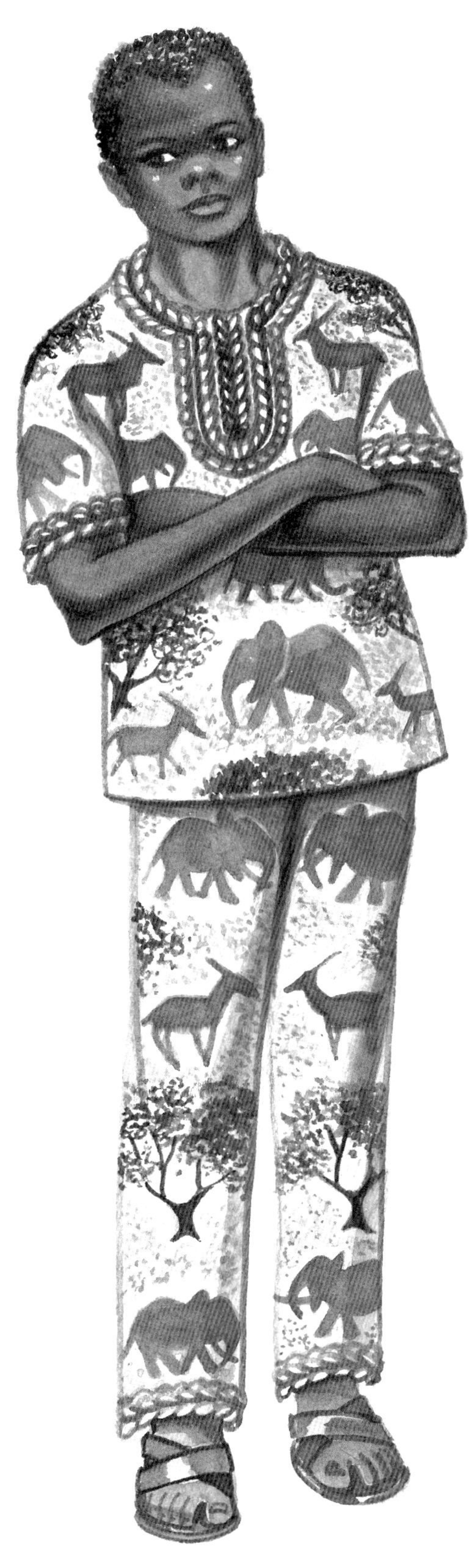

Farmer's Ethnic Dress
from Northern Ghana

One of the largest markets in Abidjan, in the Côte d'Ivoire, is named Treichville, called 'Trashville' by discriminating shoppers. It is due to chance that one of our outstanding examples of ethnic dress came from here. It was hanging in an outdoor market, and as we wandered past, a bell rang in my memory...a picture from an excellent book I had read, *African Weaving,* by Venice Lamb. The salesman had no idea what he was selling, and I did not fully realize what I was buying until I got home and studied the costume. The cost was minimal and the bargaining fun. Maymi of Mandalay, Burma, who scolded me for paying the asking price, would have been proud of me that day at Trashville. But I was not proud of myself later, to have walked away with a tunic, trousers and hat that were worth many times the pittance that unknowing salesman received. As it turned out the costume was from Ghana.

Farmers in the Bawku area of northern Ghana still wear this kind of clothing. The 'fugu,' or knee-length tunic, trousers and hat are made locally of handspun four-inch cotton stripweaving. The strips, sewn together, are vertical on the tunic and trousers but diagonal on the hat. Strip weaving is centuries old, and a hat made exactly like the one in the collection was found in a cave site along the edge of the Bandiagara Massif in Mali. The date of that find is estimated to be 11th century A.D. The Tellem textiles recovered from the caves in Mali are now in the Ulm Museum in Germany. It is reasonable to assume that in another decade good examples of strip weaving will be difficult to find.

The background color of the textile is an off-white, with narrow stripes of blue, red and black. A machine-made braid decorates the neck and front of the tunic and the bottom of the legs of the trousers. The trousers are wide at the waist, narrowing to the ankle.

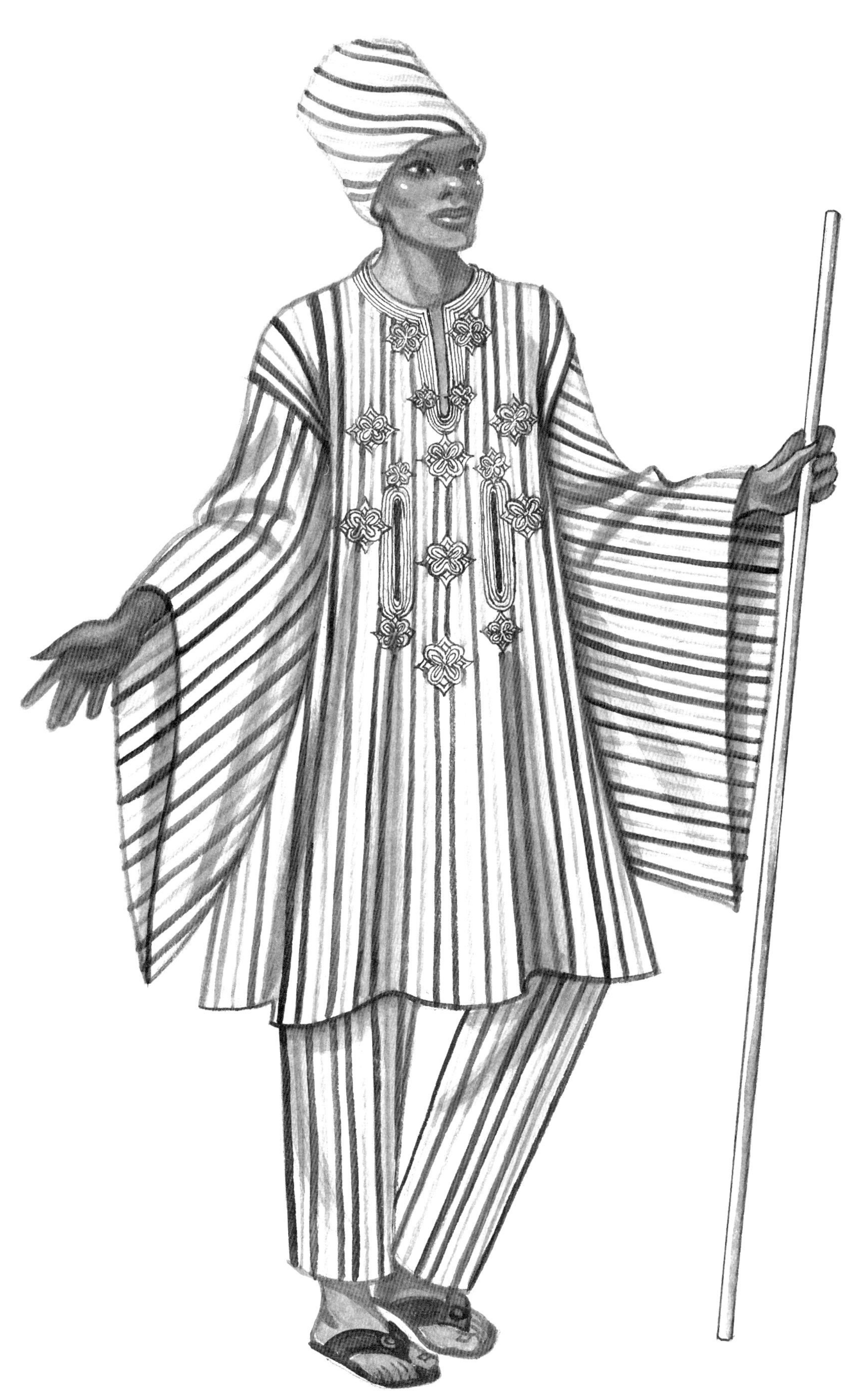

Republic of Togo

Togo is located on the southern coast of West Africa, between Ghana and Benin. It is smaller than West Virginia, with more than twice the population of that state. The capital is Lomé, the currency is the CFA franc, and literacy is 45 percent. The religions are 70 percent indigenous, 20 percent Christian and 10 percent Muslim.

The Ewe (pronounced Evy) arrived several centuries ago in south Togo. The country became a major source of slaves. Germany took control in 1884, and then France and Britain administered 'Togoland' as U.N. Trusteeships. The French sector became the Republic of Togo in 1960. In 1993, because of civil unrest, 25,000 people fled the country.

We loved Togo. The beaches are beautiful, and the people are pleasant and friendly. The cleanliness of the native compounds with their cone roofs was admirable, considering the fact that they have no running water or plumbing. The shining faces of the children in the compounds we visited attested to their ability to be clean without facilities that most travelers believe are necessities for survival.

Economically, most West African countries are in disarray, partly because existing laws do not encourage individual enterprise. However, Togo is considered the 'Pearl of West Africa,' and French and German tourists crowd the country during the winter season.

Our guide was an Ewe, and his family were weavers. He took us to his home to see their work and an Ewe example of 'kente cloth,' a masterpiece of four-inch weaving strips, now part of the textile collection of Sun Cities Museum of Art.

There is an excellent market in Lomé where we found the 'Nana Benz,' women traders known throughout Africa. They are thus called because so many own Mercedes Benz cars. This market is a handicraft village for makers and sellers of all the arts of the country. Togo sandals are famous in that part of West Africa. They are of heavy leather and hard on tender feet, but their satisfied buyers are legion, especially among trekkers.

Although many of the natives consider themselves Christian, they still believe in voodoo. An interesting fetish market sells skulls of monkeys and birds, porcupine skins, wart hogs' teeth, bones of all sizes and traditional medicinal ingredients, all labeled for various diseases. There was no lack of medicine men, nor of buyers.

A last memory of Togo is a dance near Kpalime. The dancers were women in boubous and intricately wrapped turbans. They carried babies on their backs as they danced a traditional snake dance in a long swaying line. The babies were either smiling happily or asleep. Not one was crying.

Republic of Benin

Benin is located in West Africa on the Gulf of Guinea. It is about the size of Pennsylvania, with less than half of that state's population. The capital is Porto-Novo, and Cotonou is the most important city. The currency is the CFA franc, literacy is 28 percent and the religions are 70 percent indigenous, 15 percent Muslim and 15 percent Christian.

This country used to be the Kingdom of Abomey. Because of its slave trading it became very powerful and was known as the `Slave Coast.' The palace at Abomey had a court of 10,000 people. King Glele (1858-1889) was said to have 800 wives, 1,000 slaves to care for the wives, 10,000 soldiers and 6,000 Amazonian women guards. Convicts and prisoners of war were buried with the kings, providing an entourage in the monarchs' afterlife.

Abomey became part of French West Africa in 1904 under the name of Dahomey and in 1960 became independent, changing the name to Benin in 1975. After independence it had the second largest number of coups in Africa, surpassed only by Nigeria. For 15 years, until 1989, it was a Marxist-Leninist state. Benin is now one of the most stable countries in West Africa. Among the most popular and easily portable souvenirs of Abomey are primitive appliqued figures of the panther god, Agassou, and of animals and hunting scenes. They are made of colored cloth on a black background.

Ganvie is a city of 12,000 people who live in bamboo huts built on stilts in Lake Nakoue. Fishing is the only industry here. The men plant branches in the muddy bottom of the lagoon, and when the leaves begin to decompose the fish come to feed and are caught in nets. The women sell the fish from their colorful pirogues, a type of canoe.

Woman's Ethnic Dress from Cotonou

Africans in general place great importance on clothing. It takes a substantial portion of their budget, and there is often a regal quality to their traditional dress. The woman's 'boubou' is long and sometimes embroidered. For everyday wear a loose top is worn and a two-meter length of cloth called a 'pagna' is wrapped around the body and tied at the left side of the waist to form a skirt. It takes three pagnas for one complete boubou.

Cotonou, Benin, is a quiet town with an excellent folkloric village, a storehouse of traditional marvels, including its well-dressed saleswoman, who made all of her own boubous. She would be happy, for a price, to make a dress exactly like the one she had on, which was lovely. We all went to a fabric shop where she found the right 'waxed cloth' from Holland, printed in the Côte d'Ivoire. An interesting note is that many of the designs were of feet, all shapes and sizes, mostly bare. We chose a more dignified design. It had diagonal stripes on a medium blue background, with red and green in the design. The stripes met in a pattern in the front of the garment. The random figures might have been meant to look like eyes.

In four hours a charming boubou and hat were delivered to the Benin Sheraton Hotel. The hat is a turban, which like so many articles of ethnic dress, is best when tied or arranged by a native of the country. It is amazing how many attractive headdress configurations can be created from these pieces of cloth. This garment is worn all over Africa, even in South Africa, and is seen in the U.S. at African gatherings. It is the favorite attire of South Africa's Winnie Mandela.

The name for men's elaborate outfits worn over trousers and shirts is 'grand boubou.' A less ornate version of the same costume is called a 'kaftan,' spelled with a k, not a c, as it is in Morocco. We saw many beautiful grand boubous worn by conference delegates at the Hotel Internationale Ivoire in Abdijan.

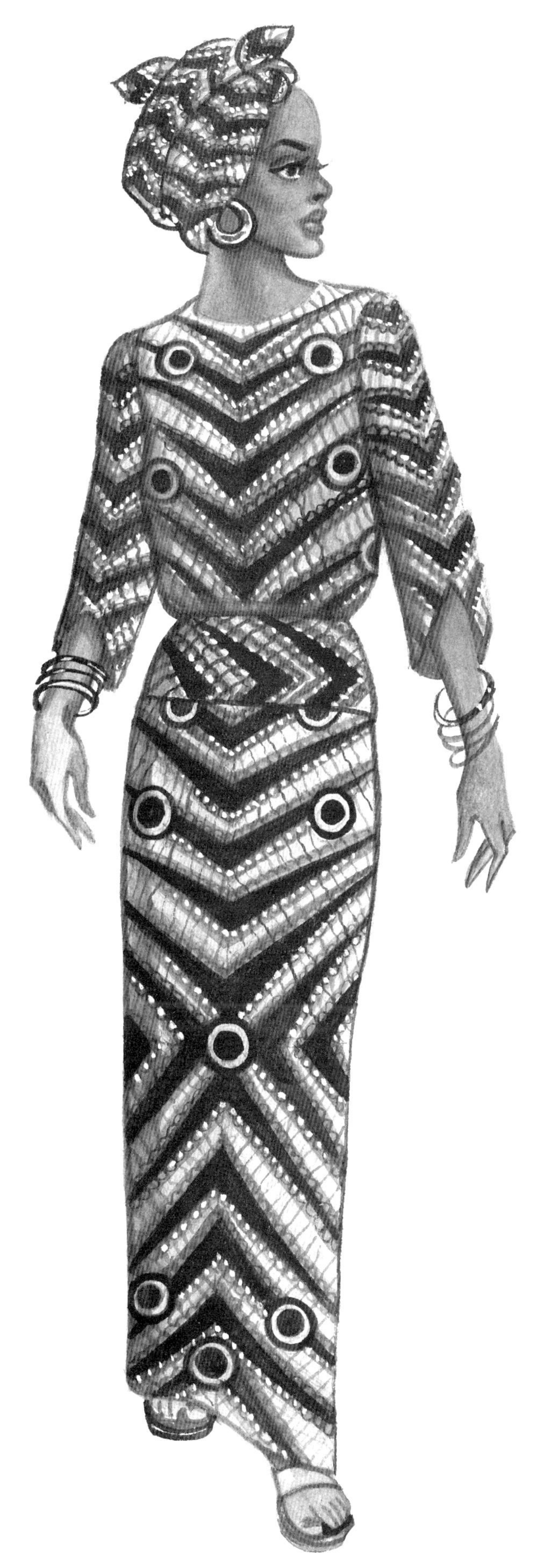

I've never sailed the Amazon,

I've never reached Brazil,

Yes, weekly from Southampton,

Great steamers, white and gold,

Go rolling down to Rio.

(Roll down - roll down to Rio!)

And I'd like to roll to Rio

Someday before I'm old.

Rudyard Kipling

Chapter Ten

South of the Border

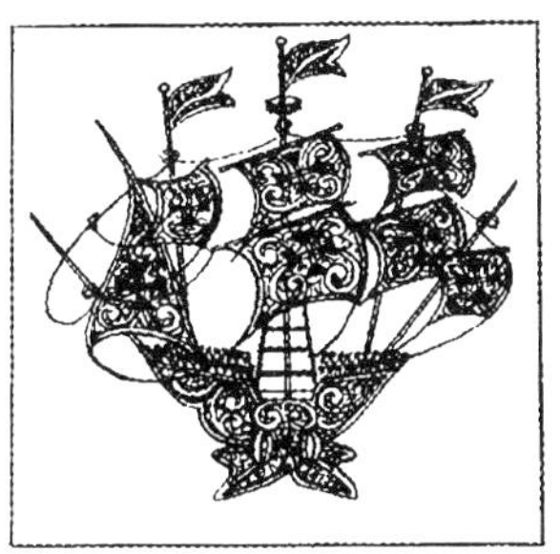

Brazil
Argentina
Chile
Bolivia
Peru
Guatemala
Mexico

Federative Republic of Brazil

Brazil occupies the eastern half of South America and is the largest country on that continent. It is larger than the contiguous United States, and has more than one and one-half times as many people. The capital is Brasilia, the monetary unit the cruzeiro, literacy is 81 percent and the religion is 90 percent Roman Catholic. The official language is Portuguese.

The Amazon River flows for nearly 4,000 miles across northern Brazil to the Atlantic Ocean, and is all navigable. It is second only to the length of the Nile.

The first European to reach this country was Pedro Alvarez Cabral, a Portuguese navigator, in 1500. Not many Indian tribes lived there, and the few that are left now live mostly in the Amazon basin. Portuguese colonists pushed their way inland, bringing many African slaves. Slavery lasted until 1888.

When Napoleon decided to move into Portugal, Prince Regent Dom Joao VI took refuge in Brazil. This was the first time a colony was made the seat of government for a mother country, and the people welcomed the prince because Brazil then became a kingdom, co-equal with Portugal. Dom Pedro, the son of Dom Joao, became king when his father was obliged to return to Portugal. When Dom Pedro was later ordered to Portugal he refused, and proclaimed Brazil independent and himself emperor. War with Argentina caused a deteriorating situation and Dom Pedro was forced to abdicate in favor of his son, Pedro II. Brazil prospered greatly under this emperor, but in 1889 he was also forced to abdicate. The government collapsed and a republic called the United States of Brazil was formed.

In 1960 the capital was moved from Rio de Janeiro to the planned, modern city of Brasilia, and in 1967 the country was again renamed, becoming the Federative Republic of Brazil. President Collor de Mello was impeached in 1992, and in 1994 Fernando Cardoso was elected president with a wide popular majority.

Inflation, recession and debt have plagued Brazil, and in 1982 there was an international outcry about the destruction of the Amazon's ecosystem. That same year Brazil hosted 178 countries for the Earth Summit, at which international ecological concerns were brought forward and discussed.

Around South America

What was I doing, lying motionless in bed, too sick to work the television set's remote control, waiting for the doctor, in Rio de Janeiro? Why hadn't I seen a doctor back home to prescribe for my painful throat and ear? It hadn't seemed too serious, but that day-and-night flight from Phoenix felled me. I knew I was in trouble when our descending flight caused me to fear a ruptured eardrum. Jo paid no attention to my protests and found the name of a doctor at the hotel desk.

Whatever I had, he said, I had brought from home. There was no sign of cold or flu, just an infection. Some strong antibiotics, fever medicine and cough medicine, along with lots of bed rest should get me up and going again in a few days. Bed rest? In Rio? A few days? We only had three days left. I hadn't been here for 30 years and I promised A.S.U.'s theater department an exotic, flashy carnival costume.

"Take the medication with fruit juice," cautioned the doctor, while telling Jo how to get the prescriptions filled without getting the hotel into the act. One in-room order of toast and hot chocolate had taught us to take our meals with the group since those were included in the price of our tour. I was there to get a costume, not to pay off Brazil's national debt.

Jo did everything exactly right . . . almost. I began taking antibiotics and would soon be on the road to recovery. Following doctor's orders Jo brought three large bottles of juice from a supermarket near the pharmacy. No one spoke English there, but she found an aisle of bottles with pictures of fruit on them. "Fruit juice, perfect!" she reasoned. She even purchased three different kinds of fruit pictures, thinking that some might taste better than others. As it turned out, they were all vinegars! The maid for our room received a real bonanza in vinegar the next morning.

Our Brazilian guide had found some telephone numbers to call about carnival costumes, and I soon discovered that one second-hand dress would cost as much as my costume budget for the entire trip. Oh, well, I rationalized, a carnival costume wasn't real ethnic dress, anyway. I would get a real 'gaucho' outfit in Buenos Aires, and my top priority was Peru and costumes of the colorful Incas.

Jo, who had never been to Rio, enjoyed the group trip to Petropolis, a mountain resort that was the site of the former summer palace of Emperor Dom Pedro II. They also went by cable car to the summit of the 1,300-foot Sugar Loaf Mountain and to Mount Corcovado's 2,300-foot-high peak, on top of which is the enormous monument named 'Christ the Redeemer,' shortened by popular usage to 'The Cristo.' A special trip was to dinner and a samba show. Many schools have been formed just to teach this dance, and at carnival time the streets are full of people sambaing to this exciting music in their exotic, flashy and very expensive costumes.

Our hotel was on the ocean with a manicured beach on which to stroll and enjoy views of the world's most spectacularly beautiful harbor. From my sickbed I could see a green foliage-covered hill with all kinds of homes.   There were recently-painted villas and tiny, tumble-down shacks. Obviously there is not much zoning in Rio. I found some interest in watching the lights come on at dusk, with people wending their way up the hill on foot, some carrying chickens, and with all kinds of dogs in tow. The view from my window and CNN on television aided somewhat in getting through my days of bed rest.

Republic of Argentina

Argentina occupies most of southern South America. It is four times the size of Texas, with less than twice Texas' population. The monetary unit is the peso, literacy is 95 percent and the religion is 90 percent Roman Catholic.

The Andes are to the west, with Aconcagua, at 22,834 feet, the highest peak in the western hemisphere. East of the Andes in the north are the wooded plains called the Gran Chaco, with the fertile, treeless pampas in the central part of the country. To the south is bleak and arid Patagonia, and to the east is the Rio de Plata (River of Silver) which is a 170-mile by 140-mile body of fresh water. Ships must be guided by Argentine pilots up this river for the 150 miles from the Atlantic to the port of Buenos Aires, which is the capital. However, the senate has recently approved the moving of the capital to Patagonia. Ushuaia, on the Beagle Channel, has the distinction of being the southernmost city in the world.

When the Spaniards arrived in 1515, nomadic Indians were roaming the pampas and, by the late 19th century, most of them had been killed. A great surge of European immigration followed. So many Italians settled in Buenos Aires that Spanish is spoken with an Italian accent.

From 1946 until his exile in 1955 General Juan Perón, with his wife Eva, headed the government. He returned in 1973 with his second wife, Isabel, and was again elected president, but died 10 months later. Isabel Perón became vice-president but was ousted in 1976 by a military junta.

In 1982 Argentine troops seized control of the Falkland Islands, which belonged to Britain. Three weeks after British troops landed on East Falkland Island, Argentina surrendered. President Galtieri resigned, and democratic rule was returned to the country.

Inflation reached 6,000 percent and President Carlos Saul Menem, who was elected in 1989, implemented drastic economic measures. At the time we were in Argentina, one peso was worth one U.S. dollar. The nation was in mourning while we were there, as the oldest son of President Menem had been killed in a helicopter accident.

Buenos Aires is one of the world's most beautiful cities. Its Pink House, the presidential palace, is magnificent. The city's divided avenues are many lanes wide and its parks rival those in other world capitals. This is a city of superlatives!

The Gaucho

As early as the 17th century, cowboys of mixed Spanish and Indian blood roamed the pampas of Argentina. Author John White, in his *Life Story of a Nation,* expressed the belief that it was the gauchos who made Argentina what it is today. They fought the Indians for the Spaniards, and later formed mounted militias against Spain, fighting alongside General José de San Martín, winning freedom not only for their own country, but also for Uruguay, Chile, Bolivia and Peru.

Gauchos are now considered national heroes and were immortalized in an epic poem by Jose Hernandez, *El Gaucho Martín Fierro.* Most Argentines can quote at least part of this poem. It depicts the gaucho as the personification of liberty, manhood and justice. However, according to Walter Owen, the poem's translator, the gaucho was a mixture of vice, virtue, savagery and culture. His law was his knife, or 'facón,' and his poncho was wrapped around his left arm in battle and used as a shield.

It was a cruel, brutal country out on the plains in no man's land, beyond the frontier of the Argentine army. The settlers pushed west, as did those in the U.S. In 1832 Charles Darwin visited a military camp whose purpose was to exterminate the Pampas Indians. The young Englishman was fascinated by the gauchos, their mustachios, long black hair falling about the shoulders of their scarlet ponchos, their wide riding trousers, boots with large spurs, and knives tucked into their waistbands. Their `bolas' were three heavy metal balls attached to ropes that were whirled and thrown to upend their enemies, who were fighting with bows and arrows.

From every point of view, the gauchos of the Argentine pampas played an important role in the formation of their country, and they are remembered in folk music, dance, poetry, novels and legends. Many believe the ghosts of the vanished Indians of the pampas ride on as South American gauchos.

The criollo, the horse of the gaucho, played an important role in Argentine history. It is a descendant of the Andalusian horse of Spain, which the Spaniards brought by the hundreds to Buenos Aires. Many of these criollos escaped and within 50 years thousands roamed the pampas. The gauchos captured these horses and they soon became invaluable to their masters.

This horse stands at about 14 hands, is strong, stocky, agile and tough. So tough, in fact, that in 1925, when the breed was losing popularity, two of these horses, Mancha and Gato, were ridden from Buenos Aires to New York City to prove their great stamina. The criollo suits the needs of present-day gauchos, and when it is said that the gaucho is half man and half horse, this is undoubtedly the breed of the horse half.

Ethnic Dress of the Gaucho of Argentina

Argentine gauchos, when working with cattle, wear a special attire that, embellished for special occasions, is known all over the world. This example was found in a folkloric shop in Buenos Aires that is known for its excellent line of gaucho clothing.

The basic 'chaleco,' or vest, and 'bombachos,' or trousers, are made of black cotton fabric, embroidered in a flower and leaf pattern in red, green, white and brown. The chaleco is sleeveless and has this design on each front panel. It is worn with a conventional man's shirt, and a black silk scarf is jauntily tied around the neck of the shirt. The bombachos are pleated in the front and outside of each leg, fitted at the waist and fastened at the ankles with a button and buttonhole. The same design as that on the chaleco is on the outer side of each leg of the bombachos.

A black and white handloomed belt about three inches in width is called a 'faja.' It is several yards long and is wound tightly around the waist to give extra support to the horseman's back. Over this belt a black leather coin-and-chain-decorated belt called a 'rastra' is worn. The coins on this belt are silver, but often they are gold, depending upon the wealth of the wearer. The 'facón,' a single-blade knife, in its ornamental silver case, is fastened to the leather belt at the back of the right side of the waist so that it is instantly available. This knife has many uses, including that of taking the place of a fork at mealtime. A long, narrow, cream-colored heavy leather whip called a 'rebenque' is used to control the horse and move the cattle.

The 'sombrero' is a black felt hat with a brim that is rolled on the sides. It has a flat top and is sometimes held on the head by a black cord. The boots, or 'botas,' are very special. They are of heavy black leather with tops that are crushed and kept that way by a retainer brace until worn. Silver 'espuelas,' or spurs, are fastened to the botas.

Some gauchos wear a red woolen 'poncho' with a vertical black strip over each shoulder. It is trimmed with a three-inch black wool fringe all around the garment, and it has an opening in the exact center for the head. This type of poncho is worn as a memorial to Juan Martín Guames, a hero killed in a battle against Spain.

This wonderful costume has a pièce de résistance, a lariat with three equal lengths of heavy rope, each having at its end a metal leather-covered ball. It is called a 'boleadora,' and its primary use is to throw at a running animal's legs in order to bring it down. It is also used in exhibitions in which the balls are struck on a wooden floor in a manner that results in the sound of thundering drums. When wielded by a skilled performer, the effect when seen and heard is electrifying. We saw a demonstration of this skill in Buenos Aires that left our entire group breathless.

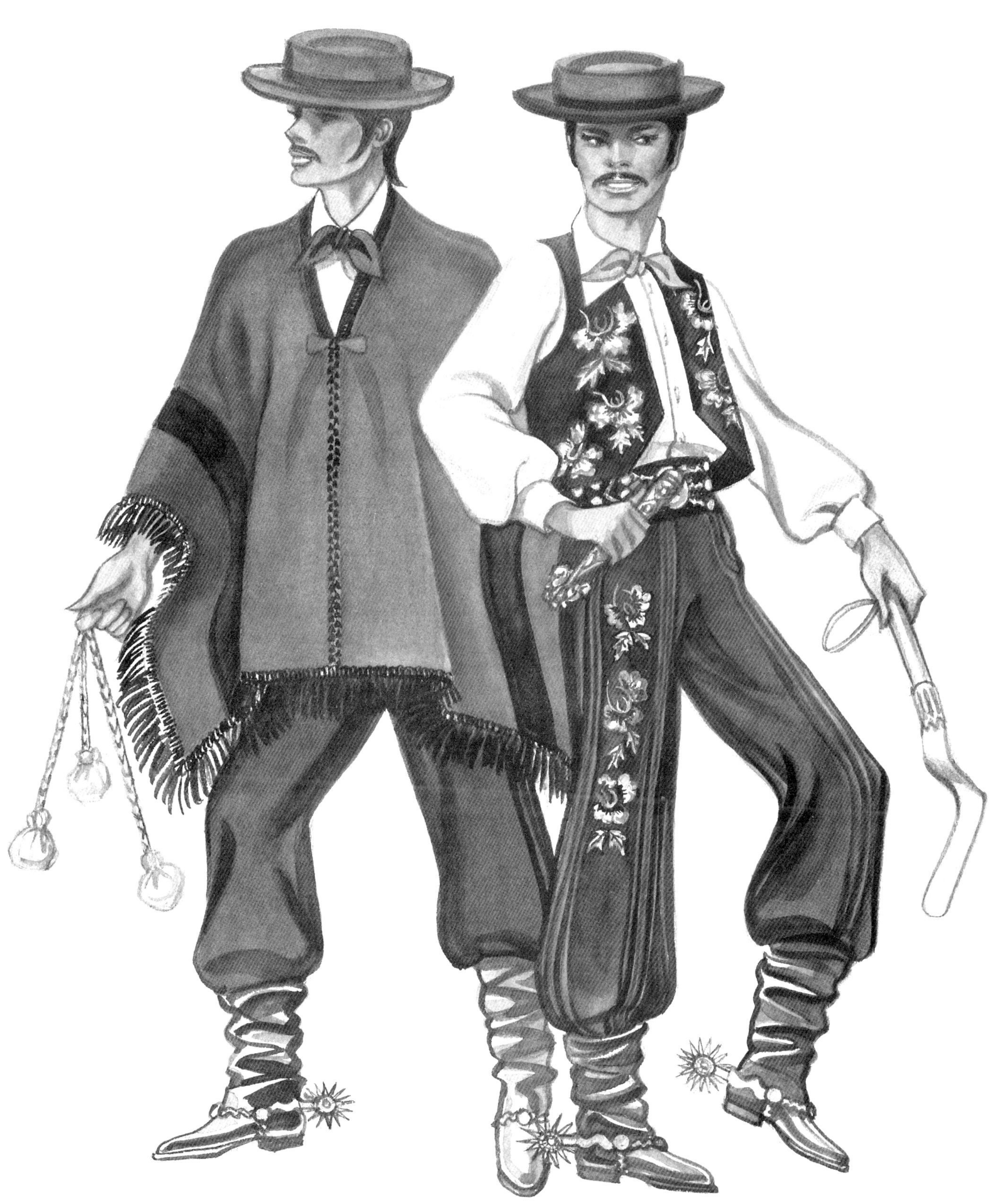

Enroute to Iguassu Falls, Argentina

On the flight to Iguassu Falls from Rio de Janeiro, I sat next to a clinical hypnotherapist. She assured me that the way I felt was all in my mind, that she could change my thinking, and I could begin to enjoy the trip. The process was going well. Her voice was low and soothing.

Before leaving home I had made an appointment to have a clogged tear duct repaired, and until that surgery could take place I 'cried' a lot, out of my left eye. As a tear rolled down my cheek, I heard her gasp. So that my benefactor did not misread the situation, I came out of what she must have considered a near-hypnotic state in order to let her know that a physical problem, not an emotional one, had caused the tear.

Her demeanor changed immediately. She lost interest in her patient, and I was left to get well as best I could. My illness had developed into a cough that made me the Typhoid Mary of the group, and now I had ruined my chance for a quick recovery.

Being in a weakened state, at airports I took advantage of a wheelchair service offered to elderly travelers. It was wonderful! As I sailed by the rest of the group, who were struggling with extra luggage, Jo was asked if I was really sick enough to need a wheelchair.

She answered, tongue in cheek, "Oh yes, her clogged tear duct has been bothering her." With that soft, southern drawl Jo can make anyone believe anything.

Iguassu Falls is made up of 275 individual falls and is located on the part of the Rio Iguassu that forms the boundary between Brazil and Argentina. The falls are in the shape of a horseshoe, are four times the width of Niagara Falls and average 230 feet in height. Some of them drop 270 feet, and a mist rises almost 500 feet into the air, creating a colorful rainbow effect.

This area rivals Niagara Falls as a honeymoon haven. There were great numbers of loving couples wandering around enjoying the scenic wonders . . . and each other. When my husband and I visited these falls 29 years earlier, it was the dry season, so we missed the full magnitude of their magnificence.

Republic of Chile

Chile, on the western coast of South America, is twice the size of California, with less than half the population of that state. It is bordered on the west by the Pacific Ocean for 2,650 miles, and varies in width from 100 to 200 miles for the entire length of the country. On the east are the Andes Mountains, with some of the highest peaks in the world. The mountain areas are well known for their excellent skiing and modern resorts.

The Indian population of Chile is only three percent, the rest being European and mestizo. The capital is Santiago, the currency the peso, and literacy is 92 percent. The religions are 89 percent Catholic and 11 percent Protestant.

Northern Chile was ruled by the Incas before the Spaniards arrived in 1530. Independence was gained in 1810 under José de San Martín and Bernardo O'Higgins. Chile won wars against Peru and Bolivia twice, gaining land in the north. In 1970 Salvador Allende Gossens, a Marxist, became president, leading the country to political and financial chaos. A military junta came into power in 1973, claiming that Allende had killed himself. Conditions did not improve, and in 1988 voters removed Augusto Pinochet from office and elected a civilian president.

A trip through Viña del Mar along the central Pacific coastline just north of Valparaiso was a special treat, as was the drive through the vineyards. Fine wines are a major export of Chile. A multitude of sea lions sun themselves on huge rocks rising from the sea along the shore.

Tierra del Fuego is the largest island in the archipelago of the same name at the southern tip of South America. It is an area of mountains, channels and high winds. Magellan discovered the island in 1520 and named it The Land of Fire because of its many Indian bonfires. Part of this island is in Chile and part is in Argentina. Below Chile is Cape Horn and Antarctica, the continent of the South Pole.

I plowed furrows in the ocean.

We have plowed the seas.

If nature is against us,

We shall fight nature and make it obey.

Simón Bolívar

Republica de Bolivia

Bolivia is a landlocked country, almost in the exact center of South America. It is approximately the size of California and Texas combined, with a population over seven million. The boliviano is the monetary unit, and literacy is 78 percent. The religion is Catholic.

Most of the people live in the altiplano, which means high country. The capital, La Paz, is the most important city in the altiplano. It is nearly 12,000 feet in altitude and is in the shadow of Mt. Illimani and on the shores of Lake Titicaca, the highest navigable lake in the world. The airport that serves La Paz is exactly the altitude of Pikes Peak in Colorado, 14,300 feet.

From 100 to 600 A.D., this part of South America was an advanced and prosperous civilization. The Aymaras of present-day Bolivia are descendents of these people. Many legends about Lake Titicaca abound, but archeologists have made little headway in verifying stories of underwater cities and hidden gold. There is no evidence of written pre-Spanish records of the Incas, but it is known that there was a state religion of the sun, presided over by Inca priests.

In the 13th century the Incas conquered this region and were responsible for substituting the Quechua language for the variety of dialects used by the people. Spanish rule began in the early 1500's and lasted until 1825, when Simón Bolívar liberated Bolivia and six other South American countries from Spanish control. The name Bolivia comes from its liberator.

Under the Spaniards the cult of the Sun God was suppressed, and a major effort was made to convert the people to Catholicism. Although Bolivia is considered a Catholic country, vestiges of the paganism of the Aymaras and Incas remain. Aymara, Quechua and Spanish are all spoken now in Bolivia.

Ethnic Dress of a Cholita

The cold, arid, windswept altiplano is populated by farmers and herdsmen of llamas, alpacas and sheep. To wrest from such a stubborn land enough food, fuel and wool to maintain life is a constant struggle. However, the most expensive wool in the world comes from an animal native to the area, the vicuña, and likewise the costliest fur from an animal raised here, the chinchilla.

The Indians, descended from the Aymaras and the Incas, are colorful in their native costumes. They are easily distinguishable from the residents of the cities, who dress in fashions as modern as can be found in London, Paris or New York.

'Cholos' are mestizos, who share Indian and Spanish ancestry; they are often bilingual, serving as interpreters between the Indians and the Spanish-speaking Bolivians. They are the miners, artisans and merchants.

This costume of a 'Cholita,' or young native girl of the altiplano, consists of a bright blue 'pollera,' a very full skirt with horizontal pleats that is worn with many petticoats of differing colors. A fancy pink 'blusa,' or blouse, has many tucks and gathers and is trimmed with white lace. Over these a pink 'manta,' or shawl, is worn. It is embroidered with bunches of grapes and has very long, hand-tied fringe.

This colorful outfit is topped by a smart, black felt bowler hat, designed by Borsalino of Italy. The shoes are shiny white leather, made as they were in 1850, with the soles secured with wooden pegs.

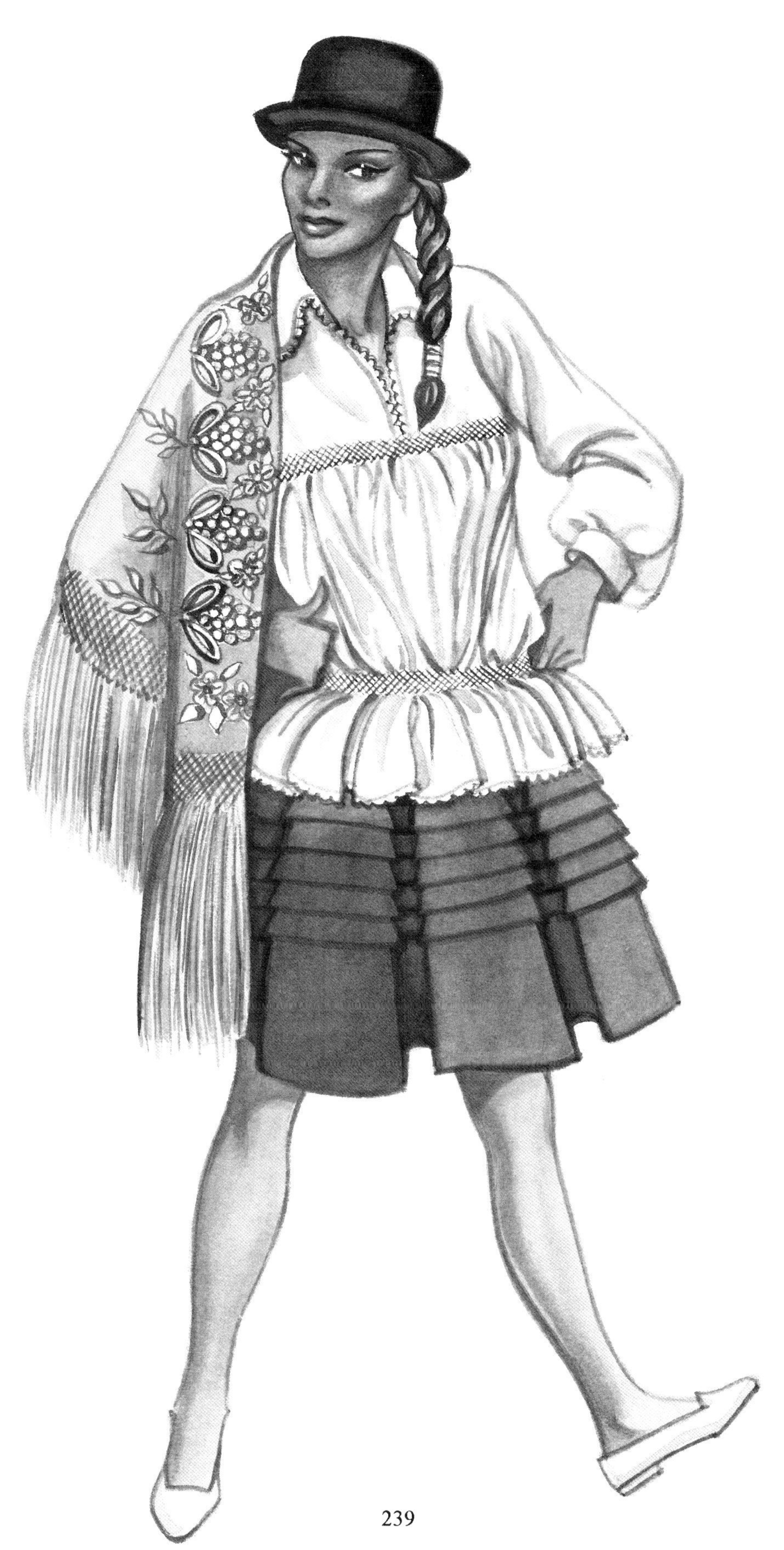

239

The Dance of the Devil

The towering Andes hide untold mineral wealth in tin, gold and silver, twisted deep in the convolutions of the high peaks. Only the Indians, adapted for centuries to the rarefied atmosphere, seem able to work in the mines at these altitudes. The Spaniards used forced Indian labor to bring up the silver, and they brought Christianity to replace paganism. It is not surprising that conflicting beliefs developed in the minds of the men who worked daily in the terrifying darkness.

A fraternity exists in which membership is passed down from father to son. It is this organization that plans the yearly celebrations that have been held in La Paz since the beginning of the century . . . The Dance of the Devil. This festive event has grown into one of the most anticipated of the year.

In this dance, the Devil, with hundreds of little boisterous devils leaping around him, is followed by dancers dressed in animal skins. All are awaiting the arrival of St. Michael, who wears a dazzling crown and robe and carries a snaky sword. The dancers are followed by the musicians playing with deafening enthusiasm "March of the Devil." St. Michael banishes the Devil, and once again for another year good has triumphed over evil.

Bolivian Devil Dancer

This remarkable mask of the Devil Dancer is the masterpiece of its creator, an artist who has trained for many years for this particular job . . . maker of masks. No two masks are alike. The more lizards, toads and snakes to be found winding themselves around the mask, the better. The two pairs of eyes are glass bulbs.

The Devil is the spirit of evil. He is meant to inspire terror in the onlooker, but he is also a giver of material riches, and his clothing must show signs of great wealth. Fine fabrics are used . . . woolens, velvets, gold and silver cloth, adorned with gems, pearls, beading, sequins and fine embroideries made with green, pink, yellow and red heavy yarns.

An undergarment of black consists of trousers and a top. There is an elongated dragon on each knee of the trousers. A magnificent cape has two solid silver gold-trimmed panels with dragons on each front panel. There is a large dragon on the heavy black velvet of the back of the cape, and under the dragon, on a wide silver band, is a golden sun. This sun is doubtless a tribute to the sun god of the Incas. A yellow-fringed heavy piece like a breastplate hangs from the neck, which is encircled by an elaborate, fringed collar. Three embroidered, fringed panels hang from a black belt, which is trimmed with 36 ten- and fifty-centavo pieces.

Red woolen gloves assure that no human flesh will be seen. Under the mask a red, jersey-knit, chin-strapped cap has long, stiff, blonde hair.

This amazing creation took three months to complete and is a testimonial to the imagination of the descendants of the Aymaras and Incas. Bringing it into this country would have been very difficult if the person who agreed to expedite the acquisition had not had a diplomatic passport.

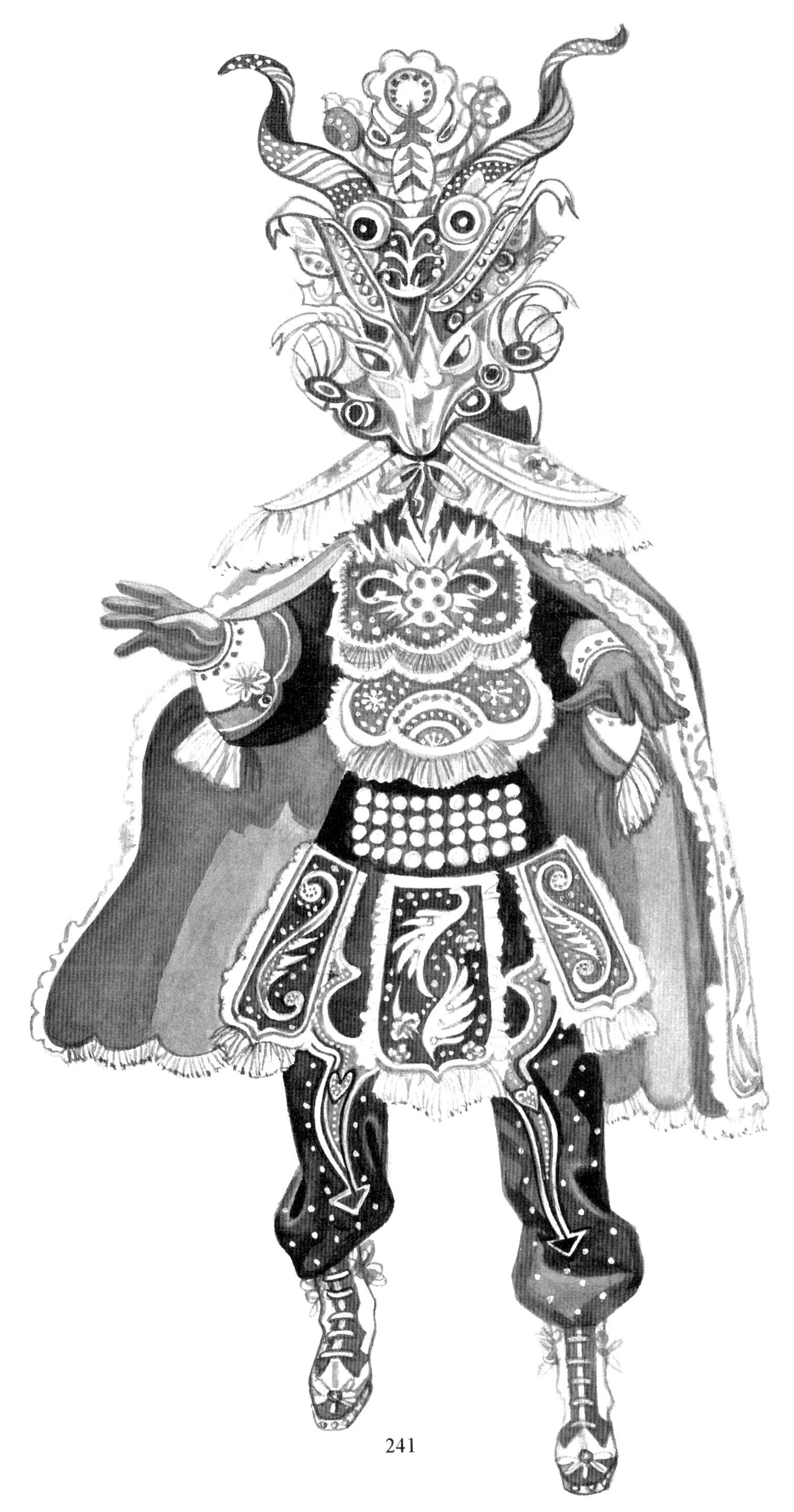

Republic of Peru

Peru is slightly larger than Alaska, with almost 40 times the population of that state. It lies on the Pacific Coast of South America and 27 percent of its land area is covered by the towering Andes mountain range. Lima is the capital, the nuevo sol is the currency and literacy is 85 percent. The religion of the country is 90 percent Roman Catholic, although the religion of the Indians, the largest ethnic group, comprising 45 percent of the population, is Roman Catholic infused with paganism.

Lima was the seat of the Spanish viceroys until the Argentine liberator, José de San Martín, captured it in 1821 and, with Simón Bolívar and Anton de Sucre, defeated Spain. In 1824 the independence of Peru was recognized.

In 1968 a military coup ousted President Belaunde Terry and another coup followed in 1975. After 12 years of military rule Peru returned to democratic leadership, re-electing the deposed Terry in 1980. In 1990 Alberto Fujimori, a Peruvian of Japanese descent, took office. He accomplished the capture of the leader of the 'Sendero Luminosa,' or Shining Path guerrillas, who had caused great disruption in the country. Because of this he enjoyed great popularity and in April of 1995 was re-elected to the presidency for another five years, with a two-thirds majority vote. Reliable sources report that by 1994 Peru became one of the world's fastest developing nations, economically.

The Empire of the Incas . . . Its History

Archeology has confirmed that the Inca empire was formed in the valley of Cuzco in the 12th century. It has also been ascertained that the lands of the Quechuas were seized by the Incas, its people absorbed into that empire, and after 1439 Pachacuti, the ninth Inca, proclaimed the Quechua language the language of all the Incas.

The Incas were the organizers rather than the creators of Peruvian civilization. The rest of the history of these people is vague, a combination of myth and memory. Both the Incas and the Spaniards purged any known records, creating their own official history, and all pre-Inca history was lost.

Victor W. Von Hagen, the distinguished American explorer of ancient western hemisphere cultures, writes in *Realm of the Incas:*

"In the early beginnings of the dynasty the ruler was often married into other tribes, but later, when his supremacy was unchallenged, his oldest sister became his principal wife, or 'coya.' This was meant to insure that his descent and divinity could not be questioned. However, he was allowed as many as 700 secondary wives, or concubines. There were numerous descendants with royal blood."

The most popular legend of the creation of the Inca empire involves the highest navigable lake in the world, Lake Titicaca, which forms a border between Bolivia and Peru. The Inca empire was believed to have been created on the Island of the Sun in this lake. Manco Capac and his sister, Mama Ocalla, were brought up from the waters of the lake by the sun god Inti. The pair was told to go out into the world, carrying a golden staff. Wherever the staff sank into the ground would be the seat of the empire of the Incas. That place was Cuzco, a valley high in the Peruvian Andes. The Lord Inca was to teach the men how to grow crops and his sister was to teach the women weaving and how to handle domestic affairs.

One hundred years after beginning a series of conquests in the early 15th century, the Incas controlled 12 million people in an area covering most of Peru, Bolivia, Ecuador and parts of Colombia, Chile and Argentina. These conquests were accomplished with the use of six-foot-long spears, short swords and very accurate slingshots, cleverly made from plaited llama wool.

The Spaniards, under Francisco Pizarro, arrived in 1532 with 130 foot soldiers, 40 cavalry and one small falconet cannon. The Incas were exhausted from civil war and had no knowledge of the world outside their experience. They were tricked by Pizarro into paying a 'roomful of gold' for release of their leader Atahuallpa, whom he had captured. When the ransom was received the Spaniards tried and executed Atahuallpa. The slingshots of the Incas were no match for the weapons of the Spaniards, and their empire became an appendage of Spain.

The People

The Incas of today are the people of the Cuzco area of Peru, descendants of the Quechua Indians. They still speak the Quechua language. The real Inca was the leader, believing himself to be god and man, above all other mortal beings. Gold and silver were considered his private property. Taxes were paid in labor, and laziness was punishable by death. The class system was very strong. The lower classes wore their tunics until they were threadbare. The Inca's tunic was burned after one wearing. The lower classes were monogamous. They had a charming marriage ceremony that consisted of holding hands and exchanging sandals.

When not working in the fields or cooking, an Indian woman of today can often be seen moving at a half-walk, half-trot with a wool distaff under her arm, spinning wool on a spindle stick. There is usually a baby wrapped in a shawl on her back, and she is often followed by a llama.

Llamas are not only pets, they have multiple uses in the life of the Indian, and the Spaniards were very impressed with them. The llama is a member of the camel family, has a long neck, long legs and a small tail. Its head resembles that of a camel, with a split nose, a harelip, and no upper teeth. It can grow to a weight of 400 pounds, is slender, can leap like a deer and run as fast as a train (an *Andean* train). It is covered with a coarse fleece, and supplies wool, hides, tallow for candles and dung for fuel. Like a camel, it spits and hisses when annoyed, and lies down and refuses to get up if overloaded or exhausted. Just as the camel was the animal of transit on the Old Silk Road, llamas serve that purpose on the Inca highways.

Another important animal is the guinea pig. It is a domesticated species of the South American rodent and lives in Indian homes. It is a family pet as well as a source of food. Guinea pigs of Peru have long, silky fur. In a church in Cuzco it was interesting to see a painting of 'The Last Supper' in which a baked guinea pig is shown on the platter in front of Christ.

An amusing custom that seems to have some meaning for the Cuzco Indian is that of plucking several hairs from his eyebrows and blowing them into the air while reciting a prayer. Although the Spaniards carried on an intensive campaign against idol worship, the Catholicism of the Incas is laced with pagan deities, particularly the sun god.

In Indian communities today there is only one trained physician per 1,000 people. The local shaman, known for his wide knowledge of medicinal plants, is used to care for the sick.

The following poem is chanted at festivals. The ideas, repetition, cadence and imagery are completely Inca.

The Inca

Beautiful Princess,	*But Princess,*	*The maker of the earth*
Thy dear brother	*thy water,*	*Pachacamac*
Thy cup	*dropping, rains,*	*Viracocha*
Is now breaking.	*where sometimes also*	*for this duty*
So for this there is thunder,	*there will be hail,*	*has placed thee,*
lightning, lightning,	*there will be snow.*	*has created thee.*
thunderbolts falling.		

Inca Ingenuity

Inca Roads

The Incas were highly skilled engineers and architects, and one of their outstanding feats was the construction of a network of roads extending along the western coast of South America and inland for a total of 10,000 miles of all-weather highways. They were designed for foot travelers and pack animals and had many short tunnels and suspension bridges. There were the Coastal Road, the Andean Road, and roads leading to all of the towns in their empire. All were 24 feet wide and began in the center of Cuzco's main square. They led to the west, east, north and south and were said to cover the 'four corners of the earth.'

Couriers and the 'quipu' were used to keep track of everything going on in the empire. The quipu was a long rope hung with 48 secondary cords, with tertiary cords in different colors. This instrument was used instead of writing, which was unknown to the Incas. The tying of knots in the cords provided a complete accounting system which only trained readers could decipher. Runners, called 'chasquis,' carrying the quipu, could run 250 miles a day. There were small chasquis stations every half league, or one-and-one-half miles. Travelers stayed in 'tampus,' built every eight miles. In his palace in Cuzco the ruling Inca could have fresh fish from the ocean in two days, brought with 200 miles of running. This excellent road system was the main reason the Spanish were able to conquer the Incas with so few men in such a short time.

A suspension bridge on one of these roads achieved fame in Thornton Wilder's book *The Bridge of San Luis Rey.* This swinging bridge, built by the Inca Roca around 1350 was 148 feet in length, hanging above the raging waters of the Apurimac River, one of the headwaters of the Amazon. It hung from fiber rope cables as thick as a man's body, made from the maguey plant. These cables were replaced each year. In 1890 the bridge was still hanging, but no longer in use. Hiram Bingham, who discovered Machu Picchu, has written that it was this bridge that first inspired his interest in Peru.

Weaving

Backstrap looms, found mostly in the graves of women, were very much like those of the Mayans of Central America. The upper part of the loom is tied to a strap or belt and the loom is then tied to a tree or it stands upright. The belt for tension is around the back of the weaver. A method of weaving the fine wool of the vicuña into textiles was perfected to a point where the Spaniards thought it was silk.

Sacsayhuamán

This is a fortress on a hillside overlooking Cuzco. It has been described as one of the greatest structures ever erected by man. Construction is of huge stones, some of which weigh as much as 20 tons. Each stone fits another so perfectly, without mortar, that a knife blade cannot be pushed between them. How the Inca mason achieved this perfection, when each stone had to be lifted many times to be made to fit, still cannot be explained, but we do know that the work force numbered 30,000 Indians. We do not know how they measured, but like the Egyptians, they must have used body parts. Our Cuzco guide suggested that we could better remember the name of this engineering marvel by calling the fort 'Saxy Woman,' which is close to its correct pronunciation.

Machu Picchu, Lost City of the Incas

Machu Picchu lies in a topographical saddle between the Peruvian peaks of Machu (old) and Hayna (new). A train covers the distance of 50 miles from Cuzco through the beautiful Urubamba River valley to the foot of the mountain, at the top of which lie the ruins of the lost city. A waiting coach takes visitors on a road that winds around the mountain to the hotel through which they can enter this ancient walled fortress.

Originally there was only one heavy wooden gate through this wall. The strongly constructed houses were most probably defense units. There are polished granite homes for the rulers, houses for the common people, barracks for soldiers and even a prison. Terraces, following the contours of the mountains like a gigantic flight of steps, provided food for the inhabitants. The Inti-huatana (stone clock) sundial is celebrated for its accuracy.

A large building is believed to have been the living quarters for the 'chosen women.' These women who served the Incas were called 'virgins of the sun.' At a hair-combing ceremony at the age of puberty, girls who were beautiful, talented and of high lineage were selected. They were then sent to special schools, one of which was in Cuzco. They were given a chance to either marry into the nobility or to serve the Inca. An important task was the weaving of garments for the Inca and his legal wife. The women serving the Inca took a vow of chastity. If this vow was broken, the penalty was to be buried alive. The accomplice and all his relatives were hung. Even his llamas were killed.

It was suggested by Hiram Bingham of Yale University that sequestering these chosen women could have been the reason for Machu Picchu's construction. He wrote that he found the city in 1911 in the "most inaccessible corner of the most inaccessible section of the central Andes." Nine out of ten of the skeletons recovered were women, thus establishing a belief that the many-roomed building in the ruins could have been a type of convent to house these special women.

Whatever the reason, Machu Picchu was never found by the Spaniards, and this monument to a lost civilization is now one of the most popular and fascinating of all tourist destinations. Guides can be heard extolling the wonders of the Lost City in Japanese, French, English, German, Italian and Spanish.

The Andes . . . A High Point for Any Trip

A 3:30 a.m. wake-up call was needed to get us to the Lima airport in time for the 6 a.m. one-hour flight to Cuzco. There was a large crowd waiting. Mingled with the tourists were Indians with their children returning to Cuzco from shopping trips in Lima, judging from the large number of parcels they were carrying. The news was bad . . . heavy rain was making landing in Cuzco difficult. So we waited, and waited. Two planes finally left, but they returned, unable to land at their destination. The morning was gone, and all flights were canceled, so we returned to our Lima hotel with tickets for the same plane the next morning. Our two days in Cuzco were now reduced to one.

We asked the desk for another 3:30 am. call. This time the plane took off as scheduled, but a heavy fog covered the entire area between mountain peaks, so we went on to Arequipa for more airport-sitting.

Finally the fog lifted enough for us to descend into Cuzco. We were too late for the train to Machu Picchu, but that didn't bother me, as I had not planned to go there. I'd been there twice, and this was my chance to get the Inca costumes that were my only reason for being in Cuzco. Adrian, our guide for the entire South American trip, informed me that I *was* going to Machu Picchu. When I objected he said he wasn't going to allow one person to spoil the trip for the rest of the group. The train was going to meet the bus at a halfway point and there wasn't even time to get me to the hotel, and that was it! He added that Cuzco was dangerous for tourists and that I would be an easy target. Even taxi drivers weren't considered a safe bet for women traveling alone. There was good reason to fear that I might not even make it to the hotel without being robbed, and he was responsible to the tour company for my safety.

What a dilemma! He added that there was just one possible solution, but he wouldn't disclose it yet. But it happened . . . Hallelujah! The Cuzco guide who met our plane was not needed, so I was handed over to her. I felt like a piece of luggage, but who cared at that point? Her car and driver took me to the hotel, where she suggested I rest a few hours while she found a responsible driver to take me around that afternoon. Since we were at an altitude of 12,200 feet and my head was aching, I was grateful for her suggestion and went to bed.

My driver José arrived, and he turned out to be exactly what I needed, which meant he had connections. His poor English even matched my poor Spanish. There was hope now; luck had not entirely deserted me. The first shop was a large folkloric place filled with uninteresting tourist items, and it was about to close for siesta. Oh, no! I had completely forgotten about that three-hour nap everyone has to have so that they can stay up all night and have dinner at an outrageous hour.

Perhaps the Indian market was open? José didn't even answer my question, so I relaxed and enjoyed the drive through ancient, historical, charming Cuzco's narrow streets. Vestiges of Spanish culture were everywhere in this Indian and colonial city. We came to a dead end in front of a high gate. José got out and pounded on the gate until a child appeared and guided us inside to HEAVEN!

We were in a factory that made mestizo clothing for fiestas. The display was dazzling. Gorgeous full skirts embellished with colorful embroidery, hats of all kinds, and accessories, too! Furthermore, since this was siesta time, we were the only shoppers in the entire factory. The owner, his wife and three children devoted their afternoon to helping me. They brought maté de coca for my headache. This is a weak tea made from coca leaves, used in high countries to provide relief from altitude sickness. Two cups of this steaming potion dissolved all pain, and we settled down to business. The entire front of the factory was glass, allowing for a superb view of the city and mountains. The next two hours made up for everything that had gone wrong on this trip.

While the dress of the Indians, except for interesting hats, is rather drab, the dress-up clothing of the mestizos, with its strong Spanish influence, is spectacular. Choosing surprisingly reasonably-priced treasures made for an unforgettable afternoon. The models were the teenaged children of the owners. Their jeans and T-shirts, worn under the beautiful costumes, added emphasis to my feeling of amazement. The family's enthusiasm grew with my delight and soon, articles that had been in the family for years were brought out. Every item had to have its use and proper wear carefully explained. I was a willing and enthralled audience. South America was wonderful, and my trip was a success, after all. José seemed to enjoy the afternoon and, if he got a commission, he deserved it. The factory owner even threw in a knitted bag in which to carry all purchases home.

My traveling companion Jo was equally enchanted with her trip to Machu Picchu. This had been a perfect day for everyone.

This visit rekindled memories. Thirty years before, I had come to Cuzco with my stewardess daughter. We found it so interesting that my husband and I returned the next year. We spent a few days in Cuzco and Machu Picchu, before our hydrofoil trip to the Islands of the Sun and Moon in Lake Titicaca. Cuzco had no train station, as such, and a group of people were gathered at the boarding area, waiting for the train to show signs of leaving for Puno, on the lake's edge. Men in laborers' clothing were talking excitedly in groups and waving their arms. We couldn't understand a word, but were told that the workers were threatening to go on strike. Some were carrying large sticks. There was nothing to do but wait, although somewhat anxiously, since our bags were already on the train. Soon, a conductor motioned to the travelers to get on board. We did so, uneventfully. When the train left the station area, the men began to chase it, brandishing their sticks in a threatening manner. They held back a bit until the train picked up speed, running faster only when we had no problem outdistancing them. We steamed comfortably and merrily on to Puno, with no idea of what was going on in Cuzco's labor relations with their railroad department.

Mestizo Man's Fiesta Costume of Cuzco, Peru

This man's sleeveless black wool vest is called a 'chaleco,' and is worn under a green wool 'chaquet,' or jacket. The inch-wide white tape, made of embroidered bands that trim all edges of both garments, have the same designs in green, yellow and red. The pockets of the vest are designed to look like flower pots, from which grow a red and white stylized flower with white leaves. There is a six-inch opening in the back of the chaquet. At the bottom of this opening and at each side of the garment and on each side of the front of the chaquet there is a white, red-centered flower with yellow fronds and green leaves. The small stand-up collars are an interesting feature. They are two inches high and about four inches wide and heavily embroidered in the colors of the rest of the trim.

'Pantalones,' or trousers, are of black wool. On the outside of each flared trouser leg there is a strip of embroidery which widens from a narrow point ten inches above the cuff to two inches at the hem. The yarn colors are white and orange.

A cream-colored fitted knit cap with brown trim is made of alpaca wool, and there are ear flaps with strings that hang to below the chin. This hat, called a 'chullo,' is worn all over the high altitude areas of the Andes Mountains and has become popular as a ski cap in fashionable, modern ski resorts. It is a direct descendant of the Inca head covering.

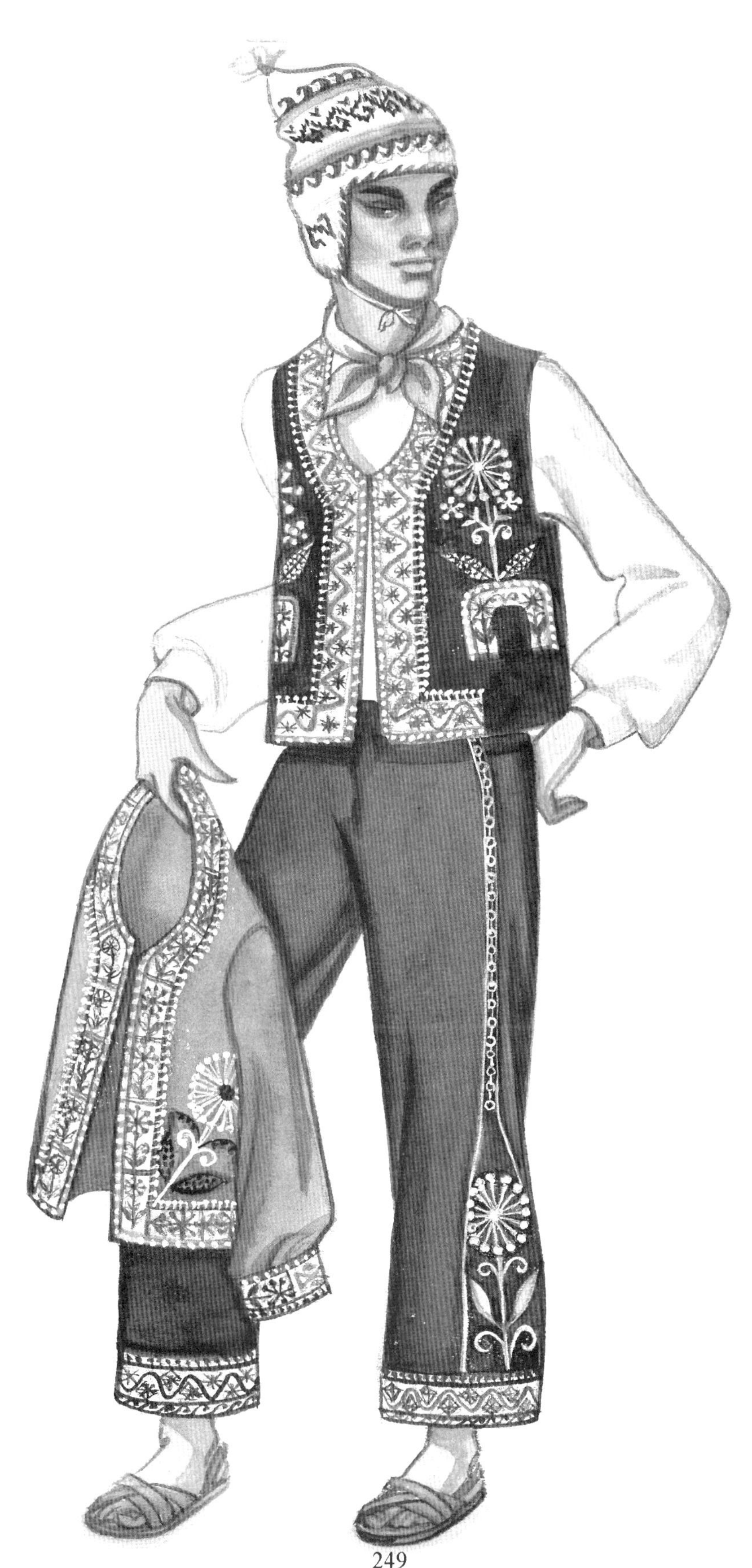

Mestiza Woman's Dress of Cuzco, Peru

The woman's chaqueta is red wool with long sleeves. There is an embroidered tape border like that on the man's vest and jacket, which trims the front, sleeves, cuffs and pockets.

A full black wool skirt called a `pollera' is lavishly decorated with four horizontal bands varying from two to three inches in width.

The large, flat hat, a 'montera,' is 14 inches in diameter. It is made of black wool, decorated with red, green, yellow and white embroidery. It shows signs of having survived many fiestas. A woolen strap hangs loose under the chin of the wearer. The montera is worn perched atop a beautiful 'manta,' or shawl, which is three by four feet long, with a decorated border of stylized flowers in each corner, like those on the man's vest and jacket.

Black leather sandals called 'zapatas' still have the red sand of Cuzco on their soles. This dress was that of a dancer in a fiesta, and a feathery string of pompons in all of the popular Cuzco colors is carried.

Mestiza Child's Dress

As in many ethnic groups, Cuzco children's clothing closely resembles that of their parents'. A black wool skirt, short and very full, is banded with a six-inch edging of embroidery and rickrack. A tiny, red, long-sleeved chaqueta is trimmed with braid similar to that used to decorate the clothing of this little girl's parents. It fastens in front, and there are two insets of embroidered red wool at the waist.

A miniature manta of green wool is 11 by 18 inches in size. It is also banded around the edges and has narrow wool braid on the inside of the edging. A wonderful hat has a flat top of black wool, 10 inches in diameter, trimmed with triangular pieces of red, green and yellow wool around the outer edges. There is a four-inch brim, broadening to the size of the flat top.

A small bag is made of black and red wool, with one red and two black tassels at the bottom. Three green buttons close the top. Two bright-colored wool elastic bands worn around hair braids add the finishing touch to this excellent example of ethnic dress of a child of Inca-Spanish descent.

Each of these costumes is appropriate to be worn at the Great Sun Festival of Inti-Raymi, god of the sun.

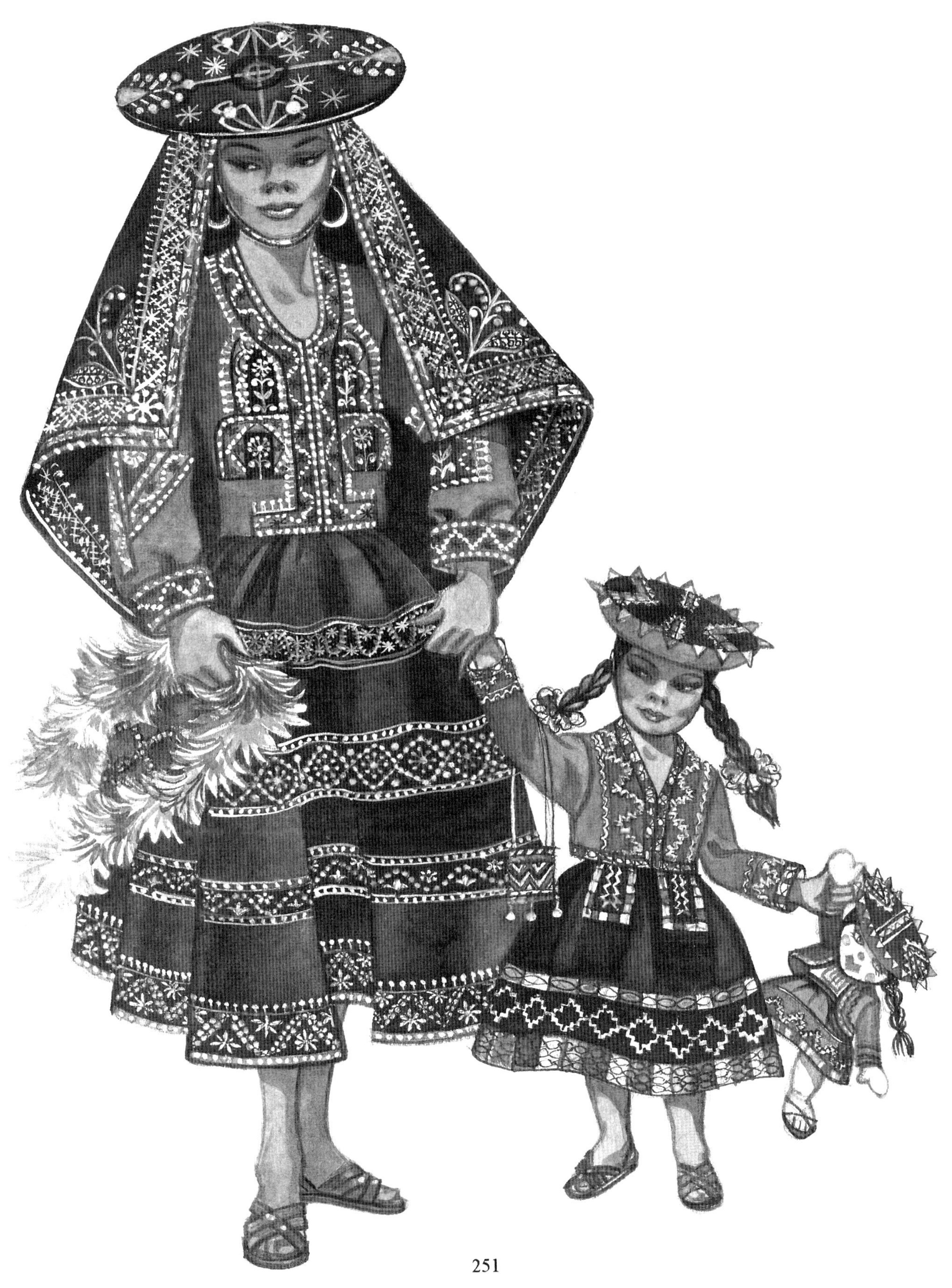

Republica de Guatemala

Guatemala is in Central America, south of Mexico. It is the size of Tennessee, with more than twice the population of that state. The capital is Guatemala City, the monetary unit is the quetzal, which is also the name of the national bird. Literacy is 55 percent. The people are 44 percent Indian and 56 percent mestizo. The religion is mostly Roman Catholic, with some animism and pagan worship.

The old Mayan empires flourished in Guatemala for a thousand years before the Spanish came. The Spanish controlled this country from 1524 to 1821. It was then briefly a part of Mexico, then of the United States of Central America, and in 1839 it became a republic. There was a swing toward socialism, an armed revolt, renewed attempts at social reform, a military coup and civilian rule, all before 1986. The president was ousted by the military in 1993 and the congress elected a new president.

Guatemala, as I see it, after 14 visits:

Imagine a country with plains, deserts, lowlands, mountain ranges with 13,000-foot-high peaks, canyons 2,000 feet deep, 30 volcanoes, plateaus, great rivers and lakes, thermal springs, waterfalls and tropical jungles, with both an Atlantic and Pacific seaboard. Spread color freely among butterflies, birds and flowers, give perpetual spring to the plateaus and highlands and tropical temperatures to the lowlands, snow-covered mountains on winter mornings, all topped with electric-blue skies and foamy white clouds. This small country has a beauty and mystique unmatched by any other country I have visited.

In this land three civilizations exist side by side, Mayan, Spanish colonial and modern. The early Mayans created a culture that proves them to be, according to historian Dr. Sylvanus Morley, "The most brilliant aboriginal people on the planet." They were astronomers and developed a calendar which in precision was better than that of either the Greeks' or the Egyptians'. They discovered a system of arithmetic which predated comparable systems in Europe, Asia and the Middle East by 2,000 years. Their simple numerical system of dots and dashes stands as "one of the most brilliant achievements ever conceived by the mind of man," again according to Dr. Morley. They developed writing to a high level. Their road system was second only to the Incas' until the Lancaster Turnpike opened in North America in 1792. The Mayans were using a sewage system when Europe was still throwing waste out the windows. Magnificent cities were erected.

In 1523 a captain of Cortés' army in Mexico set forth to subdue Guatemala. His instructions from Cortés were to "endeavor with the greatest care to bring the people to peace without war and to preach matters concerning our own Holy Faith." The expedition was a series of massacres of Indians who preferred death to submission.

Excursions Extraordinary: Antigua

Ciudad Vieja, or Old Capital, on the outskirts of present-day Antigua, ranked with Mexico City and Lima, Peru, as one of the great centers of Spanish culture during colonial times, but it was fraught with disasters of floods, volcanoes, pestilence and earthquakes. In 1775 Guatemala City became the new capital, Antigua having been destroyed by earthquake. It was rebuilt and has been declared a national monument. There is an aura of antiquity to this city that makes it an increasingly popular place for visitors.

In January of 1976 we went on a family holiday to Antigua with two of our children and their children, ages 3, 5, 6 and 7. Everything was perfect, the weather, the private cottages with fireplaces, the food and the scenery. The children loved Beatriz, the young Guatemalan girl who helped with their care. They even had the opportunity of seeing everyday Guatemalan life in Beatriz's home. Molly had seemed to stop eating, but her chubby three-year-old body showed no signs of malnutrition. The other children reported that she ate tortillas all the time she was there and that the family enjoyed watching the little 'gringa' stuff herself with their favorite food.

Had our trip taken place a week later, our memories would not have been so pleasant. Guatemala was rocked by 500 measurable earthquakes, killing 22,000 people countrywide. While the hotel we stayed in wasn't damaged, we learned that the guests slept out-of-doors in surrounding hills, for fear of being trapped in their rooms.

Before leaving Antigua I placed a large order for weavings at my favorite shop, where a dozen men worked on 35-foot footlooms, very much like those brought to Guatemala on Columbus' ships. Because of the earthquakes the textiles disappeared in the mail. I had already paid for them, but I wrote the shop owner telling him not to worry, that I understood he had enough problems at that time. I learned that tragedy had not spared him. He lost a family member and much of his business.

His reply is printed here, unedited. There is a poignancy to his letter that gives an insight into the fortitude of these talented and courageous people.

"My Dear Señora,
I feel a shame of myself for not been able to answer your very affectionate letter due to our tragedy. Thanks God, we are back on our Wheels, and thanks to all people like you in all over the U.S. for such wonderful help we have recieved from all of you. God bless you. I think the earthquake business is all over the hemisphere and God is a wonderful driver, just trust Him, and let Him drive your destiny, this is what I have learn lately."

Amatitlán

The trip just described was not the last of Guatemala for us. Another time we traveled with friends, pulling our two Airstream travel trailers. There had been problems in Mexico for visitors using this mode of transportation, and we would not have dared go by ourselves, but our friend was a Marine Corps general with four stars on his windshield. Also, he had worked for a year with the president of Mexico on a drug case, and an official stamp was next to the stars on his windshield. That did it! No one would dare touch us, and they did not, as long as we were with our friends.

We parked in a surprisingly modern and comfortable trailer park in Amatitlán, 16 miles south of Guatemala City. This park had a hot springs swimming pool that was scoured thoroughly and often, making a delightful bathtub in the cool evening air of the nearly mile-high area. The water was scalding as it rushed into the pool. Within easy view of the park was the cone of Pacaya, the 8,346-foot-high active volcano, which threw sparks high into the air. Every night was like the Fourth of July.

When not swimming or roasting wieners (on very *long* sticks) over the hot lava flow that crept down the mountain from its fiery cone, I amused myself by riding the aging local bus to the Indian market at the end of the line in Guatemala City. This method of transport was not recommended in any travel books, but once the seats with broken springs were located and avoided, it was an excellent way to observe the descendants of the Mayan empire. Since the rest of the group, including my husband, preferred to find other ways to study local culture, I went alone. On one of my bus excursions a little girl piped up, "Mira, Mama, como nieve." (Look, Mama, like snow.) Her embarrassed mother scolded her. Once again my white hair attracted attention. When an iguana slid his head and snaky neck out of the basket on the rack overhead, my reaction caused the whole bus to break into laughter. This was the only time I have ever heard the stoical Mayan laugh. As I leaped from my seat, how was I to know the ugly beast was tied in the basket? The other passengers were obviously doing a cultural study, too . . . of me!

The time finally came, all too soon, to leave our idyllic spot. We made arrangements, in case we were separated, to meet at a recommended trailer court in Tapachula, just across the Mexican border. Our companions, with the stickers on their windshield, were waved across the border. We were not so lucky. When it was our turn the Mexican officials closed the barrier and said, "Siesta time." Two hours later a guard entered our trailer, saw a pile covered with a blanket and yanked it off. "This is illegal. Where are your permits?" he demanded. Permits for a dozen three- and four-yard pieces of weavings? The blanket was not for secreting purposes, it was to keep the dust off. We would have been happy to pay duty, although it was under the limit. No way! They said we needed a permit, and the closest place to get it was in Mexico City, 500 miles away.

This was not the Mexican government's policy; it was some customs officials practicing "la mordita," (the bite). We parked our rig and were led into a room that looked more like a barracks than a waiting room. No one spoke English. An hour later, when a group of Canadians came into the room, I told them in a loud voice about our predicament. The guard signaled to me. (I was glad it was me rather than my husband, as he would have let them have the weavings.) Stepping behind a wall, the guard held out his hand. I placed all the pesos I had in his hand, and he bowed and pointed toward the exit. We crossed the border and joined our friends at the trailer court. We had just lost three hours and $80.

Tikal

Tikal is located in what is now the northeastern region of the Department of Petén in Guatemala. It is the largest pre-Columbian Mayan city and ceremonial center, and one of the most impressive ruins to be found on this continent. As one approaches by air, five great pyramid roof crests appear through the enormous mahogany, cedar and chicle trees. These pyramids soar from 184 feet to the height of temple #4 which is 210 feet, the tallest in the Americas. The north end of the plaza is dotted with stelae and altars, some of them beautifully carved. There is evidence of human sacrifice. A central acropolis of palace structures, with 42 buildings and hundreds of rooms that were residences for the aristocracy, covers about one square mile.

In 900 B.C., Tikal was a small village, developing into an area of great plazas by 900 A.D. At its peak there was a population of about 10,000 in the center core, with about 50,000 in the surrounding countryside. After the farming season, everyone was expected to join in building and renovating the center. This was a public works program that continued over a thousand years. All endeavors were directed to enhance the city, glorify the gods and amass wealth for the ruling classes. Then, somewhere around 900 A.D., Tikal was abandoned for reasons that have never been conclusively determined.

This site was discovered in the 17th century. In 1956 the University of Pennsylvania began a program of excavation and rebuilding, concluding their work 13 years later. When they left, most of Tikal was still buried under the jungle. Guatemalans took over the project and today, 222 square miles form a national park, preserving the archeological zone.

Little authentic information remains from the exodus of the Maya to the arrival of the conquistadors, since the latter destroyed every vestige of Indian culture they could find and killed off the ruling houses. Only three Mayan books survived destruction. The costumes of the people are their culture and the weavings their history.

Guatemalan Textiles

By the time Columbus arrived in Central America, Indian textiles had reached a high degree of art Elaborate costumes of chiefs and priests are carved on the walls of ancient Mayan temples. The textiles of the Indians are their books, and each weaver writes his own story According to ancient tradition, a textile was begun with a prayer and required many months to complete. Each figure of the design had its own significant position on the fabric and, if it was to be made into clothing, ultimately on the body. Nobility and aristocracy had exclusive, elaborate designs of their own.

The wearer's biography was for all to see. His social and official rank, profession, age, marital status, the happiness of his marriage and even whether his generative powers were waxing or waning were woven into his clothing. Museums and universities are collecting representative tribal costumes, but examples are fast disappearing. It is not unusual to see a foreigner bargaining for a piece of clothing an Indian is wearing, faded as it may be from many washings.

The footloom, introduced by the Spaniards, made it possible to share these beautiful weavings with the rest of the world. These looms are nearly as primitive as the handlooms, and they may occupy most of the space in Indian huts, turning out modern textiles that are truly amazing.

Chichicastenango

Chichicastenango is the site of the most colorful and famed Indian fair in Central America. Held every Thursday and Sunday, it is a center for surrounding Quiché villages. This area is so traditional that nearly every boy in 'Chichi' is named Tomás, after the town's patron saint.

We stayed at the Mayan Inn, a delightful hotel decorated with genuine Spanish antiques. We dined to the mellow sound of marimba music, with as many as nine musicians simultaneously playing one instrument. The music of Guatemala is euphonious and pleasant, and the players were dressed in traditional Quiché garb. Mornings, Tomás the houseboy built a mesquite fire in our room while we had coffee. Because of the bracing climate both the fire and the coffee were welcome.

The town cathedral, El Calvarío, was built in 1540 by the Dominican order. It is an excellent example of the linking of two cultures, ancient Mayan and Christian. On the steps of this church the natives swing their small pots billowing with copal smoke while chanting to their native gods. At the completion of this ceremony they climb the steps of the church to attend the Catholic service inside, scattering rose petals. They are not taking any chances with their afterlife.

Ethnic Dress of the Quiché Tribe

The 'huipil,' or blouse, of this dress is a square when opened up, embroidered with pink and aqua flowers on a darker background. The pile is velvety, made by inserting a filler yarn into the pattern with the fingers. The basic textile for this blouse has been woven on a footloom.

The floor-length skirt, called a 'refajo,' also footloomed, has a multi-colored braid around the hipline. The tightly wound belt is embroidered with flowers of many colors, symbolizing fertility. The red head scarf is wound into a cushion for the ever-present burden the Indian woman carries on her head. The basket, purchased in Amatitlán, is made by hand of local reeds, and the cloth that is carried in it matches the skirt. The señorita is on her way to the town laundry, which is probably an icy mountain stream.

Child's Dress from Santiago Atitlán: Tzutuhil Tribe

On the shores of Lake Atitlán, 100 miles from Guatemala City, is the village of Panajachel. Here are modern hotels and amenities. Across the lake are the perfect cones of three volcanoes, and in the shadow of one of them is a Tzutuhil Indian village. Each of the 17 villages around the lake have their own commercial projects. Santiago Atitlán builds the 'cayugos' used on the lake by the natives. They are made from the wood of the avocado tree, and up to 10 standing men can paddle them. This Mayan town has walled mud compounds with thatched roofs on winding streets. It is famous for beautiful costumes, especially those with many bright-colored birds, animals and insects embroidered onto the clothing of men, women and children.

This child's handloomed dress consists of a skirt with pink and brown stripes. It is long and is tightly wrapped and held up with a narrow belt. The huipil has an off-white background with navy blue stripes. The upper half of the blouse is embroidered on one side with 17 exquisite multi-colored birds, and on the other side with small figures of insects, leaves, flowers, animals and fruits. A long pink scarf adds the finishing touch.

Granddaughter Dina is the señorita here, and her sister Kara is the child.

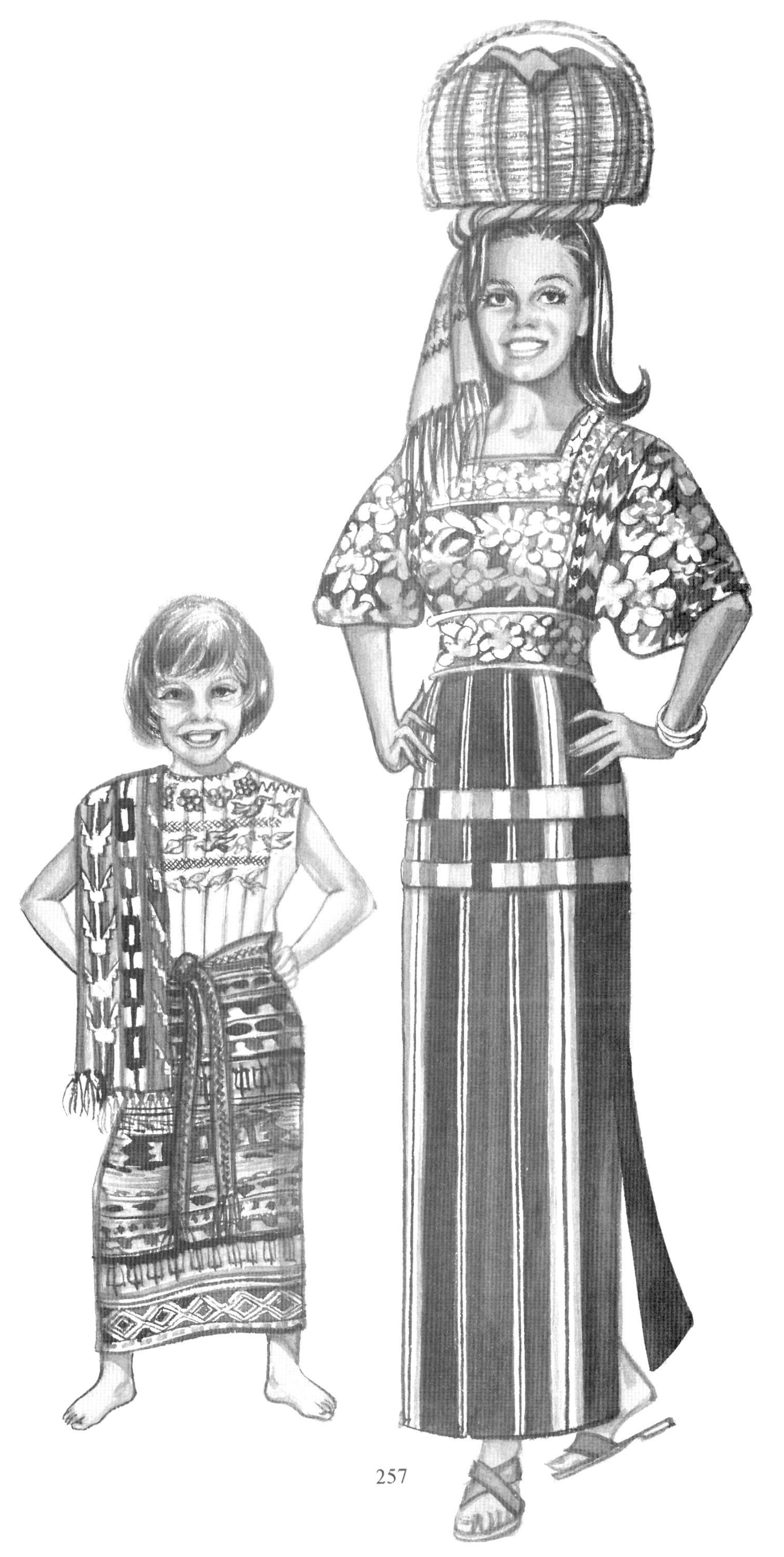

257

Miss Universe, Ixil Tribe, Nebaj

Miss Guatemala won the costume division in the 1975 Miss Universe Pageant, wearing a traditional ethnic dress like this one.

The tunic top, or huipil, has silk embroidery on three-yard-long panels on the front and back of the garment. The basic tunic is made of an off-white handloomed fabric, and the neck is trimmed with a strip of purple fabric with a design in red and yellow. The background color of the panels is red, with horizontal white bands about an inch wide. The figures in the embroidery are called 'chacs.' They represent the gods of sun, rain, wind and agriculture and are in the form of animals and birds and geometric designs. There is even a howler monkey among the animals, bringing back memories of early-morning roaring matches with neighboring monkey clans in the jungle around Tikal.

A skirt of handloomed red fabric is indigenous to Nebaj. Narrow green and white stripes are woven into the four-yard textile, which is wrapped into a skirt, with a large pleat on the left side.

The shawl is rolled and wound around the head to form a crown, with tassels tucked in the crown, making a charming headdress. The silver coin necklace has 50 'un centavo' pieces, held together with a silver chain.

The owner of a dress shop in Guatemala City was able, with her sources in Nebaj, to find this stunning example of a costume of the Ixil tribe of Guatemala.

Granddaughter Christy is modeling the Miss Universe costume.

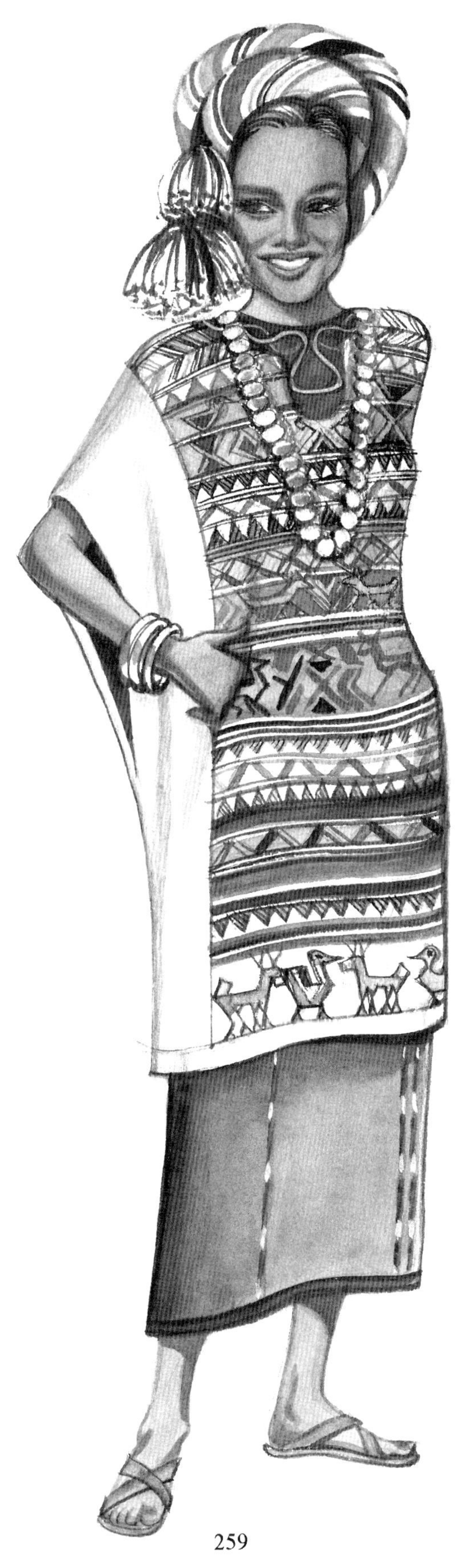

Then felt I like some watcher of the skies

When a new planet swims into his ken;

Or like stout Cortez when with eagle eyes

He star'd at the Pacific - and all his men

Look'd at each other with a mild surmise -

Silent, upon a peak in Darien.

John Keats (1795-1821)

Mexico

Mexico is located south of the U.S. border. It is three times the size of Texas, with five times the population of that state. The capital is Mexico City, the second largest city in the world. The currency is the new peso and literacy is 90 percent. The religion is 89 percent Roman Catholic. The government is a federal republic with a president as head of state.

The golden age of Mexican culture was from 200 to 800 A.D. During this time the Mayans moved into Yucatán, built pyramids and invented a calendar. The Toltecs established a flourishing culture from 900 to 1150 A.D. In 1325 the Aztecs conquered the Toltecs and founded the Aztec capital of Tenochtitlán, which is now the site of Mexico City.

The Spanish conquistador Hernán Cortés arrived in 1519 and burned his ships behind him, thereby committing his entire force to victory. By 1521 he had destroyed the Aztec empire. The Aztecs of Mexico believed Cortés was the resurrected god Quetzalcóatl, the feathered serpent. This belief minimized their resistance in the same way a similar belief influenced the Incas regarding Pizarro in Cuzco.

After three centuries of Spanish rule the people rose up and a republic was declared in 1823. Mexico seized lands in the present American southwest, resulting in the U.S.-Mexican War which lasted from 1846 to 1848. As a result Mexico lost all land north of the Rio Grande.

Austrian Archduke Ferdinand Maximilian Joseph accepted the offer of the Mexican throne, believing the people had wanted him to do so. However, this belief was false. When Juaréz and his army moved into Mexico City in 1867, Maximilian was executed, after having reigned for three years.

Since 1929 the Institutional Revolutionary Party, the IRP, has been dominant in Mexican politics, but has been contained by strong measures. In January of 1994 the North American Free Trade Agreement, NAFTA, was reached between the U.S., Canada and Mexico. After the assassination of the IRP presidential candidate in May of 1994, Ernesto Zedillo Ponce de León became president.

Mexican Memorabilia

Pyramids of the Sun and the Moon

These pyramids at Teotihuacán are flanked by lesser pyramids. The Pyramid of the Moon is at the north end of the city. To the south is the Temple of Quetzalcoátl (an important deity of ancient Mexico). It is a large complex covering 38 acres. To the east is the great Pyramid of the Sun, standing 216 feet high with five terraces. In 1971 excavation at the Pyramid of the Sun revealed steps to a cave 110 yards long, which is believed to have been considered the 'womb of the earth.' There was evidence of human sacrifice. The buildings are connected by the one-and-one-half mile Avenue of the Dead. It is said that when the Aztecs saw the pyramids they were filled with amazement at these ruins from a mystic past. The Aztecs worshiped Toltec gods. They believed that human sacrifice would gain them favor with these gods, and conducted killing orgies at ceremonial events.

Xochimilco

This is a delightful spot, famous for its 'chinampas,' or floating gardens. Indians constructed rafts on Lake Xochimilco, covered them with reeds, branches and mud, and planted them with willows whose roots anchored the floating gardens to the lake bed, making many small islands. Here, flowers and produce could be grown to be transported to the city. A 'trajinera,' a flower-covered launch, can be hired. Each boat has an arch overhead with flowers spelling out a woman's name. Our boat was Dolores. As we sailed through the canals we passed other boats with mariachis and food and drink vendors. Xochimilco is also known for the Diego Rivera paintings at the Palacio de Cortés.

Ballet Folklorico

A highlight of any trip to Mexico, especially for costume buffs, is the Ballet Folklorico at the Palacio de Bellas Artes in Mexico City. This very large marble palace was built as an opera house between 1904 and 1934. The huge stage curtain is Tiffany stained glass, showing Mexico City's two volcanoes, Popocatépetl and Ixtaccihuatl. The show is spectacular, with costumes and dances of various regions, blending pre-Hispanic and Iberian motifs. There are also Aztec ritual dances, a "Fiesta in Veracruz," and a remarkable athletic dance of a dying deer. The dancers are accompanied by mariachis, marimba players and vocalists. The Folkloric Ballet de Mexico is another example of the fine job traditional dancers are doing in sharing the history and cultures of their lands with the world. This ballet was the first of its kind I had seen, and I was privileged to see it twice in Mexico and once in the U.S. It was a wonderful introduction to the world of ethnic dress.

Taxco and Acapulco

There is a five-hour deluxe bus service from Mexico City to Acapulco by way of Taxco. Taxco is a colonial treasure, which has been declared a national monument. In 1522 Cortés discovered Taxco's silver mines, creating great excitement. The interest tapered off until William Spratling, from new Orleans, became enchanted with the town and established a center where pre-Columbian-style jewelry and other artifacts achieved a worldwide reputation. The city's silversmiths today are the descendants of Spratling's students, and their creations are exquisite.

Acapulco Bay is one of the world's best natural harbors. The weather all year is in the 80's and the beaches are a sunbather's dream. But knowledge is necessary around the sea and lack of it can quickly turn any dream into a nightmare. A member of our family was caught in an undertow. Fortunately, a lifeguard was nearby and she was rescued, but the experience was frightening. An undertow is water from the breakers finding its way back to sea, causing a rip current. Since this current is of limited width, swimming parallel to the beach gets one out of danger, but panic, added to ignorance, can be deadly. Fortunately, it was not.

Many years ago we stayed at the Las Brisas Resort while we were in Acapulco. Our casita was deluxe and private, with its own swimming pool and jeep. The cost was reasonable. Now, however, it is rated in *Fodor's* as very expensive. Everything is in pink, from the casitas, the servants'uniforms (now three per person), to the jeeps. There is even a pink line down the middle of the road leading to each casita, and a lovely touch, fresh pink hibiscus blossoms floating in the pool each morning. All of this and a panoramic ocean view from each casita!

Part of Acapulco's featured entertainment is watching young boys leap into the sea from rocky cliffs 130 feet above the water. This show used to take place once a day, in the evening. Now they leap four times daily. A breathtaking torch leap is on the program, and a moment of prayer at the small shrine on top adds gravity to the scene, reminding one that the danger involved is real.

Bullfighting

The 'Corrida de Toros' is made into an occasion of grandeur. According to some accounts the first bullfight in Mexico celebrated the return of Hernán Cortés from an expedition. During the three centuries that Mexico was ruled by Spain, many religious and civic ceremonies were commemorated by bullfights. These had the disapproval of the Catholic church, but sometimes priests were seen at the 'Plaza de Toros,' or bullring.

The 'torero,' or bullfighter, is clad brilliantly, and releasing the bull into the ring is handled with ostentation. The bull is bred for aggressiveness and is never allowed to fight more than once. If the torero has not dispatched the bull within 16 minutes, he is disgraced. If he has shown courage and the kill has been clean and swift, he is showered with flowers, hats and articles of clothing. In Valencia, Spain, El Cordobés, who was celebrated for his skill, was the recipient of bags of oranges thrown by the men and bras from the women. The torero often dedicates the vanquished bull to his ladylove. Occasionally, a spectator leaps the barrier and challenges the bull. In Spain punishment for this can be as much as 100 lashes.

Crowds often become raucous and unruly, more so in Spain than in Mexico. My husband wanted to see the most famous of all toreros in action in Valencia, and our young son begged to see a bullfight in Mexico City, so we saw those two events.

Aficionados of the bullfight ignore its dissenters, and our son practiced with an old red tablecloth, shouting 'Olé!' at each pass of the imaginary toro. Actually, bulls are colorblind and respond to movement, not color.

Ethnic Dress and Dance of Yucatán

The Yucatán Peninsula is a state in southeastern Mexico. Its capital is Mérida, and much of the population is Mayan. With roads, trains and air travel, Mayan centers, such as Chichén Itzá and Uzmal, became important tourist attractions. Colonial Yucatán was more closely connected to Europe than to Mexico.

This dress of Yucatán is made of cream-colored satin with a tunic and a long, full skirt, worn with a `rebozo,' or shawl. The tunic comes to the knee or below. The sleeves are short, and the square neck as well as the hems of the tunic and skirt are trimmed with a wide band of red and purple flowers, with green leaves and smaller flowers in blue and yellow. These are all embroidered on a white background with one edge scalloped in two shades of green. A five-inch width of lace is sewn to the embroidered band, and the entire trim is attached to the skirt and tunic with inch-wide lace. There are two rows of stitching an inch apart just above the hems of both the tunic and skirt. This is a Spanish touch found on many colonial garments.

The rebozo is two feet wide and six feet long, with six-inch silky, hand-tied orange and white fringe. The shawl is made of orange grosgrain ribbon woven with seven horizontal bands in black, white and beige in a jagged, lightning pattern.

The dancer wears her hair in a bun tied with a large, colorful bow, and she probably prefers to wear high heels.

The Yucatecan Jaraña

This dance stems from the Spanish dance and music brought to Yucatán in colonial times. The performance marks the culmination of the 'vaqueriá' or round-up. All the townsfolk gather, arrayed in their best finery, with the women in their colorfully-trimmed white tunics and full skirts.

Two drum beats announce the dance and the men and women form rows facing each other. The dance has a fast hop alternating with a slower one, which adds a melancholy note to the pattern. The men and women maintain a discreet distance from each other, changing positions as they dance. Sometimes the man uses his handkerchief to imitate a torero enticing the bull, and the woman weaves back and forth, imitating the animal. Or the man may raise his arms, pretending to have castanets. The music makes sudden stops, at which time everyone shouts 'bomba, bomba,' and a dancer will then improvise a verse such as this one:

> In that dress very precious
> You're so charming and dear
> That while I am near
> I am caught in your meshes.
> It's decidedly clear
> Your mother must bless us.

After the recitation, the musicians strike up once more and the dancing continues until dawn, often becoming a marathon to see who can last the longest.

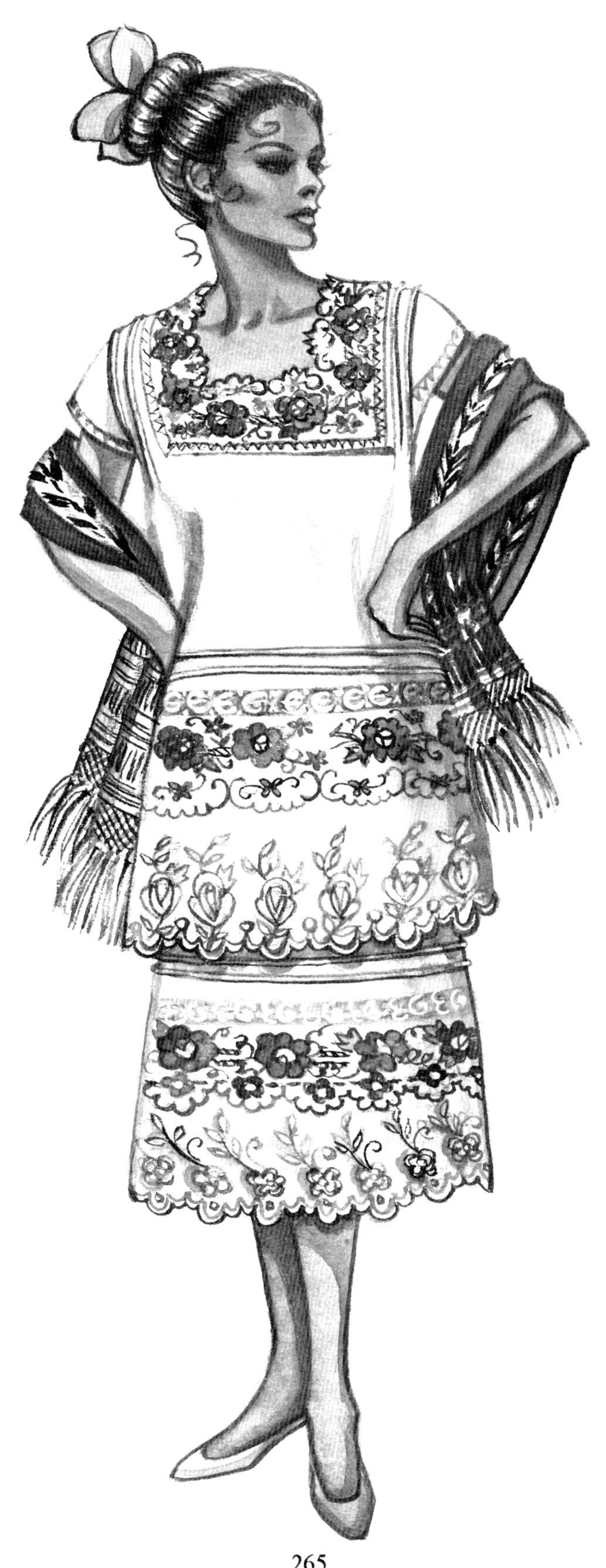

Woman's Jarabe Tapatío of Jalisco

Jalisco is a state in west-central Mexico. Its capital is Guadalajara, Mexico's second largest city, with an exploding population nearing six million. It is one of Mexico's most traditional and socially conservative cities. Its citizens are called Tapatíos.

This dress is made of green satin, elaborately embellished with red, yellow, white and navy narrow bands of satin ribbon sewn onto the fabric. The inch-high collar is red satin covered with white lace. A V-shaped ribbon and lace-trimmed bodice is 11 inches wide across the shoulders, coming to a point at the waistline. A narrow belt is made of the same material as the dress. The puffy elbow-length sleeves are edged with ruffled white lace, and the bottom of the nine-yard-wide spectacular skirt is finished with white lace over a red satin flounce. This dress is worn for many dances, among them that most popular from Jalisco, the Mexican Hat Dance.

All of the Mexican costumes in the collection were acquired from Laura Moya's Institute for Spanish Dance in Phoenix, Arizona. She has studied and taught Mexican dance and has an extensive wardrobe of traditionally correct ethnic dress of that country. I was able to persuade her to part with three attractive examples.

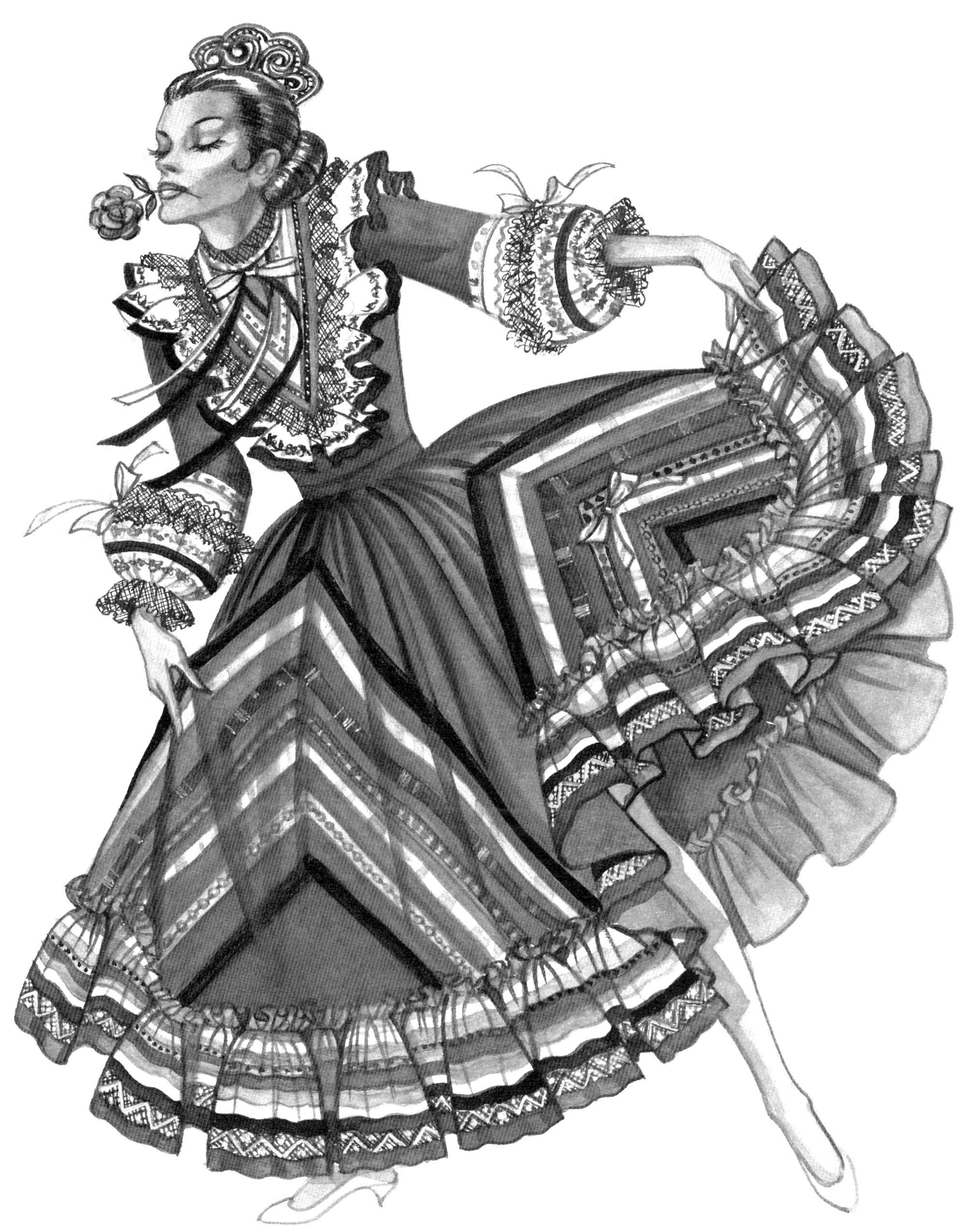

The Man's Mariachi Costume

The word 'mariachi' comes from the French word 'mariage.' In the early 1800's French aristocrats hired groups of street singers to entertain at weddings. Today, for a small fee, one can be serenaded in the musicians' own plazas in both Mexico City and Guadalajara.

This mariachi outfit has a black jacket and trousers, both made of a synthetic fabric, and trimmed with silver braid. Inch-wide silver braid trims the narrow rolled collar and the edges of the sleeves and outlines the entire short jacket. It is worn over a traditional man's shirt and is fastened with a chain and two large buttons made of silver cording. The trousers fit tightly and two-inch silver braid outlines the pockets and the outer seam of each pant leg.

A long, red, silk tie may be tied into a bow or have loose ends, and a red, four-inch-wide belt with a foot-long silky fringe at each end ties around the waist.

The black felt sombrero, lavishly decorated with gold and silver braid and sequins, is a thing of wonder. Its overall diameter is 24 inches, with a brim that turns up in front and back. There is a gold strap with a red silk tassel that hangs 17 inches below the chin.

This popular costume is worn by musicians, and the 'charros,' or Mexican cowboys, have adopted it for festive occasions. They wear it with riding boots which have raised heels. They can be seen on Sunday mornings at 'charreadas,' or rodeos, at Mexico City's Rancho del Charro. Dashingly dressed, they practice rope tricks and parade their steeds along the bridal paths of huge Chapultepec Park.

Mexican Music

Guadalajara, in the west central state of Jalisco, has given mariachis their own square, the Plaza of the Mariachis, where visitors are rarely without entertainment. Today's mariachi groups are composed of from three to twelve musicians. They are string orchestras with violins, guitars (both large and small), harps, mandolins and double basses. Sometimes brass wind instruments are included. These groups play both folk and popular music and the instrumentation changes from performance to performance.

The musical traditions of Mexico have their roots in pre-Columbian Indian and Spanish culture. Before the conquistadors arrived, the music of the Aztecs was a part of their religious rituals, under the Goddess of the Five Flowers. Pre-Hispanic Mexican music was performed in a plaza, on a platform or on a pyramid. Priests, nobles and even kings took parts. Many of the songs dedicated to the gods have survived. The manuscripts of Spain's Friar Bernardina de Sahagún, in the 16th century, were the first examples of scored music in the Americas.

Musicians who served in Aztec temples were employed in Spanish churches after the conquest. Ranchero music goes back to Spanish chivalric ballads and romances, becoming 'corridos,' songs of heroes and villains, politics, current events and, of course, love.

On the Spanish galleons came rhythms and musical forms that blended Latin, Mediterranean, Arab, African and Indian music. From all of this came the tango, the rumba, the fandango, the bolero and other exciting rhythms of Latin America.

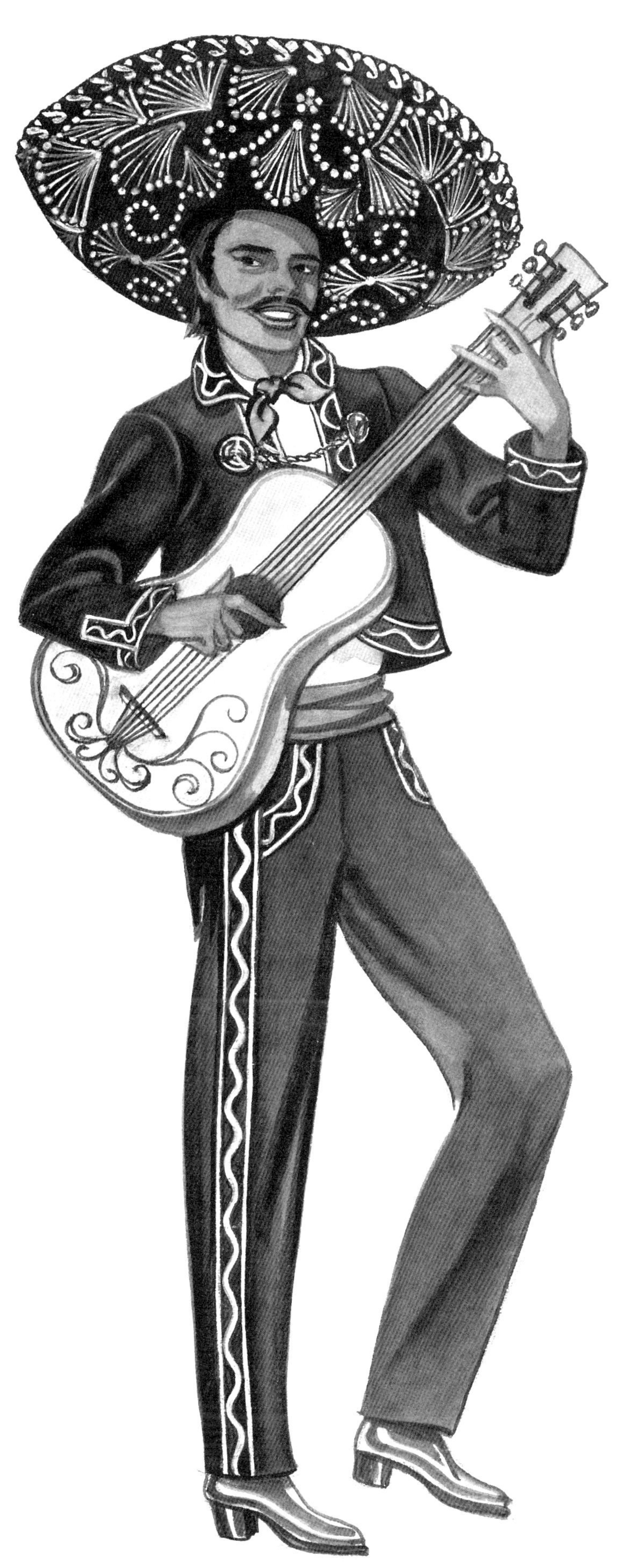

Homeward Bound

Round the world and home again,
    That's the sailor's way!
We've traded with the Yankees,
    Brazilians and Chinese;
We've laughed with dusky beauties
    In shade of tall palm-trees;
Across the line and Gulf-Stream
    Round by Table Bay-
Everywhere and home again,
    That's the sailor's way.

William Allingham

Postscript

Costume historics in general have concentrated on the ever-changing fashion of the European elite through the years, and have tended to pay little attention to the folk order. What is the folk order? It is personal, as well as traditional. In the folk order, clothing represents the past, the present and the future. A peasant wearing the costume of his ethnic background is showing his pride in his past; he is showing that he is an important part of his present environment, and that he has hope for the future through his children, who will carry on the traditions and customs of his people.

Whole books have been written on just one country, one tribe or native group, but comprehensive studies of the story of costume are few. Several years ago the Univeristy of Hawaii claimed to be the only university to offer a course in Asian costume for credit. While the folk order is still existent in parts of South America and Africa, as well as on some Pacific islands, its greatest strength is to be found in Asia and Southeast Asia.

Ethnic dress is regional, not national. National boundaries are imposed by governments long after native cultures were developed. Much of the unique beauty of the arts and clothing of these cultures is disappearing. In areas where ancient traditions have enriched man for centuries, 'progress,' or more correctly 'conformity,' is taking place.

Conformity is not new. It has always been a strong force in the adornment of the body. For example, feet have been bound, waists constricted, necks elongated by the wearing of metal bands, ears and noses pierced, and discs inserted in lips and earlobes. Style is tyrannical!

Folk societies are working to preserve the clothing traditions of their backgrounds, and folk dancing and theatrical groups are cooperating in this endeavor. It is possible today for performers or collectors to purchase new, authentic examples of the ethnic dress of many countries in folkloric shops.

Museums are springing up to house acquisitions, and old costume and embroidery patterns are being renovated. For example, many young people in the Phoenix, Arizona, area are becoming more aware and are taking pride in the study and preservation of their cultural heritages. Cambodians, who were unable to get many of their national treasures out of their country because of the desperate political situation, are getting together with their elders to share their knowledge and memories. Thai, East Indian, American Indian, Mexican, Japanese, Senegalese and Israeli dancing groups are also working to achieve similar goals.

It is to be hoped that these legacies of the costume world that are still being worn in the countries of their origin will serve to enhance understanding and enrich appreciation of their individual uniqueness.

Western fashion, through television and tourism, is making strong inroads on habits of behavior and dress everywhere. Let us hope that examples of the beauties of great and ancient cultures can be preserved for the grandchildren of our grandchildren.

Bibliography

The following are just some of the many very useful books used in my continuing study of the world and its ethnic dress.

Bhutto, Benazir. *Daughter of Destiny, an Autobiography,* Simon & Schuster, Inc., New York, 1989.

Blair, Lawrence. *Ring of Fire,* Bantam Books, New York, 1988.

Buckley, Michael and Strauss, Robert. *Tibet, a Travel Survival Kit,* Lonely Planet Publications, Berkeley, California, 1986.

Dhar, Sheila. *This India,* Government of India, New Delhi, 1973.

Davenport, Millia. *The Book of Costume,* Crown Publishers, New York, 1948.

Fairservis Jr., Walter A. *Costumes of the East,* The Chatham Press, Inc., Riverside, Connecticut, 1971.

Forman, Bedrich. *Borobudur, The Buddhist Legend in Stone,* Octopus Books Limited, London, 1980.

Harrold, Robert and Legg, Phyllida. *Folk Costumes of the World,* Blandford Press, London, New York, Sydney, 1981.

Lamb, Venice. *West African Weaving,* Old Piano Factory, London, 1975.

Macedo, Justo Caceres. *The Prehispanic Cultures of Peru,* Guide for Examination in Peruvian Archaeological Museums, 1988.

Meisch, Lynn. *A Traveler's Guide to Eldorado and the Inca Empire,* Penguin Books, New York, 1977.

Newton, Alex. *West Africa, a Travel Survival Kit,* Lonely Planet Publications, Berkeley, California, 1988.

Pattersen, Carmen L. *The Maya of Guatemala, Their Life and Dress,* Ixchel Museum, Guatemala City, 1976.

Reeves, Richard. *Passage to Peshawar,* Simon and Schuster, New York, 1984.

Von Hagen, Victor W. *World of the Maya,* New American Library, 1960.

Von Hagen, Victor W. *The Realm of the Incas,* New American Library, 1961.

Xun Zhou and Chunming, Gao. *5000 Years of Chinese Costume,* The Commercial Press, Ltd., Hong Kong, 1984.

Yarwood, Doreen. *The Encyclopedia of World Costume,* Crown Publishers, New York, 1986.

Reference Books

Encyclopedia Americana, Grolier, Inc. Danbury, Connecticut, 1991.

Encyclopedia Britannica, Encyclopedia Britannica, Inc., 1979

Ethnic Dress: Origins and Influences, The Costume Society of America, 15th Annual Meeting and Symposium, Denver Art Museum, Denver, Colorado, 1989.

The World Almanac and Book of Facts, Funk and Wagnalls, Mahwah, New Jersey, 1995. Reprinted with permission from The World Almanac and Book of Facts 1995. Copyright © 1994 Funk & Wagnalls Corporation. All rights reserved.

World Book Encyclopedia, World Books, Inc., Chicago, Illinois, 1992.

Credits

All of these costumes have been donated by Dorothy Owen Knop to two museums:

Sun Cities Museum of Art has the majority of them.

Arizona State University, Department of Theater has those shown on the following pages: (7, 153, 155, 163, 165, 171, 173).

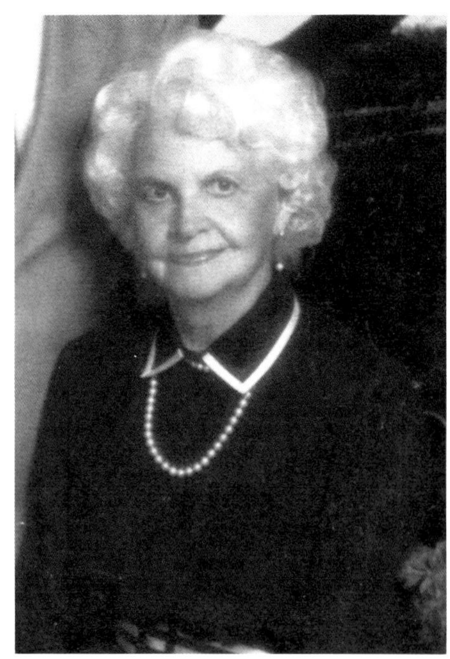

Dorothy Owen Knop graduated from Northwestern University in Evanston, Illinois, with a Bachelor of Science degree and majors in Spanish and English.

She obtained her teaching credentials from Milwaukee Downer College in Milwaukee, Wisconsin, and taught high school English in the Florida schools.

Her extensive traveling and collecting began after her two sons and a daughter were grown. The study of the history and development of ethnic dress gave focus and purpose to her travels and resulted in a collection of traditional costumes that has responded to the growing interest in world cultures.